PATIENT POSITIONING AND IMMOBILIZATION IN RADIATION ONCOLOGY

SSN = T_2
Carina = T_4 - T_5
Trachea = C_6 - T_5

PATIENT POSITIONING AND IMMOBILIZATION IN RADIATION ONCOLOGY

Gunilla C. Bentel, R.N., R.T.T.
Chief Dosimetrist and *Clinical Associate*
Department of Radiation Oncology/Physics Division
Duke University Medical Center
Durham, North Carolina

With contribution from

Lawrence B. Marks, M.D.
Associate Professor
Department of Radiation Oncology
Duke University Medical Center

McGraw-Hill
Health Professions Division

New York St. Louis San Francisco Auckland Bogotá Caracas
Lisbon London Madrid Mexico City Milan Montreal
New Delhi San Juan Singapore Sydney Tokyo Toronto

McGraw-Hill
A Division of The **McGraw-Hill** *Companies*

PATIENT POSITIONING AND IMMOBILIZATION IN RADIATION ONCOLOGY

234567890 QPK/QPK 12 11 10 09

ISBN 0-07-134158-7

This book was set in Times Roman by Digitype.
The editors were James Morgan III and Muza Navrozov.
The production supervisor was Catherine H. Saggese.
The cover was designed by Marsha Cohen/Parallelogram.
The index was prepared by Irving Condé Tullar.
Quebecor/Kingsport was printer and binder.

This book is printed on recycled, acid-free paper.

Library of Congress Cataloging-in-Publication Data

Bentel, Gunilla Carleson.
Patient positioning and immobilization in radiation oncology / author, Gunilla C. Bentel.—1st ed.
p. cm.
ISBN 0-07-134158-7 (alk. paper)
1. Radiotherapy—Positioning. I. Title.
[DNLM: 1. Radiotherapy—methods. 2. Posture. 3. Immobilization.
WN 250B477p 1999]
RM855.B46 1999
615.8′42—dc21
DNLM/DLC
for Library of Congress

Contents

Foreword

Gunilla Bentel has done it again. Her current offering, *Patient Positioning and Immobilization in Radiation Oncology,* is the third in her series of practical, insightful, and useful texts. Herein she extensively discusses the importance of patient positioning and immobilization, a topic frequently overlooked by physicians, physicists, and dosimetrists. She systematically addresses each major body site. The reader is methodically taken through the positioning and immobilization process, aided by approximately 200 clear illustrations.

This book is timely, since there is increasing recognition of the importance of immobilization with the more widespread use of conformal radiation therapy. When smaller field margins are used, greater attention is typically paid to positioning and immobilization. However, appropriate patient positioning and field placement are desirous irrespective of the field margins. Even if a large margin around the target is desired, it is generally preferable to have this margin placed as *intended* about the target.

It is particularly important for physicians to appreciate the importance of appropriate patient positioning and immobilization. Physicians need to be intimately involved in the treatment planning process, be familiar with how immobilization devices are created, and learn to utilize the techniques described in this book to improve treatment. Selecting the appropriate position and immobilization device should not be left solely to the dosimetrist/physicist. Rather, the physicians need to be integrally involved, as they are in a unique position to assimilate the physical and clinical aspects of each particular case. Since each position/immobilization device has differing benefits and risks, the clinician and the physicist/dosimetrist need to work together in the treatment planning process.

Ms. Bentel is a pioneer in the use of immobilization devices during radiation treatment planning, which has been the object of her studies for several decades. This work culminates her multiple publications and frequent lectures on this topic. This book will serve as an important reference for radiation therapy technology students, dosimetrists, physicists, and physicians.

LAWRENCE B. MARKS, M.D.

Preface

Effective repositioning of patients in the same position throughout a course of radiation treatments is a fundamental requirement of fractionated radiation therapy. The need for effective patient immobilization has become more widely recognized in recent years with the use of smaller margins facilitated by conformal treatment techniques. In general, such conformal techniques are more vulnerable to geometric errors than are fields with larger margins. Nevertheless, the benefits of improved patient repositioning should apply to all patients.

The objectives of this book are to present a practical guide to patient positioning and immobilization and to facilitate a better understanding of the geometric relationship between the radiation beam and the target. The first three chapters address general aspects of patient positioning and immobilization, while the other eight chapters are site specific and focus on the practical aspects of patient immobilization. Most chapters include a literature review of treatment accuracy, and each chapter concludes with a question and answer section.

The book is intended as a clinical guide for radiation therapists, dosimetrists, physicists, and physicians.

Acknowledgments

The writing of this book would not have been possible without the contribution of many coworkers. I am particularly grateful for the enormous efforts made by Dr. Lawrence B. Marks. He made invaluable editorial comments and offered many useful suggestions during the development of this text. I would also like to recognize the efforts of all the physicists and technical staff in the Department of Radiation Oncology at Duke University; the Durham Regional Hospital; the Memorial Hospital of Martinsville and Henry County, Virginia; and Moore Regional Hospital, Pinehurst, North Carolina. Some staff members have contributed with suggestions and advice, while others have posed for or taken pictures used in this book. I would especially like to recognize the efforts of physicists Shiva Das, Ph.D., Michael Munley, Ph.D., Curtis Whiddon, Ph.D., and Beverly Steffey and technical staff Lori Absalom, Kim Light, Kevin Smith, Kathy Temple, and Denise Torain. Without the expertise of two of the world's greatest computer system managers, Phil Antoine and his assistant Jacques Perrolle, this manuscript would never have materialized. I would also like to recognize the invaluable secretarial assistance of Jane Hoppenworth and the efforts by the skillful staff in the Department of Educational Media Services at Duke University.

PATIENT POSITIONING AND IMMOBILIZATION IN RADIATION ONCOLOGY

CHAPTER

1

Treatment Geometry

INTRODUCTION

The goal of radiation therapy is to irradiate a predefined target volume while avoiding adjacent radiosensitive structures. These goals often conflict and can be difficult to achieve. Thus, treatment planning and delivery can be complex and requires the expertise of a team of caregivers, including radiation oncologists, medical physicists, dosimetrists, and radiation therapists.

A treatment course is usually preceded by a simulation procedure where the patient's position, field sizes, and beam directions are determined. The setup parameters are recorded and marks are made on the patient and immobilization device to facilitate patient/beam alignment during each treatment.

Repeatedly reproducing the geometric relationship between the treatment unit and the target is essential. This relationship is often described using a standardized coordinate system. An in-depth understanding of the coordinate system, standardized anatomic reference planes, and motions of the treatment machine is needed.

COORDINATE SYSTEM AND PLANES

The coordinate system allows one to describe the location of any point with respect to another known point (origin). Three axes (x, y, and z) transect this known point (Fig. 1-1). The location of any point with respect to the origin is described by the distance measured along each axis and by indicating on which side of the axis the point is located. The latter is indicated by a positive or negative sign in front of the measured distance. The following conventions usually apply in radiation therapy (Fig. 1-2): the x-axis represents the patient's right-to-left direction, with a negative sign indicating a location on the left of the origin when facing the patient (e.g., the patient's right). The y-axis represents the cephalad-to-caudal direction, with a negative sign indicating a location caudal to the origin. The z axis represents the anterior-to-posterior direction, with a negative sign indicating a location posterior to the origin. The orientation of the transverse (or axial), sagittal, and coronal planes is shown in Fig. 1-3. Rotation about the x-, y-, and z-axes can also be referred to as rotation in the sagittal, transverse, and

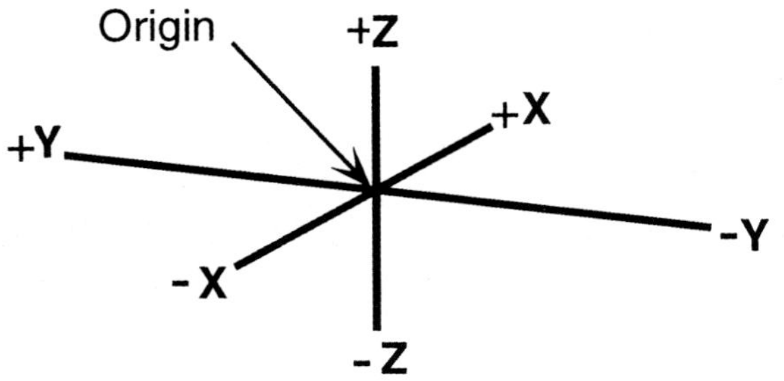

Fig. 1-1 The location of any point with respect to the origin can be described by the distance measured along the *x*-, *y*-, and *z*-axes and a plus (+) or minus (−) sign indicating at which side of the axis the point is located.

coronal planes. With the patient lying straight and supine on the treatment couch, these three axes correspond to the three anatomic planes.

To aid in realigning the patient with the radiation beam, a laser alignment system that casts long lines (> 1 m), indicating three orthogonal planes, is often used (Fig. 1-4). The system is mounted such that the point where the lines intersect (origin) corresponds to the common point of all machine rotations (isocenter). With the patient supine and straight on the couch, the lines coincide with the patient's three planes (Fig. 1-5). A vertical line coincides with the in/out motion of the treatment couch when at 0° and is parallel with the sagittal plane. Two horizontal crosshairs (right and left) cast a transverse line that coincides with the right/left and up/down motion of the couch and is parallel with the transverse plane—i.e., perpendicular to the sagittal line—and a coronal line that is perpendicular to the transverse line and is parallel with the coronal plane. Patient alignment systems should be used in simulator/computed tomography (CT) and each treatment room. For accurate patient repositioning, it is essential that the projection of the lines from these systems be identical and that they coincide with the axes of rotation of the couch and the gantry. Frequent verification of their accuracy is recommended.

It is not sufficient to realign the patient based on the central axis marks alone, since rotational errors may not be detected. Even a rigid box (Fig. 1-5) can be twisted or rotated when it is aligned with the central axis only. Failure to realign the patient distant to the central axis may cause tissues intended for treatment to be displaced out of the beam and other tissues to be moved into the beam; thus the treatment is not delivered as planned (Fig. 1-6). The resultant

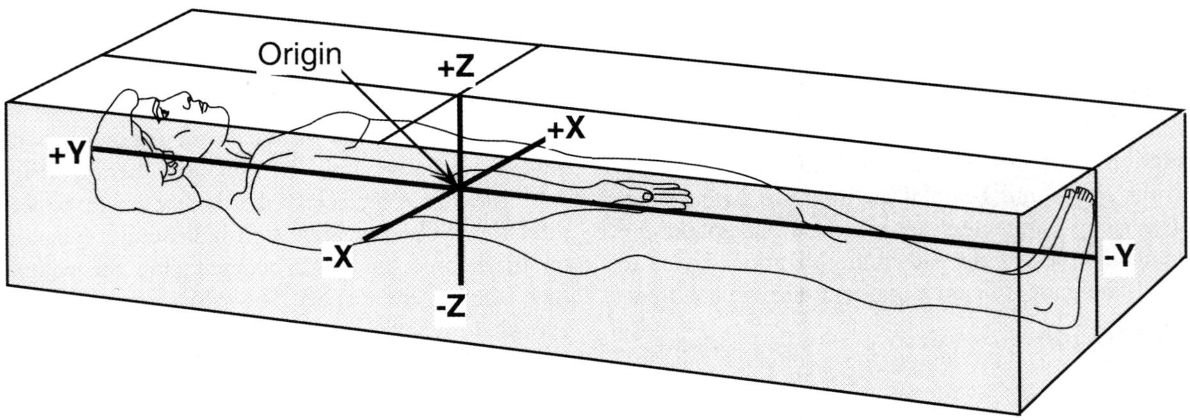

Fig. 1-2 The coordinate system as it is usually applied in radiation therapy. The *x*-axis represents the patient's right-to-left direction, with a negative sign indicating a location on the left of the origin when facing the patient (e.g., the patient's right). The *y*-axis represents the cephalad-to-caudal direction, with a negative sign indicating a location caudal to the origin. The *z*-axis represents the anterior-to-posterior direction, with a negative sign indicating a location posterior to the origin.

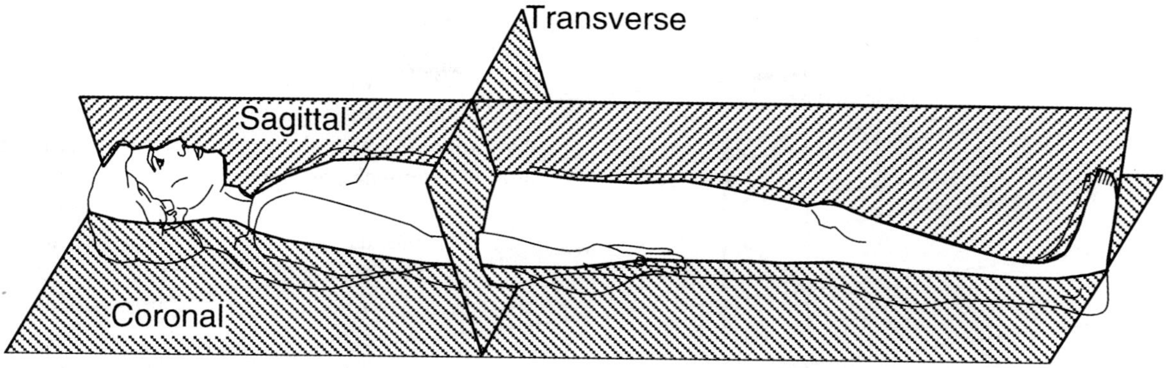

Fig. 1-3 The orientation of the transverse (or axial), sagittal, and coronal planes with respect to the patient.

deviation from the intended treatment increases at farther distances from the isocenter (rotational pivot point) (Fig. 1-7). Aligning the patient based on marks at *and* away from the isocenter will reduce such rotational errors.

An analogy has been made by Reinstein[1] between the patient's position on the treatment couch and an airplane on its landing approach. Knowing the *x, y, z* center of mass coordinates of an airplane on its landing approach (isocenter in radiation therapy) does not adequately describe the plane's position situation: The pilot must also know its roll (lateral tilt), pitch (longitudinal tilt), and yaw (rotation on vertical axis) to land safely. If the treatment couch is flat and horizontal and the posterior surface of the box (patient) is flat, there is no "roll" or "pitch." The problem of "yaw" (patient rotation on the vertical axis) may still exist. To eliminate this problem, the rigid box (patient) needs to be aligned with the long laser alignment lines such that the tissues away from the isocenter are also repositioned correctly with respect to the treatment field (Fig. 1-5).

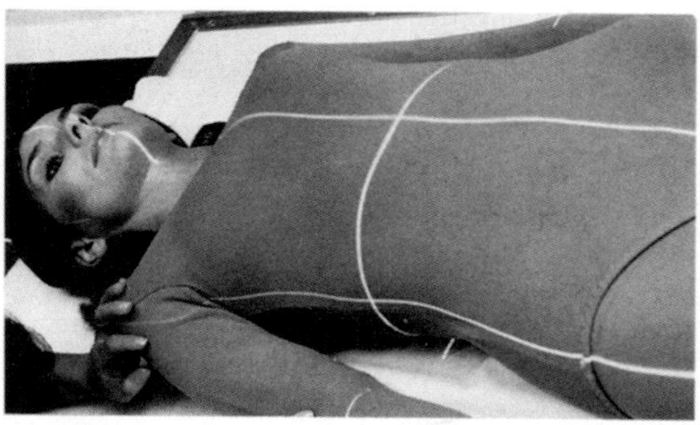

Fig. 1-4 To aid in realigning the patient with the radiation beam, a laser alignment system that casts long lines (> 1 m) indicating the three planes is usually used. The system is mounted such that the point where the lines intersect (origin) corresponds to the common point of all machine rotations (isocenter). (Courtesy of Gammex RMI, Middleton, Wisconsin.)

Once the patient's appropriate position has been secured for simulation or CT imaging, the long alignment lines need to be reliably marked on the skin and/or on the positioning device to facilitate repositioning for each treatment. On a CT unit, where there is no isocenter, the alignment system is often mounted such that the three lines intersect at a point corresponding to the center of the reconstruction circle. Since it is difficult to reach into the CT aperture to adjust the patient's position, this system may be mounted outside the tunnel to facilitate patient alignment. The alignment system represents an important tool to reproduce the patient/beam relationship from the simulator/CT to treatment and from treatment to treatment.

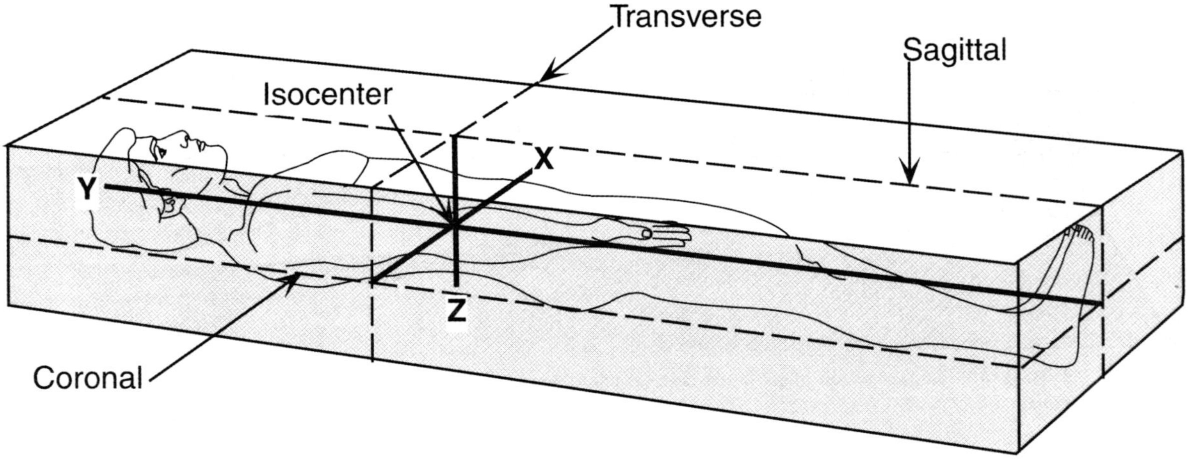

Fig. 1-5 Sagittal, transverse, and coronal alignment lines and the *x*-, *y*-, and *z*-axes displayed on an imaginary box containing the patient. The sagittal alignment line lies parallel with the *y*-axis and with the in/out motion of the treatment couch when at 0°. The two transverse lines (right and left) lie parallel with the *x*- and *z*-axes and with the right/left and up/down motion of the couch, i.e., perpendicular to the sagittal line. The two coronal alignment lines (right and left) lie parallel with the *y*-axis and with the in/out motion of the treatment couch and perpendicular with the transverse line. The alignment lines need to be long to facilitate patient (box) alignment even at long distances from the isocenter.

MACHINE MOTIONS

Radiation treatments are most commonly delivered using a linear accelerator. Before a treatment course begins, the treatment fields are usually "simulated" using a simulation unit. This unit, capable of producing diagnostic-quality radiographs, is also capable of mimicking the motions of most treatment machines. Thus, the motions described here for treatment machines also apply to simulator units. For clarity, the terminology used herein assumes that the patient is lying straight, flat, and supine on the treatment couch.

Most radiation therapy machines have three rotating parts: gantry, collimator, and couch (Fig. 1-8). The gantry rotates 360° on a horizontal axis (*y*-axis) that is parallel to the long axis of the treatment couch position (when at 0°), and the couch rotates about the *z*-axis. Since the collimator is fixed to the gantry, the axis on which it rotates changes with gantry rotation. When the gantry is at 0°/180° (vertical) or 90°/270° (horizontal), the collimator rotates about the *z*- and *x*-axes, respectively. The collimator is capable of rotating about the beam's central axis regardless of gantry angle. To deliver the treatments, any of these rotations can be used alone or in combination. When the angles are combined, beam directions are limited only by collision between the couch/patient and the head of the machine. Some of these limitations are discussed in Chap. 3.

Field sizes and shapes are defined by motor-driven collimators that produce rectangular fields. Other field shapes can be achieved by using multileaf collimators or inserting customized shielding blocks in the beam. The radiation field is indicated by a light field that projects the shadow of two perpendicular wires across the field—e.g., a crosshair (Fig. 1-9). The two wires intersect at the center of a radiation field (central axis) defined by symmetrical collimators. With the collimator at 0° and the patient in the conventional position on the treatment couch, one wire casts a shadow from head to foot and the other from right to left.

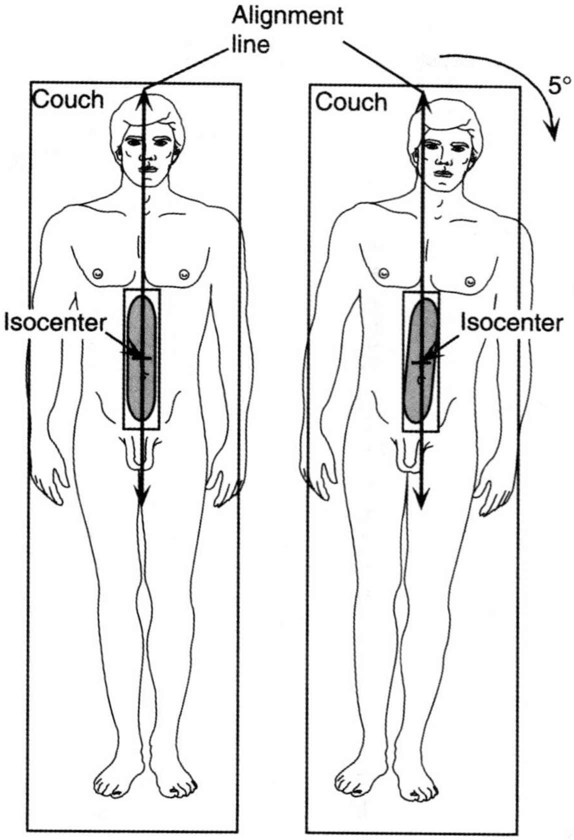

Fig. 1-6 It is not sufficient to align the patient with the isocenter marks only. When the patient's body is rotated on the *z*-axis (vertical), the target may be missed and normal tissues moved into the beam. A similar misalignment occurs on a lateral field if the patient is rotated on the *x*-axis (transverse). In this example, the patient is rotated; however, a collimator or couch rotation would have the same effect.

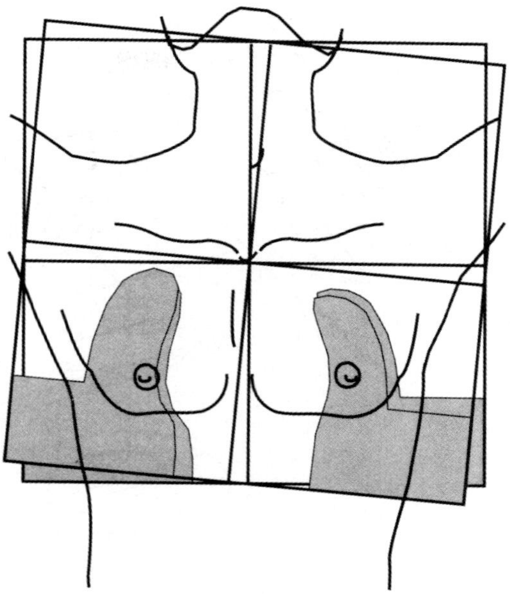

Fig. 1-7 A field can be misaligned even when the isocenter is placed correctly. Such misalignment becomes larger as the distance from the isocenter increases. In this illustration, the collimator is rotated; however, a patient or couch rotation would have the same effect.

The center of rotations of the gantry is called the *isocenter*. The distance between the radiation source in the gantry head (called the *beam target*) and the isocenter is typically 100 cm. The beam's central axis passes through the isocenter at all gantry angles, forming a transverse vertical plane (Fig. 1-10). The patient support assembly consists of a tabletop that can be translated along the three major axes and rotates about the vertical *z*-axis (passing through the isocenter). The motions of the couch are used to move the patient such that the intended target lies within the treatment field.

SETUP MARKS

Careful marking of the "prescription" position is an important element during simulation/CT. When target localization or treatment simulation is accomplished on a simulator unit, the isocenter is usually set in the center of the target and the beam's direction is set by machine rotations. The patient's position and the location of the isocenter are documented by marking the alignment lines on the skin and/or an immobilization device (Fig. 1-11). When the target localization and treatment plan are based on CT imaging, the situation is different because an isocenter has not yet been established when the CT scan is obtained. The alignment lines during the CT position are therefore usually set and marked at an arbitrary location and labeled "CT" to avoid confusion with subsequent

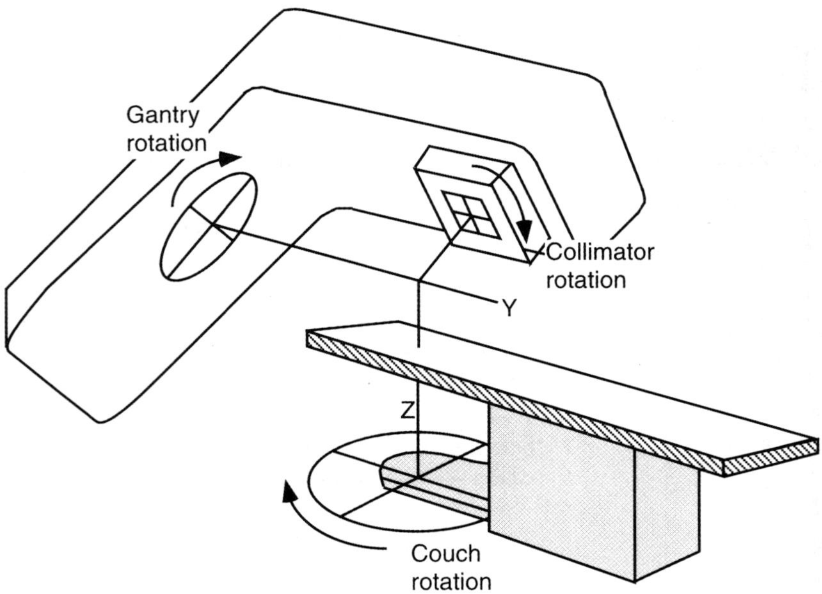

Fig. 1-8 The gantry rotates on a horizontal axis (*y*-axis) that is parallel to the treatment couch position when at 0° and the collimator and couch on a vertical axis (*z*-axis).

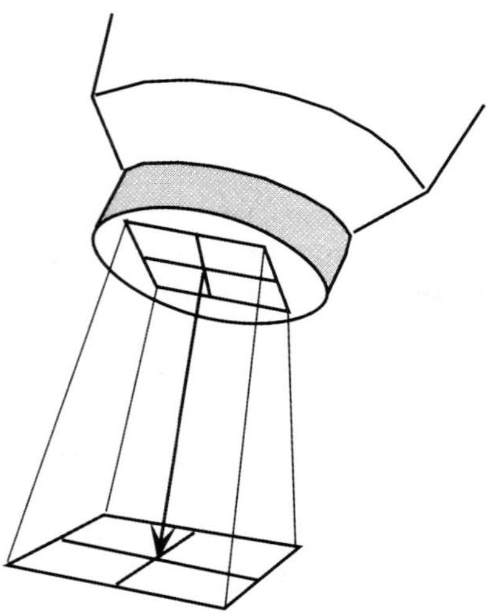

Fig. 1-9 The radiation field is indicated by a light field that projects the shadow of two wires that intersect at the center of a radiation field (central axis).

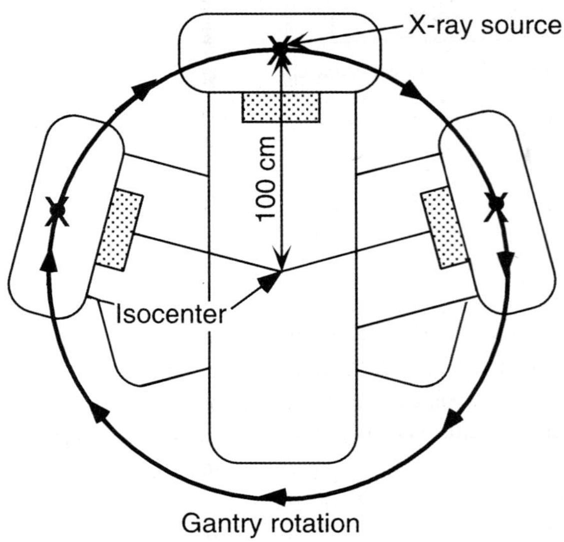

Fig. 1-10 The gantry is capable of 360° rotation about a point referred to as the isocenter. Most modern treatment machines are constructed such that the isocenter is located 100 cm from the x-ray source (beam target).

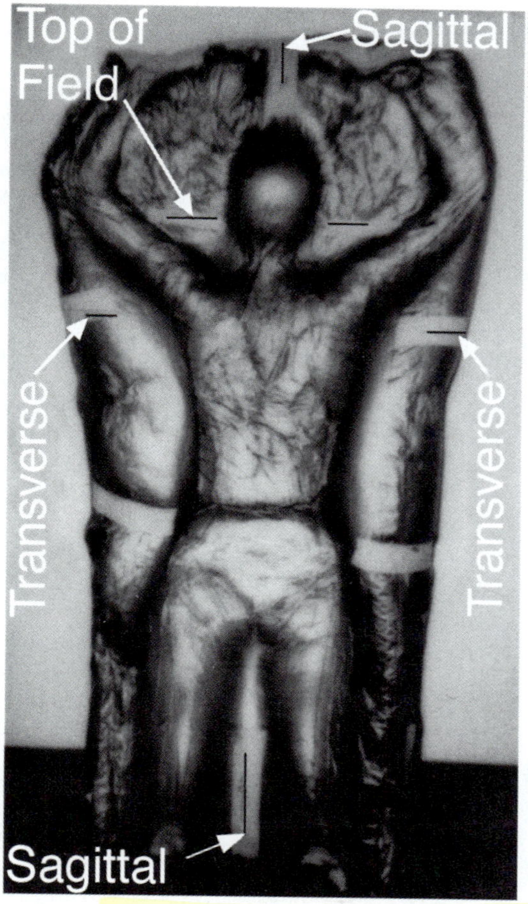

Fig. 1-11 The patient's "prescription" position should be clearly marked and documented during target localization and/or treatment simulation. An extended immobilization mold aids in reproducing the position and facilitates reliable setup marks.

treatment marks. The three-dimensional treatment planning (3DTP) computer software uses the intersection of the alignment lines as the origin in the coordinate system. The location of the planned treatment isocenter with respect to the origin is calculated and recorded by the software. When the patient returns for the first treatment, he or she is aligned with the CT marks. The couch is then moved until the isocenter location, measured from the CT marks, has been achieved. The alignment lines at this new location are marked and labeled "treatment" and are used for setting up subsequent treatments.

It is not sufficient to mark the isocenter alone (e.g., the patient-airplane analogy). Even when the isocenter is set up correctly, discrepancies between the planned and treated fields may still be present (Fig. 1-7). This discrepancy becomes more evident farther from the isocenter. Therefore, the alignment lines should be marked at long distances away from the irradiated area. This can take the form of either a long solid line or two short lines at opposite sides of the isocenter—e.g., the sagittal line above the head and between the thighs and the transverse on the patient's right and left sides. In our own experience, setup reproducibility improved when extended immobilization devices were implemented and the alignment marks were made on the device at long distances (about 20 to 40 in.) from the isocenter.[2–4] Such devices and setup markings are described in most chapters of this text. Marking of field outlines and central axes is technically not absolutely necessary. However, such marks may be useful to verify that field sizes, beam directions, beam-shaping blocks, and so on are correct.

In most areas of the human body, skin moves over underlying tissues; thus, setup marks on the skin may be unreliable. This is particularly evident in areas where there is a thick layer of mobile soft tissue under the skin. For example, skin overlying breast tissues can move several centimeters with respect to the underlying chest wall. To alleviate this discrepancy, skin marks can be made in areas where the skin is taut and relatively immobile. For example, instead of being placed at the isocenter on the breast, the sagittal alignment mark (indicating the left/right position of the isocenter) can be made cephalad and caudal to the breast; similarly, the transverse reference line can be marked over the sternum.

Skin marks tend to smear and fade and are therefore reinforced many times during a treatment course. The marks may migrate as they are re-marked, giving rise to changes in the skin mark/target relationship. When a rigid immobilization device is used, making the realignment marks on the device may eliminate some of the problems with skin marks and thus facilitate a more reliable setup. Marks on the immobilization device do not move with respect to the target (assuming the patient is repositioned correctly in the device); they do not smear or fade, and hence the problems of re-marking and migration are eliminated. Since marks on an immobilization device are usually easier to see than those on the skin, a fine-tipped pen can be used, possibly reducing the small variations in setup caused by thick lines. Setup marks on the immobilization device may be used together with skin marks. When there is a discrepancy between these marks, it is likely that the marks on the rigid device are correct, since skin marks may have shifted with respect to underlying deeper tissues.

REFERENCES

1. Reinstein LE: Patient positioning and immobilization, in Khan FM, Potish RA (Eds): *Treatment Planning in Radiation Oncology.* Williams & Wilkins, Baltimore, 1998.
2. Bentel GC, Marks LB, Sherouse GW, et al: The effectiveness of immobilization during prostate irradiation. *Int J Radiat Oncol Biol Phys* 31:143–148, 1995.
3. Bentel GC, Marks LB, Krishnamurthy R, Prosnitz LR: Comparison of two repositioning devices used during radiation therapy for Hodgkin's disease. *Int J Radiat Oncol Biol Phys* 39:791–795, 1997.
4. Bentel GC, Marks LB, Krishnamurthy R: Impact of cradle immobilization on setup reproducibility during external beam radiation therapy for lung cancer. *Int J Radiat Oncol Biol Phys* 38:527–531, 1997.

PROBLEMS

1-1 The coordinate system is used to
(*a*) align patients each day for treatment
(*b*) describe a point in space
(*c*) describe the isocenter
(*d*) confirm that all alignment lines are parallel

1-2 In the usual orientation of the *x*-, *y*-, and *z*-axes with respect to the patient
(*a*) the *y*-axis represents the right/left direction
(*b*) the *x*-axis represents the anterior/posterior direction
(*c*) the *z*-axis represents the cephalad/caudal direction
(*d*) the *x*-axis represents the right/left direction

1-3 In the usual orientation of the three planes with respect to the patient
(*a*) the transverse plane lies across the patient
(*b*) the sagittal plane lies across the patient
(*c*) the coronal plane lies parallel with the *x*-axis
(*d*) the sagittal plane lies parallel with the *z*-axis

1-4 On a CT unit, where there is no isocenter,
(*a*) the alignment lines usually intersect at the center of the reconstruction area
(*b*) the alignment lines always intersect at an arbitrary point inside the center of the aperture
(*c*) the three alignment lines always intersect at a point outside the CT aperture
(*d*) alignment systems are usually not available

1-5 On most radiation therapy machines
(*a*) the gantry rotates on a vertical axis and the couch on a horizontal axis
(*b*) the collimator and gantry rotations are always on the same axis
(*c*) the couch rotates on a vertical axis and the gantry on a horizontal axis
(*d*) the gantry and couch rotations are always on the same axis

1-6 The treatment couch can
(*a*) be rotated 360° and be moved left/right and in/out from the gantry
(*b*) be rotated to any position and moved up/down only
(*c*) not be rotated but can be moved left/right and in/out from the gantry
(*d*) be rotated and moved up/down, left/right, and in/out from the gantry

1-7 Setup marks on the skin
(*a*) are the most reliable aids to repositioning the patient
(*b*) are usually unreliable because they tend to move over underlying deeper tissues
(*c*) should never be used
(*d*) never need to be re-marked because patients are told not to bathe during the treatment course

1-8 Marking the isocenter only is
(*a*) sufficient for accurate realignment of the patient
(*b*) adequate when the target margins are small
(*c*) adequate when small fields are used
(*d*) insufficient for patient realignment

CHAPTER

2

Treatment Accuracy and Precision

INTRODUCTION

Most treatment fields are designed to treat the target volume plus "a margin" to account for treatment uncertainties. The size of the margins depends on the magnitude of the uncertainties and should be as small as possible without compromising target coverage. Inadequate dose to the target may lead to failure to control the disease, and excessive dose to normal tissues may lead to complications. The dose that can safely be delivered to the target is often limited by the tolerance level of normal tissues in the vicinity. Attempts to improve the therapeutic ratio are often made by limiting the volume of normal tissues being irradiated incidentally. In general, it is thought that using three-dimensional treatment-planning (3DTP) tools improves the ability to determine the target volume and to direct the beams such that normal tissues are avoided. However, these benefits may be lost if the treatment is not implemented as planned or reproduced from treatment to treatment. Methods to address these issues are presented in this book.

When the margins are small, as is often the case when 3DTP tools are used, the risk of missing the target is increased. Precise and effective immobilization techniques are especially important in these settings.[1] The need for effective patient immobilization has become more widely recognized in recent years, and many immobilization devices have therefore been developed.[1-20] Although the impetus for improving patient immobilization has been the ability to reduce the margins of certain tumors, the advantage has extended to include other treatment sites as well. For example, an immobilization device developed for the treatment of brain tumors can also be used in patients with head and neck tumors.

UNCERTAINTIES

The topic of treatment uncertainties is not straightforward; some of the issues are addressed in the following paragraphs. It is widely recognized that there inevitably are uncertainties in the planning and delivery of radiation therapy. Uncertainties associated with the delivery of a prescribed radiation treatment can be divided into two groups: those of dose (i.e., inhomogeneities, dose calculations, variables in machine output) and those of patient/beam geometry (spatial). Spatial uncertainties can be broadly divided into those inherent to mechanical inaccuracies in the equipment (simulator, treatment machine, alignment systems, and so on) and those related to the patient. Some discrepancies may be both mechanical and patient-related.

There are many sources of target/beam misalignment, and it is often difficult to determine the root of the problem. Some of these sources are listed below. The magnitudes of the uncertainties given in the following sections are approximate and may vary from machine to machine and from patient to patient. The range of mechanical inaccuracies of equipment is usually specified by the manufacturer; however, larger errors may be caused by extensive use.

MECHANICAL UNCERTAINTIES

- *Field size settings:* Mechanical dials, where the scale is often in 0.5-cm increments, may be in error by ~2 mm. For digital settings, the error may be smaller.
- *Rotational settings:* Mechanical dials, where the scale is often in 1° increments, may be in error by ≤1°. For digital settings, the error may be smaller.
- *Crosshairs:* Wires may become displaced (~2 mm).
- *Isocenter:* Deviations (~2 mm) may occur due to sagging of the machine.
- *Light-beam congruence:* May be in error by ~1 to 2 mm. Misalignments may be caused by small shifts in the mirror or light bulb.
- *Alignment system:* Lines may not intersect at isocenter (<5 mm) or may not be perpendicular; some systems display relatively thick lines (~3 mm).
- *Couch top:* Differences in sag among couches (5 to 10 mm). Simulator and computed tomography (CT) couches are often solid. In the treatment room, a tennis-racket-type insert is often used, causing differences in sag. With extensive use, couch tops may become tilted (side to side or end to end).
- *Beam-shaping blocks:* May be in error (<5 mm) if the Nichrome wire is too hot or is moved too fast around a corner when the Styrofoam is cut.

Many of these uncertainties can be reduced by rigorous quality-assurance testing of the treatment equipment and alignment systems. Other discrepancies are inherent in the machine and cannot be eliminated (isocenter accuracy, width of the alignment lines). To eliminate discrepancies between couch tops, the surface should be identical in the simulation/CT and treatment rooms.[21] Small discrepancies between the simulation and treatment conditions are inevitable because the patient is not a rigid object and elimination of all inconsistencies between the simulator and treatment unit is unlikely.[22–29]

PATIENT-RELATED UNCERTAINTIES

- *Target delineation:* Errors (≤5 mm) may occur as a result of difficulties in determining the extent of tumor and in transferring anatomic information from CT and/or magnetic resonance imaging (MRI) to simulation radiographs.
- *Organ motion:* Organ motion (e.g., respiratory, cardiac) and changes in the size and shape of an organ (e.g., stomach, bladder, rectum) may cause uncertainties on the order of about 5 to 10 mm.
- *Skin marks:* Skin marks may shift relative to deeper tissue, often ~5 mm, and such shifts can be greater in areas where there is an increased thickness of soft tissue. The width of the setup lines may cause variations in how a field is set up.
- *Repositioning:* Discrepancies in reproducing the position may occur and may be reduced by using an immobilization device.
- *Patient motion:* Some patients, especially children, may move (~5 mm) during treatment (owing to pain or an uncomfortable position or because they are uncooperative, demented, or restless).

The magnitude of patient-related uncertainties may vary depending on treatment site and the patient's general condition (age, weight, mobility, and so on). In general, patient-related uncertainties cannot be eliminated; however, efforts should be made to reduce them.

One of the greatest challenges in radiation therapy is accurate delineation of the target volume. Uncertainties may be reduced by advances in diagnostic imaging and the ability to outline the target on CT images that are used for 3DTP.

Uncertainties associated with organ motion and changes in organ size are difficult to eliminate. Respiratory motion may be decreased by having the patient breathe quietly during treatment. Consistency of an organ size/location may be maintained by asking the patient to comply with certain guidelines—having a full or empty bladder, not eating immediately prior to treatment for stomach/upper abdomen treatments, and so on.

Accurate beam/target realignment relies on external marks being fixed relative to the target; however, due to the probability that the target or the skin marks may move, it is unlikely that this relationship will be reproduced for each treatment (Fig. 2-1). Measures to improve the odds that it will occur have been addressed in Chap. 1. Suffice it to say that when the marks are extended well beyond the treatment area and are made on a rigid immobilization device, setup reproducibility, in our experience, appears to be improved. The ability to *reposition* the patient and the patient's ability to *maintain* the position during treatment may be improved with the use of immobilization devices.

In everyday practice, we accept the fact that not all discrepancies can be corrected; therefore, a margin is added around the tumor. It is important to recognize that the effect of uncertainties may be cumulative or offsetting; however, it would be impossible to know how they relate. It has been suggested that displacements caused by machine inaccuracies, even when they are within the specified minimum requirements, can be <5 mm, while uncertainties of setup and positioning of the target volume due to patient or organ motion can cause errors of up to 8 mm, resulting in a combined uncertainty of <10 mm.[30] Variations in the day-to-day setup are difficult to contend with because patients tend to move, and there are inaccuracies in the alignment of the treatment beam with the setup marks. The American Association of Physicists in Medicine (AAPM) recommends <5-mm spatial uncertainty.[31] Several studies show that in present practice, without the use of immobilization devices, these recommendations are not met.[1,26,32,33] Rosenthal et al. report a mean variability of 0.6 cm in prostate patients treated without immobilization.[1] Rabinowitz et al. showed, in a study of 71 patients, that in 20% of setups, the spatial error was more than 10 mm.[26] Rosenthal et al. found a total uncertainty (random and systematic) of 0.7 cm in a retrospective review of 318 port films in 51 patients treated for head and neck malignancies using a bite-block immobilization system.[33] Byhardt et al. found, in a study of port films of 337 patients, that setup errors of ≥5 mm occurred in 15% of the setups; in 10% of the setups, the error was ≥10 mm.[32]

TARGET MARGINS

While it is impossible to eliminate all of the causes of uncertainties, it is essential to develop an understanding of their source and magnitude and to recognize the impact that they have on treatment delivery so that they can be reduced and adequate margins applied.

TERMS AND CONCEPTS FOR VOLUMES AND MARGINS

The International Commission on Radiation Units and Measurements (ICRU) has recommended definitions of terms and concepts for volumes and margins in radiation therapy, as follows (Fig. 2-2):[34]

The *gross tumor volume* (GTV) denotes the demonstrable tumor.

The *clinical target volume* (CTV) denotes the GTV and subclinical disease (volumes with suspected tumor).

The *planning target volume* (PTV) denotes the CTV and includes margins for geometric uncertainties. The final plan requires an additional margin that takes into account the penumbra of the beam.

The *treated volume* is the volume of tissue enclosed by an isodose surface, selected and specified by the radiation oncologist as being appropriate to achieve the purpose of the treatment. Because of limitations in treatment delivery, it is often impossible to design a treatment plan that limits the prescribed dose to the PTV only. Unintentionally, some tissues near the target are also irradiated to the same dose as the target. The treated volume is therefore always larger than the PTV and usually has a simpler shape.

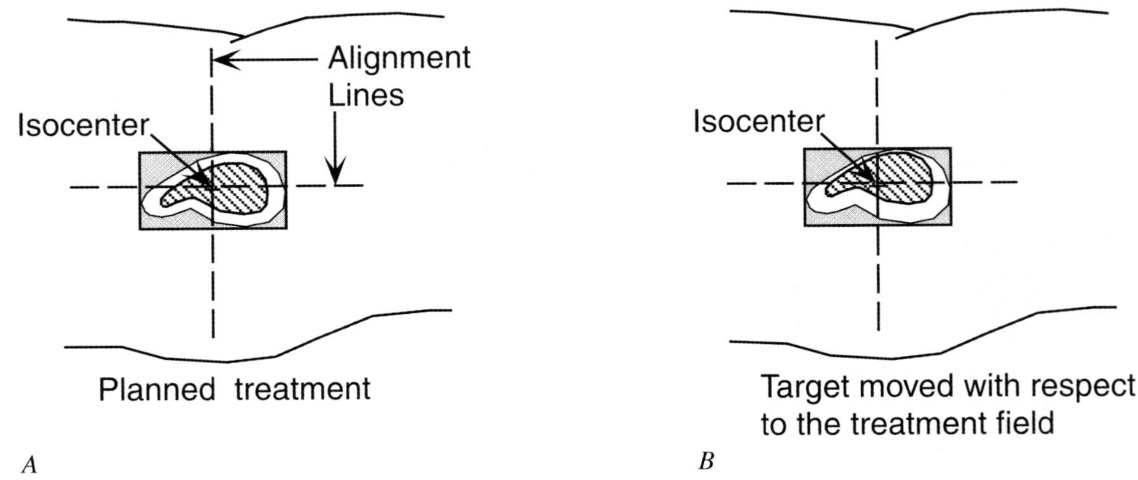

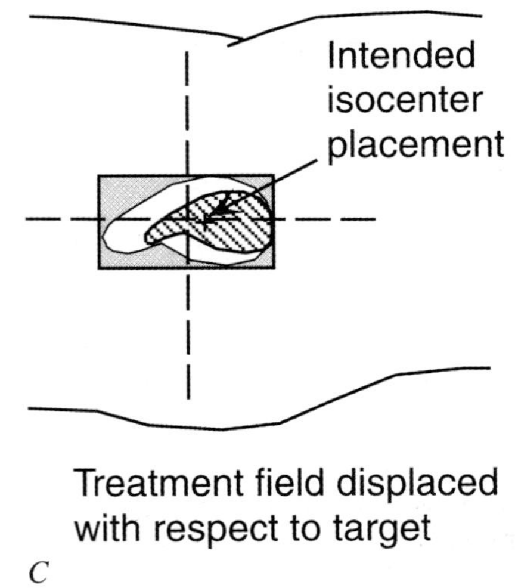

Fig. 2-1 The planned beam/target alignment (*A*) may not be reproduced when the target moves (*B*) or the setup marks are displaced (*C*).

The *irradiated volume* is the volume of tissue that receives a dose considered significant in relation to tissue tolerance—for example, tissues in the exit region of unopposed beams or in the penumbra region of a beam.

A corresponding approach should be used in defining margins around organs at risk, leading to the concept of *planning organ-at-risk volume* (PORV). In many situations, the PTV and PORV may overlap (or compete for space); thus certain

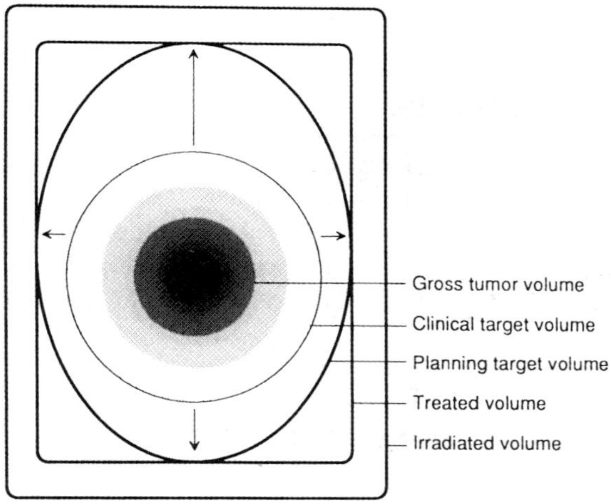

Fig. 2-2 Schematic illustration of the different volumes recommended by the *ICRU Report #50.* (Courtesy of The International Commission on Radiation Units and Measurements, Bethesda, Maryland.)

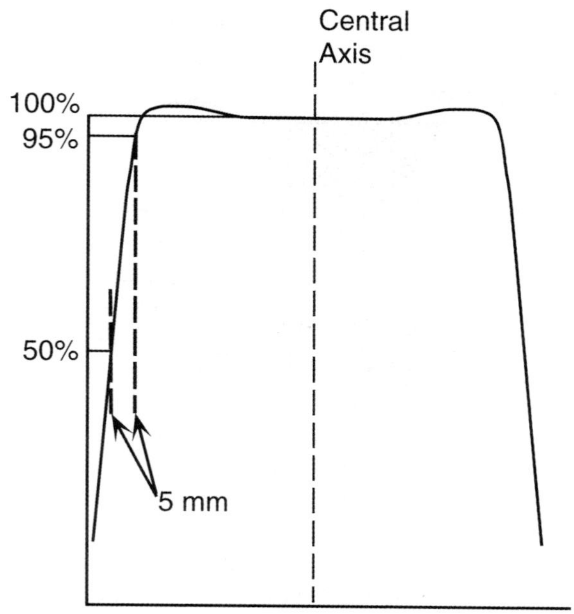

Fig. 2-3 A dose profile illustrating the distance (5 mm) between the 50% isodose level (beam-defining field light) and the 95% line, where the dose often is prescribed.

compromises of the margins may be needed. For example, it may be impossible to treat a brain tumor with a 1.5-cm margin while at the same time achieving a 0.5-cm margin around the optic chiasm.

Uniform application of these terms when radiation treatments are prescribed, recorded, and reported promotes comparison of treatment results from different centers.

MARGIN SIZE

There is no rule for the size of the margins; however, often 1.5-cm physical margins are set around the CTV to account for the uncertainties and the penumbra of the machine.[35] To account for uncertainties in target determination, a minimum value of 5 mm is often used, given the difficulties of interpreting conventional diagnostic images and transferring this information to the simulator films. To account for inconsistencies in the reproducibility of the geometric patient/beam alignment and the probability of organ and patient motion, many radiation oncologists add a modest 5-mm margin. Sometimes the target margin within the same field may be different, depending on the direction of greater uncertainties. For example, a lung tumor may move more in the cephalad/caudal direction and consequently requires larger margins in these directions. Finally, a margin is added for the penumbra of the beam. The edge of the beam-defining field light usually coincides with the 50% isodose level (Fig. 2-3). The distance from this geometric field margin to the 95% line, where the dose often is prescribed, varies from machine to machine but is often ~5 mm on a linear accelerator. Under optimal circumstances, including the use of rigid patient immobilization and three-dimensional treatment-planning systems, this margin may be sufficient. In the absence of these technologies, however, larger margins may be necessary.

NORMAL TISSUE CONSIDERATIONS

Since radiation-induced complications do not occur in tissues that are not irradiated,[36] it is beneficial to minimize incidental irradiation of normal tissues.

Keus et al.[37] and Letschert et al.[38] showed that decreasing the volume of irradiated normal tissue reduced the complication rate. Letschert et al. also found that by decreasing the volume of irradiated small bowel by a factor of 2, the total dose could be increased by 17% while the incidence of small bowel complications remained unchanged. Reduction of the complication rate afforded by reducing the volume of irradiated normal tissue may facilitate dose escalation and improved local tumor control rates. Goitein and Busse[39] predicted, in an idealized mathematical model, that by decreasing the field margins by 5 mm in a supraglottic field, the total dose could be increased to where a 15% improvement in tumor control probability could be achieved without increasing the normal tissue complication rate.

A modest increase of the margin can have a significant effect on the volume of normal tissues exposed. The volume of normal but exposed tissue (outside the tumor) can be calculated for different target sizes and with different margins. For example, when the margins for a typical prostate field are increased from 10 to 13 mm, a modest increase of 3 mm, the irradiated volume increases by 25%.[1]

The results of an idealized calculation are shown in Table 2-1 for a patient treated with a single field for a rectangular target volume irradiated with margins of various size. The target is assumed to involve the entire 20-cm thickness of the patient. The target sizes of 10 × 10 and 20 × 20 cm shown in Table 2-1 represent the two dimensions perpendicular to the beam. A significant increase in the volume of incidentally irradiated normal tissue is recognized as the margin is increased. The numbers in the table are only approximate and do not reflect the effect of beam divergence or the use of multiple beams.

EFFECTS OF MISALIGNMENT

Accurate repeated reproducibility of the radiation beam/target alignment is fundamental to successful radiation therapy. Missing part of a tumor once or twice during a treatment course may reduce the control rate. Similarly, inadvertent irradiation of a critical structure may increase morbidity. Figure 2-4 demonstrates the effect of misalignments on the dose. When the fields are set up accurately for each treatment and assuming no motion during the treatment (i.e., during delivery of 100% of the dose), the distance between the 95 and 50% isodose lines is small (approximately 0.5 cm) (Fig. 2-4A). When the treatment fields are accurate during delivery of one-fifth of the dose and in error by 0.5 cm in four

Table 2-1 Effect on Normal Tissue Volume When Target Margins Are Changed

	Target Size			
	10 × 10 cm		20 × 20 cm	
Margins Used, mm	Total Volume, cm³	Normal Tissue Volume,[a] cm³	Total Volume, cm³	Normal Tissue Volume,[a] cm³
5	2205	205	8405	405
10	2420	420	8820	820
15	2645	645	9245	1245

[a]Normal tissue volume was found by subtracting the target volume from the total volume.

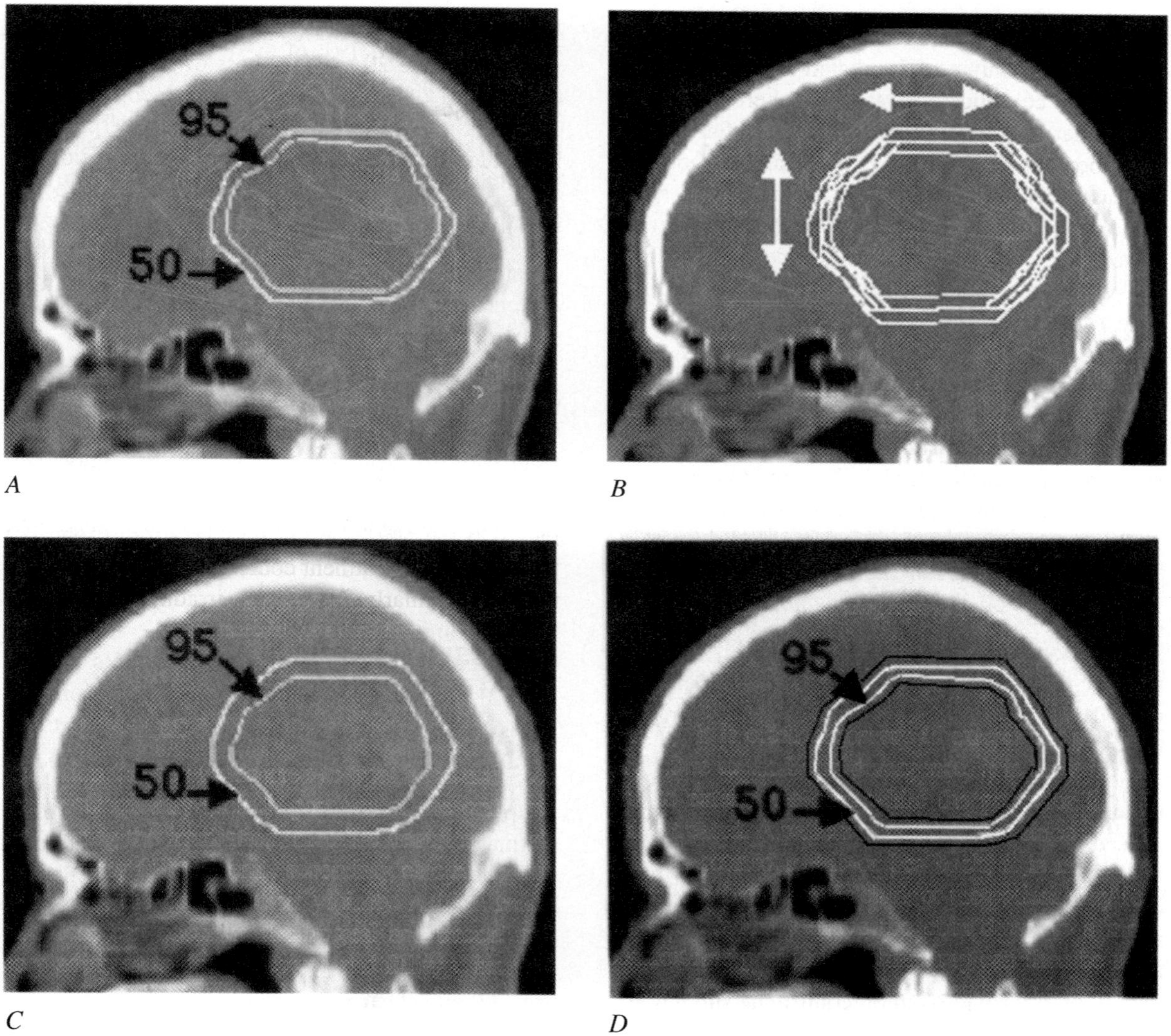

Fig. 2-4 When treatment fields are set up accurately for each treatment and there is no motion during the treatment (i.e., during delivery of 100% of the dose), the distance between the 95 and 50% isodose lines is small (approximately 0.5 cm) (*A*). When the treatment fields are accurate during delivery of one-fifth of the dose and in error by 0.5 cm in four different directions (*B*) during four-fifths of the dose, the distance between the 95 and 50% isodose lines is increased—i.e., the 95 and 50% isodose lines cover a smaller and larger area, respectively (*C*). In *D,* the isodose lines from *A* and *C* are superimposed on the same illustration for comparison. The black lines represent the dose distribution when the alignment is accurate.

different directions (Fig. 2-4*B*) during four-fifths of the dose, the 95 and 50% isodose lines cover a smaller and larger area, respectively—e.g., the distance between the isodose lines is increased (Fig. 2-4*C* and *D*). In this case, the misalignments were in opposite directions; thus the effect is offset. When the misalignment is consistently in the same direction, the distance between the 95 and 50% isodose lines in the direction of the misalignment is increased. In Fig. 2-5, the target is covered by the

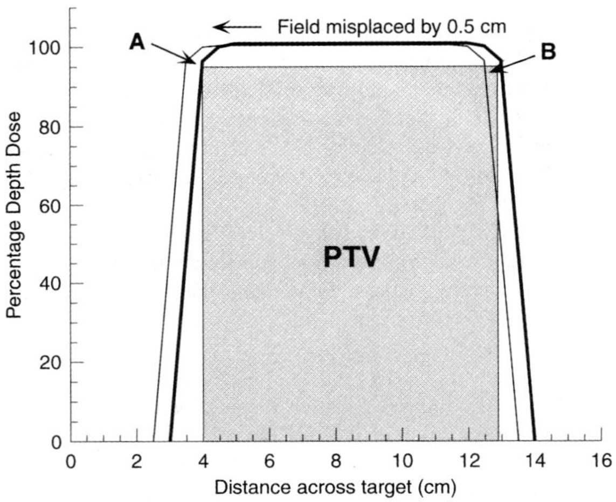

Fig. 2-5 Dose profile demonstrating the target covered by the 95% isodose line in the planned treatment (*thicker line*). When the field is misplaced by 0.5 cm *(thinner line)*, normal tissues are moved into the field (A) and part of the target is missed (B).

95% isodose line (thicker line); however, when the field is misplaced by 0.5 cm, normal tissues are moved into the field (*A*) and part of the target is missed (*B*).

Goitein and Busse studied the theoretical effect of underdosage at the perimeter of the treatment field caused by random immobilization errors.[39] They found that as much as a 12% improvement of tumor control probability could be achieved by good immobilization techniques in a supraglottic field. The authors conclude that good immobilization as a means of improving tumor control in supraglottic carcinoma is important.

Some older studies of mantle fields suggest that inaccuracies in patient setup may affect local tumor control. Maruyama and Kahn reported a 33% recurrence rate at sites adjacent to the blocked areas involving the mediastinum in patients with Hodgkin's disease.[40] Rubin et al. reported a 12% marginal recurrence rate in patients treated for Hodgkin's disease.[41] Marks et al. presented data from a retrospective review of portal films of 902 setups on 99 patients with Hodgkin's disease and malignant lymphoma and found that in 36% of the setups, the position of the shielding blocks was not duplicated as planned.[42] In 10 of 99 patients, the disease was not controlled locally. Two of these failures were at the margins of the fields and were shown by portal films to be correlated with positioning errors leading to reduced dose at the sites of recurrence. Kinzie et al. reported on the consequences of field misalignments in 155 patients treated for Hodgkin's disease in a Patterns of Care Study.[43] They found that with inadequate tumor margins, the in-field and marginal recurrence rates increased to 33% versus 7% in those with adequate margins.

From these studies, one might conclude that errors in treatment delivery, including patient positioning errors, are a significant cause of marginal recurrence. In these older studies, patient immobilization was probably less rigorous and target identification more difficult than they are today. Therefore, marginal recurrence rates are likely to be lower today.

ASSESSING SPATIAL TREATMENT ACCURACY

Portal imaging is an important quality-assurance procedure for monitoring the reproducibility of setup geometry in radiation therapy. The role of portal imaging has become more critical in recent years with the use of relatively small margins facilitated by 3DTP technology. The most common methods to monitor treatment accuracy are visual comparison of simulation film (prescription) and port film (treated) and electronic portal imaging.[9,44–49]

There are some distinct differences in how these two methods affect the treatment. Weekly port films are usually taken either immediately prior to or following a treatment and represent only a snapshot of a treatment setup; thus deficiencies occurring between port film days may go undetected for several days before being corrected. Electronic portal images, on the other hand, are usually obtained on a daily basis, often immediately prior to and/or during treatment delivery. In this situation, setup errors can be detected and corrected prior to each treatment and, in some situations, also during the treatment. Port films are often reviewed following the treatment and needed corrections are made prior to the next treatment—an obvious disadvantage. In the weekly port film method, the physician usually reviews the port films. With electronic portal imaging, the images are reviewed, often by the technical staff, at the treatment console.

Intermittent monitoring of the accuracy of the setup is prudent and may lead to discovery of errors that could otherwise go undetected. Assessing the accuracy of patient/beam alignment and the effectiveness of an immobilization device is important, and the result should be considered when field margins are designed. Thus, if port films are consistently inadequate, an increase in the field margins might be indicated.

REFERENCES

1. Rosenthal SA, Roach M III, Goldsmith BJ, et al: Immobilization improves the reproducibility of patient positioning during six-field conformal radiation therapy for prostate carcinoma. *Int J Radiat Oncol Biol Phys* 27:921, 1993.
2. Bentel GC: Positioning and immobilization device for patients receiving radiation therapy for carcinoma of the breast. *Med Dosim* 15:3, 1990.
3. Bentel GC: Positioning and immobilization of patients undergoing radiation therapy for Hodgkin's disease. *Med Dosim* 16:111, 1991.
4. Bentel GC, Marks LB: A simple device to position large/flaccid breasts during tangential breast irradiation. *Int J Radiat Oncol Biol Phys* 29:879, 1994.
5. Bentel GC, Marks LB, Sherouse GW, Spencer DP: A customized head and neck support system. *Int J Radiat Oncol Biol Phys* 32:245–248, 1995.
6. Bentel GC, Marks LB, Hendren K, Brizel DM: Comparison of two head and neck immobilization systems. *Int J Radiat Oncol Biol Phys* 38:867–873, 1997.
7. Bentel GC, Marks LB, Krishnamurthy R, Prosnitz LR: Comparison of two repositioning devices used during radiation therapy for Hodgkin's disease. *Int J Radiat Oncol Biol Phys* 39:791–795, 1997.
8. Bentel GC, Marks LB, Krishnamurthy R: Impact of cradle immobilization on setup reproducibility during external beam radiation therapy for lung cancer. *Int J Radiat Oncol Biol Phys* 38:527–531, 1997.
9. Creutzberg AL, Althof VG, Huizenga H, Visser AG: Quality assurance using portal imaging: The accuracy of patient positioning in irradiation of breast cancer. *Int J Radiat Oncol Biol Phys* 25:529–539, 1993.
10. Inoue T, Chatani M, Teshima T, et al: Immobilization and reproducibility in radiotherapy for cancer of the larynx and pharynx using simplified shell and bite-block. *Strahlentherapie* 161:642–645, 1985.
11. McCune K, Parsons L, Schoenfeld L, Maddeford A: A technique for evaluating cast foam positioning and immobilization devices used in breast cancer radiotherapy. *Med Dosim* 16:119–125, 1991.
12. Miller RW, Raubitschek AA, Harrington FS, et al: An isocentric chair for the simulation and treatment of radiation therapy patients. *Int J Radiat Oncol Biol Phys* 21: 469–473, 1991.
13. Rosenthal SJ, Gall KP, Jackson M, Thornton AFJ: A precision cranial immobilization system for conformal stereotactic fractionated radiation therapy. *Int J Radiat Oncol Biol Phys* 33:1239–1245, 1995.
14. Rudat V, Flentje M, Engenhart R, et al: The belly-board technique for the sparing of the small intestine: Studies on positioning accuracy taking into consideration conformational irradiation technics. *Strahlenther Onkol* 171:437–443, 1995.
15. Schwade JG, Houdek PV, Landy HJ, et al: Small-field stereotactic external-beam radiation therapy of intracranial lesions: Fractionated treatment with a fixed-halo immobilization device. *Radiology* 176:563–565, 1990.
16. Shanahan TG, Mehta MP, Bertelrud KL, et al: Minimization of small bowel volume within treatment fields utilizing customized "belly boards." *Int J Radiat Oncol Biol Phys* 19:469, 1990.
17. Thornton AF, TenHaken RK, Weeks KJ, et al: A head immobilization system for radiation simulation, CT, MRI, and PET imaging. *Med Dosim* 16:51–56, 1991.
18. Weller MK, Muller PL, Sugai S, Levenick J: Immobilization techniques and dosimetric aspects for pituitary tumors. *Med Dosim* 16:127–135, 1991.
19. Westbrook C, Gildersleve J, Yarnold J: Quality assurance in daily treatment procedure: Patient movement during tangential field treatment. *Radiother Oncol* 22:299, 1991.
20. Marcus KC, Svensson G, Rhodes LP, Mauch PM: Mantle irradiation in the upright position: A technique to reduce the volume of lung irradiated in patients with bulky mediastinal Hodgkin's disease. *Int J Radiat Oncol Biol Phys* 23:443, 1992.
21. Bieri S, Miralbell R, Nouet P, et al: Reproducibility of conformal radiation therapy in localized carcinoma of the prostate without rigid immobilization. *Radiother Oncol* 38:223–230, 1996.
22. Hess CF, Kortmann RD, Jany R, et al: Accuracy of field alignment in radiotherapy of head and neck cancer utilizing individualized face mask immobilization: A retrospective analysis of clinical practice. *Radiother Oncol* 34:69–72, 1995.
23. Mitine C, Dutreix A, van der Schueren E: Black and white in accuracy assessment of megavoltage images: The medical decision is often grey. *Radiother Oncol* 28:31–36, 1993.

24. Dunscombe PB, Fox K, Loose S, Leszczynski K: The investigation and rectification of field placement errors in the delivery of complex head and neck fields. *Int J Radiat Oncol Biol Phys* 26:155–161, 1993.
25. Hunt MA, Kutcher GJ, Burman C, et al: The effect of setup uncertainties on the treatment of nasopharynx cancer. *Int J Radiat Oncol Biol Phys* 27:437–447, 1993.
26. Rabinowitz I, Broomberg J, Goitein M, et al: Accuracy of radiation field alignment in clinical practice. *Int J Radiat Oncol Biol Phys* 11:1857, 1985.
27. Gildersleve J, Dearnaley DP, Evans PM, Swindell W: Reproducibility of patient positioning during routine radiotherapy, as assessed by an integrated megavoltage imaging system. *Radiother Oncol* 35:151–160, 1995.
28. Lirette A, Pouliot J, Aubin M, Larochelle M: The role of electronic portal imaging in tangential breast irradiation: A prospective study. *Radiother Oncol* 37:241–245, 1995.
29. McCullough EC, McCullough KP: Improving agreement between radiation-delineated field edges on simulation and portal films: The edge tolerance test tool. *Med Phys* 20:375, 1993.
30. Svensson GK: Quality assurance in radiation therapy: Physics efforts. *Int J Radiat Oncol Biol Phys* 10(suppl 1): 23, 1984.
31. AAPM: *AAPM Report No. 13: Physical Aspects of Quality Assurance in Radiation Therapy.* New York: American Institute of Physics, 1984.
32. Byhardt RW, Cox JD, Hornburg A, Liermann G: Weekly localization films and detection of field placement errors. *Int J Radiat Oncol Biol Phys* 4:881, 1978.
33. Rosenthal SA, Galvin JM, Goldwein JW, et al: Improved methods for determination of variability in patient positioning for radiation therapy using simulation and serial portal film measurements. *Int J Radiat Oncol Biol Phys* 23:621, 1992.
34. ICRU: *Prescribing, Recording, and Reporting Photon Beam Therapy: Report #50.* Bethesda, MD: International Commission on Radiation Units and Measurements, 1993.
35. Killoran JH, Kooy HM, Gladstone DJ, et al: A numerical simulation of organ motion and daily setup uncertainties: Implications for radiation therapy. *Int J Radiat Oncol Biol Phys* 37:213–221, 1997.
36. Suit HD, duBois W: The importance of optimal treatment planning in radiation therapy. *Int J Radiat Oncol Biol Phys* 21:1471, 1991.
37. Keus R, Noach P, deBoer R, Lebesque J: The effect of customized beam shaping on normal tissue complications in radiation therapy of parotid tumors. *Radiother Oncol* 21:211, 1991.
38. Letschert JGJ, Lebesque JV, deBoer RW, et al: Dose-volume correlation in radiation-related late small-bowel complications: A clinical study. *Radiother Oncol* 18:307, 1990.
39. Goitein M, Busse J: Immobilization error: Some theoretical considerations. *Radiology* 117:407, 1975.
40. Maruyama JE, Khan FM: Blocking considerations in mantle therapy. *Radiology* 101:167–171, 1971.
41. Rubin P, Haluska G, Poulter CA: The basis for segmental sequential irradiation of Hodgkin's disease: Clinical experience and patterns of recurrence. *Am J Roentgenol* 105: 814, 1969.
42. Marks JE, Haus AG, Sutton HG, Griem ML: Localization error in the radiotherapy of Hodgkin's disease and malignant lymphoma with extended mantle fields. *Cancer* 34: 83, 1974.
43. Kinzie JJ, Hanks GE, MacLean CJ, Kramer S: Patterns of Care Study: Hodgkin's disease relapse rates and adequacy of portals. *Cancer* 52:2223, 1983.
44. Meertens H, Van Herk M, Bijhold J, Bartelink H: First clinical experience with a newly developed electronic portal imaging device. *Int J Radiat Oncol Biol Phys* 18:1173, 1990.
45. Boyer AL, Antonuk L, Fenster A, et al: A review of electronic portal imaging devices (EPIDs). *Med Phys* 19:1, 1992.
46. Lam KS, Partowmah M, Lam WC: An on-line electronic portal imaging system for external beam radiotherapy. *Br J Radiol* 59:1007, 1986.
47. Michalski JM, Graham MV, Bosch WR, et al: Prospective clinical evaluation of an electronic portal imaging device. *Int J Radiat Oncol Biol Phys* 34:943–951, 1996.
48. van Herk M, Bel A, Gilhuijs KG, et al: Electronic portal imaging. *Bull Cancer* 82(suppl 5):601–606, 1995.
49. Mijnheer BJ: Quality assurance in radiotherapy: Physical and technical aspects. *Qual Assur Health Care* 4:9–18, 1992.

PROBLEMS

2-1 Spatial treatment uncertainties consist of
(*a*) dose inhomogeneities and patient positioning errors
(*b*) mechanical inaccuracies in the equipment and patient-related inconsistencies
(*c*) mechanical inaccuracies in the equipment and dose inhomogeneities
(*d*) patient-related inconsistencies and dose inhomogeneities

2-2 Uncertainties of treatment delivery
(*a*) are always caused by moving skin marks
(*b*) are always caused by mechanical inaccuracies of the equipment
(*c*) may be caused by mechanical inaccuracies of the equipment and/or patient repositioning
(*d*) may be prevented

2-3 When the geometric margins are 0.5 cm, the risk of missing the target is
(*a*) greater than when the margins are 1 cm
(*b*) smaller than when the margins are 1 cm
(*c*) smaller than when the margins are 1.5 cm
(*d*) the same as when the margins are 2 cm

2-4 The magnitude of patient-related uncertainties may depend on the
(*a*) treatment machine used
(*b*) penumbra of the beam
(*c*) size of the immobilization device
(*d*) treatment site and the patient's general condition

2-5 Mechanical inaccuracies of the treatment equipment
(*a*) can be eliminated by monthly quality-assurance testing
(*b*) are guaranteed by the manufacturer not to exist
(*c*) can be reduced by frequent quality-assurance testing
(*d*) are inherent to the machine and can never be eliminated

2-6 The clinical target volume (CTV) includes the
(*a*) gross target volume and the planning target volume
(*b*) planning target volume and subclinical disease
(*c*) gross target volume and the irradiated volume
(*d*) gross target volume and subclinical disease

2-7 Reducing target margins
(*a*) generally increases the complication rate
(*b*) allows higher doses to be delivered
(*c*) facilitates better targeting
(*d*) prevents the delivery of higher doses

2-8 Increasing the margin for a typical prostate field from 10 to 13 mm
(*a*) increases the irradiated volume by approximately 50%
(*b*) decreases the irradiated volume by approximately 25%
(*c*) increases the irradiated volume by approximately 25%
(*d*) increases the irradiated volume by approximately 2.5%

2-9 Monitoring setup reproducibility
(*a*) is usually accomplished by weekly port films
(*b*) is always accomplished by using electronic portal imaging
(*c*) can be accomplished by visual comparison of simulation films and port films or by electronic portal imaging
(*d*) is not necessary in most patients

2-10 The magnitude and frequency of spatial setup errors found on port film reviews

(*a*) should be disregarded but recorded in the patient's chart

(*b*) may lead to changes in the size of tumor margins

(*c*) can be used as a guide for setting tumor margins on the next patient treated for the same disease

(*d*) are usually greater when immobilization devices are used

CHAPTER

3

General Considerations of Positioning and Immobilization

INTRODUCTION

The need for effective patient immobilization has become widely recognized in recent years as the application of conformal treatment techniques, where small margins often are used, has increased. Since techniques utilizing small margins are more vulnerable to geometric target misses, precise and effective immobilization techniques are essential. Although there is need for improving patient immobilization in conformal radiation therapy, the same benefits should extend to all of radiation therapy.

PATIENT POSITIONING

Traditionally, in all radiation therapy treatments, attempts have been made to position the patients "straight" on the couch. Although this is a desirable goal, the ability to accurately *reproduce* the position is more important. In order to treat the same volume as the simulation or "prescription" radiograph indicates, it is crucial to *reposition* the patient exactly for each treatment as during the simulation procedure. That is, in order to deliver the "prescription treatment," the patient must be in the "prescription position."

In deciding a patient's treatment position, several important issues need to be considered, including comfort, reproducibility, ability to maintain the position for extended periods of time, and anticipated beam orientation. These issues are related, since an uncomfortable position may be difficult to reproduce and maintain. Patient comfort may be one of the most important considerations in choosing the position. Other parameters that may limit the choice of position are the patient's age, general health, weight, and treatment site.

In many situations, the patient's position is dictated by the beam direction. For example, to prevent incidental irradiation of the ipsilateral arm in tangential breast treatment, the arm is usually elevated. In the lower extremities, one leg may need to be displaced to avoid incidental irradiation of the uninvolved leg. In brain or head and neck treatment, it is often necessary to position the patient with a chin extension or flexion such that critical organs are outside the beam's trajectory. Such an unnatural position may not be comfortable, reproducible, or easy to maintain. A positioning or immobilization device may be especially useful in these situations.

Since reproducing the patient's position is essential in radiation therapy, the couch surface in the simulator/computed tomography (CT) and treatment room needs to be of the same shape and consistency. Hence, these couch tops are usually hard and flat. A hard surface can be uncomfortable, especially for a thin patient without "natural" padding. A thin pad is often used to provide comfort; however, for accurate repositioning, this pad must be identical on the simulator/CT and treatment couch. Repositioning the patient for each treatment on such a couch/pad is simple and unlikely to cause discrepancies in patient/beam alignment.

Patients unable to walk are usually brought to the radiation therapy clinic on a stretcher. These patients are often transferred to the simulation or treatment couch by being pulled/lifted in the bed sheet. The sheet tends to get bundled up under the patient, causing an undesirable "roll" or "tilt" (see the airplane analogy in Chap. 1). Since it is unlikely that the sheet will be causing the same roll or tilt for every treatment, it should instead be removed from under the patient prior to each treatment. The scenario with the bundled-up sheets is likely to occur in patients requiring spinal irradiation. Since these fields are often narrow and thus sensitive to a rotational error, removal of sheets and clothes from under these patients is particularly important. When some other sites are treated (e.g., head and neck, brain, extremities), a bundled-up sheet under the torso is unlikely to affect patient/beam alignment. For optimal reproducibility, a sheet and/or pad under the patient needs to be taut, not bundled up.

Setup discrepancies may result from the habit of leaving the patient's clothes on (and only moving them aside such that the field marks can be visualized) during treatment (Fig. 3-1). When an abdominal or spinal field is irradiated, clothes are sometimes moved up under the chest and down under the hips. The likelihood that these clothes will be of the same thickness and that they will be moved to exactly the same location for each treatment is probably nil; the position is therefore not reproducible (Fig. 3-2). Instead, the patient should be undressed above the waist and clothes below the waist should be moved down below the hips; thus the patient's bared chest and hips will be resting on the couch, improving reproducibility.

Ideally, all treatment fields should be delivered with the patient in the same position. There are, however, situations when this is not possible. For example, in some patients with lymphoma, Waldeyer's ring is treated through lateral fields abutting anterior/posterior mantle fields. The raised-arm position, often used for mantle field irradiation, would need

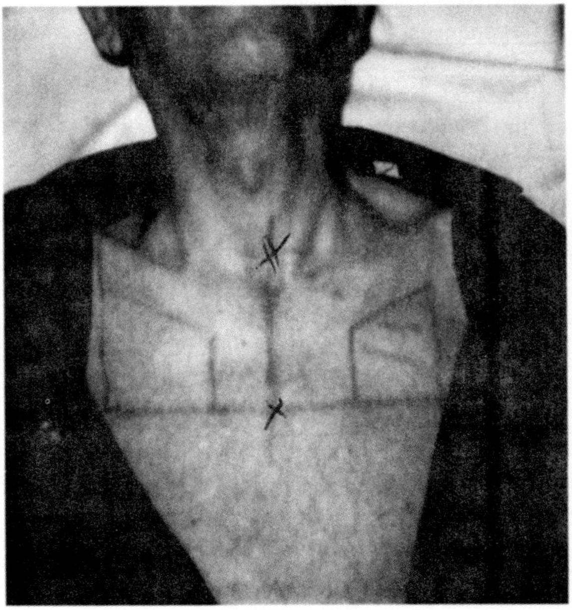

Fig. 3-1 The patient's clothes are sometimes moved aside only so that the setup marks can be visualized. It is unlikely that the patient will wear the same clothes during each treatment; thus inconsistent setup occurs. Thick layers of clothing (collars, belts) may also cause decreased skin sparing.

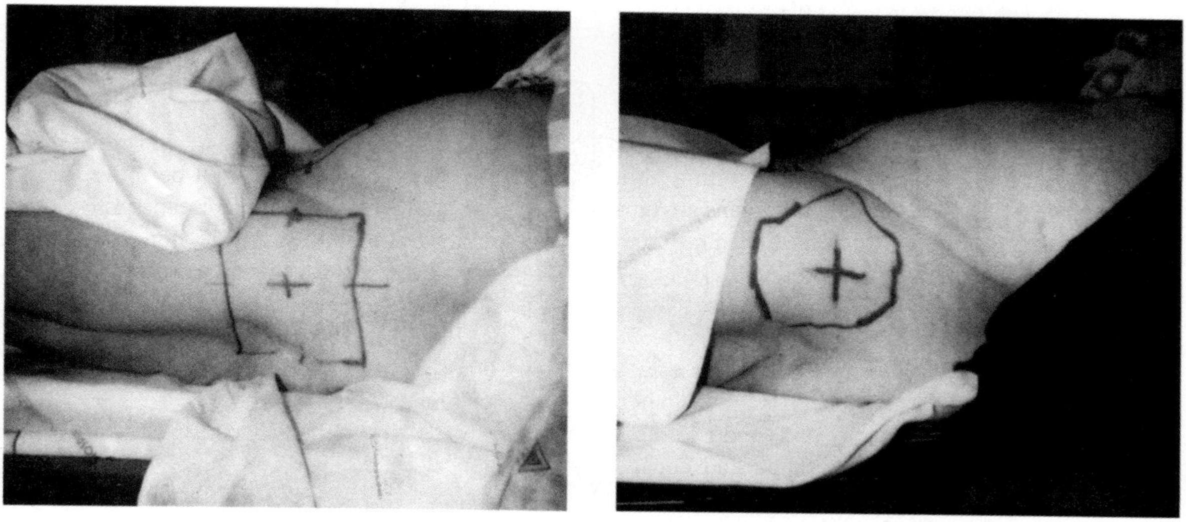

A B

Fig. 3-2 Sheets and clothes under the patient may not be of the same thickness or in the same location during simulation (*A*) and treatment (*B*) or during each treatment, causing patient/beam misalignments.

to be changed to facilitate treatment of the lateral head and neck fields. Similarly, when large fields (whole abdomen, mantle) cannot be accommodated by the couch window, it may be necessary to treat the patient in the supine and prone positions for anterior and posterior fields, respectively.

LIMITATIONS OF TREATMENT EQUIPMENT

Restrictions in treatment delivery, imposed by limitations of the treatment equipment, can be divided into two groups: (1) collimator/couch collision and (2) beam interception by portions of the couch. Both of these problems are related to the construction of the machine and, in some situations, the solution is the same.

COLLIMATOR/COUCH COLLISION

The extension of the head of the treatment machine into which auxiliary devices are inserted is frequently referred to as the *collimator* and it is so referred to here, though it is only one part of it. To minimize the risk of collisions, radiation therapy machines need to be streamlined. The couch, for example, should be as narrow as possible and provide adequate support for the patient—obviously contradictory requirements. It is important to consider the distance between the distal part of the collimator and the isocenter as well as the collimator shape/size. The distal part of the collimator should be as far from the isocenter as possible, and the outer dimensions should be as small as possible to leave maximum space for maneuvering the gantry around the patient.

Figure 3-3 illustrates the geometric arrangement of two different machines with a 100-cm source-isocenter distance. In one (Fig. 3-3*A*), the distal part of the collimator extends 50 cm from the target, leaving a 50-cm collimator-isocenter distance for maneuvering the machine around the patient (Fig. 3-3*B*). In the second (Fig. 3-3*C*), the target-collimator distance is 65 cm, leaving only a 35-cm collimator-isocenter distance (Fig. 3-3*D*). In this arrangement, the outer dimensions of the collimator must

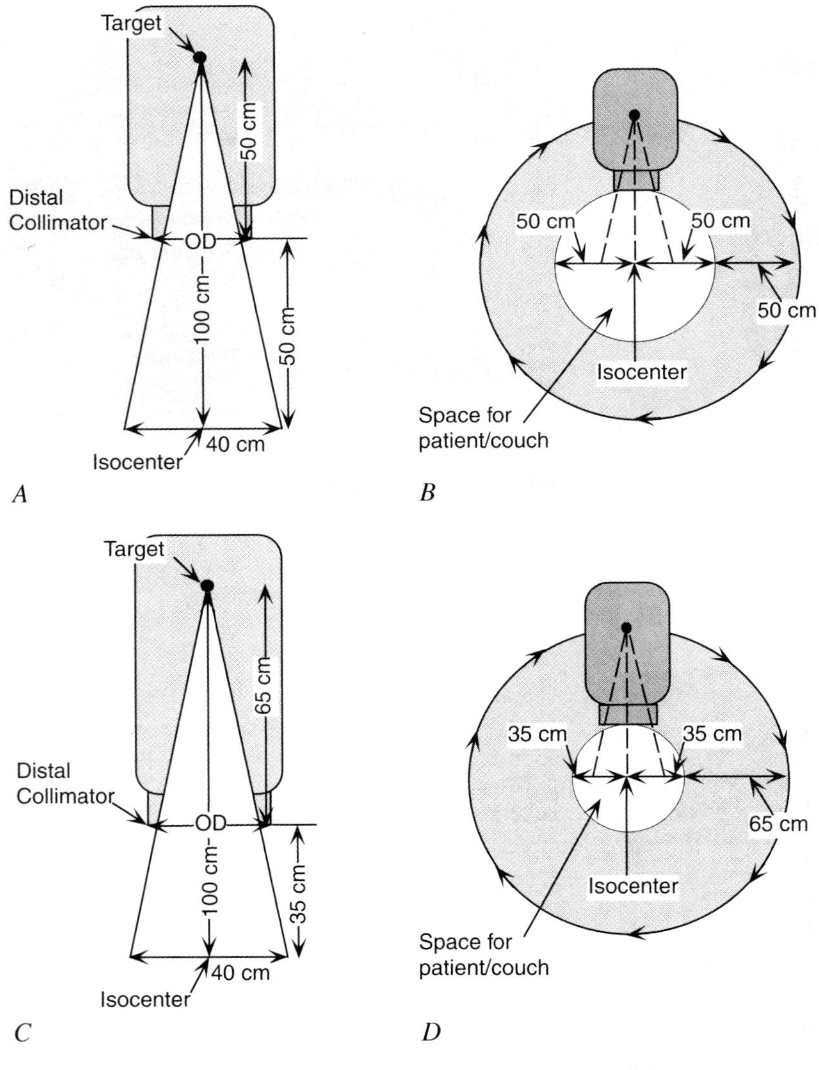

Fig. 3-3 Schematic illustration of two machines, both with 100-cm source-isocenter distance but with different beam collimation. When the distal part of the collimator extends 50 cm from the target (*A*), it leaves a 50-cm collimator-isocenter distance in which to maneuver the machine around the couch/patient (*B*). When the distal part of the collimator extends 65 cm from the target (*C*), only 35 cm of collimator-isocenter distance is available to maneuver the machine around the couch/patient (*D*).

be larger, since it is farther downstream in the diverging beam—an obvious disadvantage. There are, however, some advantages with a longer target-collimator distance: (1) the beam penumbra is sharper, though this benefit is inconsequential, since custom-made field-shaping blocks with diverging edges often are used, and (2) the accessory holder is easier to reach for insertion of accessories (e.g., shielding blocks, wedges, compensators); however, the size and weight of these are increased, since they are placed farther downstream, where the beam has diverged more.

The external shape of the collimator is also important for clearance. Since the maximum field size is square, it seems that a square-shaped collimator, conformed to the exiting beam, would be of minimal size and therefore would interfere least with the machine motions around the patient/couch (Fig. 3-4*A*). Circular collimators would appear to have unnecessarily large external dimensions (Fig. 3-4*B*).

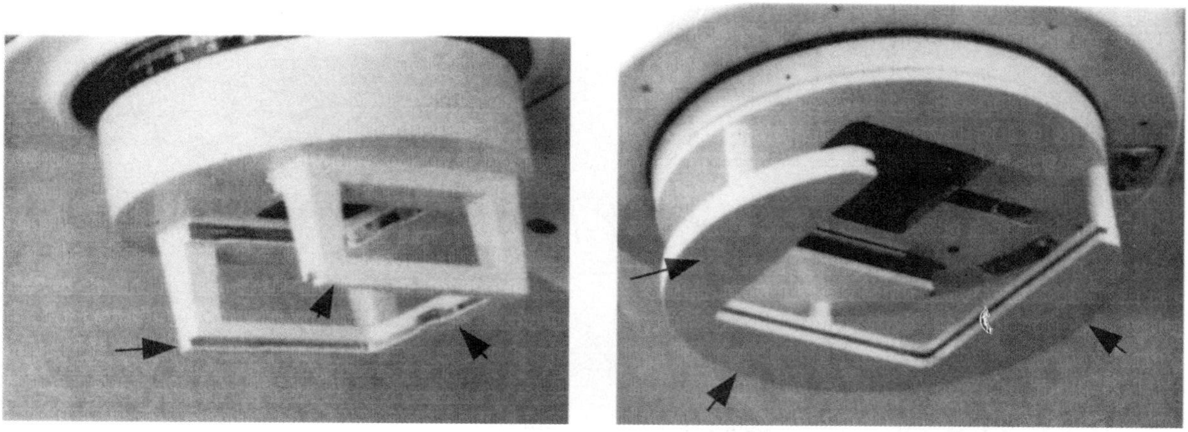

A *B*

Fig. 3-4 Since the maximum field size is square, the shape of the collimator should be square (*A*) and the external dimensions as small as possible to allow maximum space in which to maneuver the machine around the patient (*arrows*). A circular collimator (*B*) appears to have unnecessarily large external dimensions (*arrows*).

BEAM INTERCEPTION

Beam directions are sometimes limited by the presence of portions of the treatment couch in the beam trajectory. Modern treatment couches are usually designed with openings arranged such that beams can be directed from different angles without being intercepted by the couch. The openings are usually covered by a Plexiglas or Mylar sheet or a tennis racket–type insert, offering support for the patient's body (Fig. 3-5). A large "window" at one end of the couch allows posterior fields to be treated without being intercepted by the couch. The opposite end of the couch often has removable sections on each side, permitting unobstructed treatment of posterior oblique fields (Fig. 3-5), and the couch top can be reversed, such that the desired opening lies in the beam.

PROBLEMS AND SOLUTIONS

The problems of both collision and beam interception are related to the gantry angle used and the location of the isocenter relative to the couch/patient. Maximum clearance for a 360° gantry rotation is generally achieved when the isocenter is placed in the geometric center of the space occupied by the patient and the couch. This is rarely possible, since the isocenter is usually in or near the center of the target and thus can be practically anywhere relative to the patient/couch combination. Most radiation treatments are delivered via several stationary fields aimed from different directions rather than through rotational techniques. A collimator/couch collision may occur when the gantry is moved from one stationary field to another. When this occurs, the patient/couch can be moved temporarily to facilitate gantry rotation to the desired angle. Using setup marks and alignment lines, the couch is then returned to its position for treatment. In many modern machines, a digital readout displays the couch position, facilitating accurate repositioning. In another solution to avoid a collimator/side bar collision, the isocenter is shifted with respect to the target and the field shape is accomplished by using independent jaws or customized beam-shaping blocks (Fig. 3-6).

There are situations where the field is intercepted by either the side bars or the central spine (Fig. 3-7).

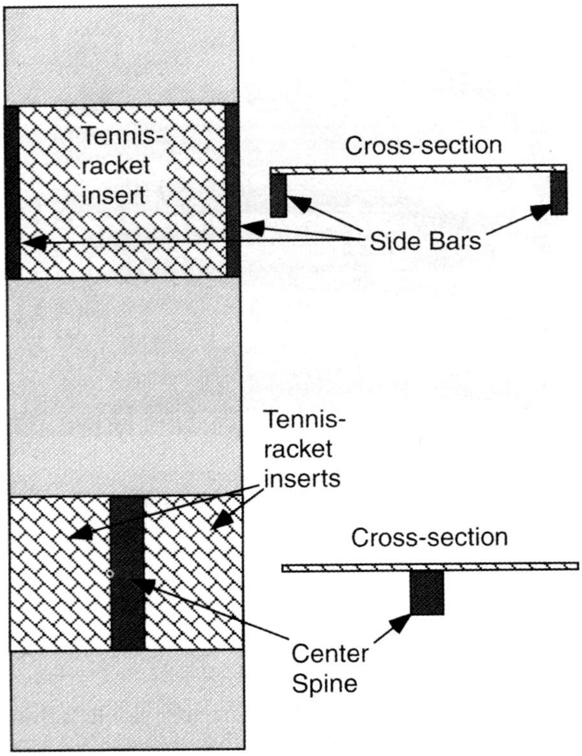

Fig. 3-5 A large "window" in one end of the couch facilitates treatment of posterior fields without interception by the couch. At the opposite end of the couch there are often removable sections on each side, permitting unobstructed treatment of posterior oblique fields. The couch top can be reversed such that the desired opening lies in the beam.

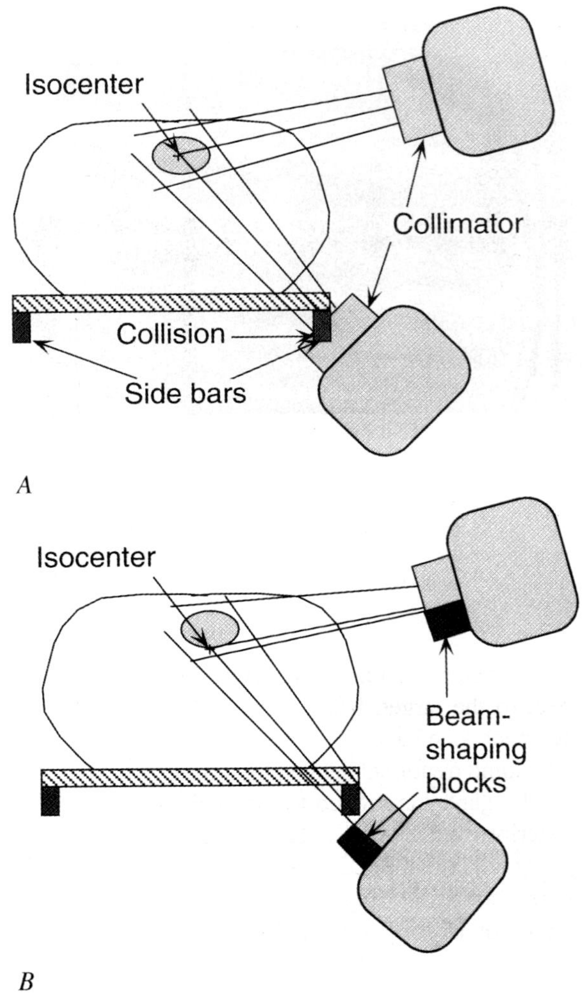

Fig. 3-6 When the isocenter is in the center of the target (*A*), the collimator may collide with the side bars on the couch. When the isocenter is shifted posteriorly and the field shape is accomplished by using independent jaws or customized beam-shaping blocks, the collimator may clear the side bars (*B*).

For example, patients with lung tumors may be treated concurrently with large anterior/posterior mediastinal and oblique off-cord fields. If the patient is positioned with the chest over the large central window, the oblique fields are likely intercepted by the side bars (Fig. 3-7*A*). If the couch top is reversed and the patient's chest positioned over the opposite end of the couch, the anterior/posterior fields are intercepted by the center spine (Fig. 3-7*B*). One suboptimal solution to this dilemma is to move the patient off the couch and reverse the orientation of the tabletop between treatment of the anterior/posterior and oblique fields. A new tabletop design facilitates treatment of all fields while the patient remains on the couch.

It might be possible to address collision and interception difficulties by moving the position of the isocenter relative to the treatment couch. Such isocenter shifts can be accomplished by moving the patient to the side of the couch (Fig. 3-8*A* and *B*) or elevating the patient (e.g., on a block of Styrofoam*) off the couch (Fig. 3-8*C*). In these methods,

*Dow Chemical, Midland, Michigan.

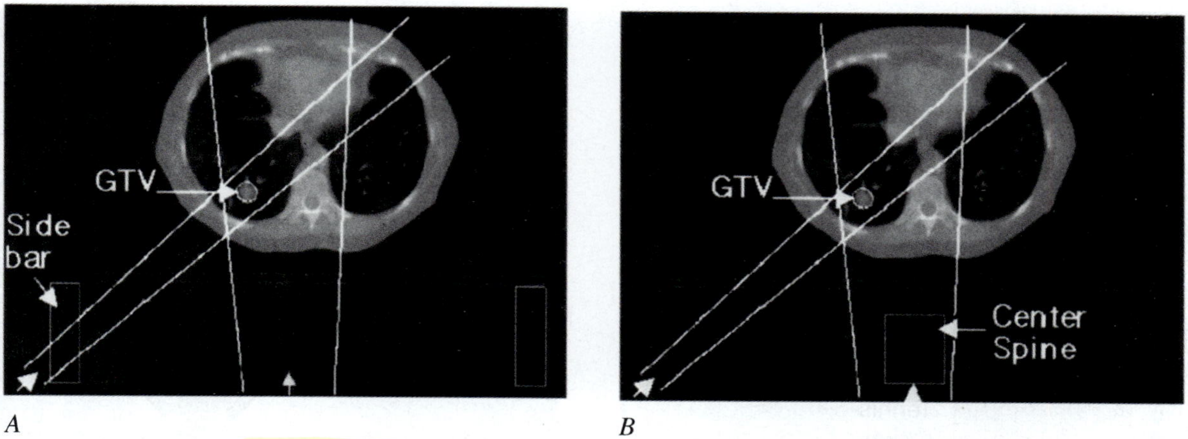

Fig. 3-7 When the patient is positioned with the chest over the large central window, the oblique fields are likely to be intercepted by the side bars (*A*). If the couch top is reversed, the anterior/posterior fields are intercepted by the center spine (*B*).

the isocenter remains in the same location with respect to the target, but it is moved with respect to the couch/side bars.

In some treatment setups, the couch is turned 90° and the gantry is rotated to the desired angle. For a posterior/caudal brain field in a supine patient, the gantry angle is limited by the pedestal of the patient support assembly (Fig. 3-9*A*). To increase the possibilities of treating a posterior/caudal field, the patient's head can be flexed (Fig. 3-9*B*).

IMMOBILIZATION

An immobilization device should serve two main purposes: to rigidly immobilize the patient and facilitate making setup marks on the device. To be effective, an immobilization device needs to extend well beyond the treatment site. When orthopedic surgeons are faced with a tibial fracture, they immobilize both the ankle and knee in a cast to prevent motion at the fracture site. The same philosophy applies in radiation therapy; when the pelvis is treated, the waist, hips, and knees need to be rigidly immobilized in one "cast"—not in three separate devices.

An unnatural or uncomfortable position can be difficult to maintain for long periods of time. To develop a better understanding of the need for positioning and stabilization devices, radiation therapy staff should practice different positions on a treatment couch. It is fundamental to successful immobilization that patients be provided with supports that allow them to relax while still maintaining the position. Such devices may also aid in reproducing the position from day to day.

A well-constructed immobilization device may have additional, less obvious benefits. For example, its use may make the patient feel more secure and less apprehensive than when lying on a narrow couch, high above the floor, alone in a room with dimmed lights. It may also reduce reliance on patient cooperation and alertness, lessen the probability of body rotation, help stabilize the relationship between external marks and internal structures, and reduce setup time. Improved setup accuracy reduces the number of port films that need to be taken, developed, reviewed, and stored.[1–5] The reduction in setup time when immobilization devices are used leads to greater throughput of patients. The cost of using immobilization devices should be weighed against the benefits described above and the more accurate and precise treatment that is achievable with casting and immobilization techniques.

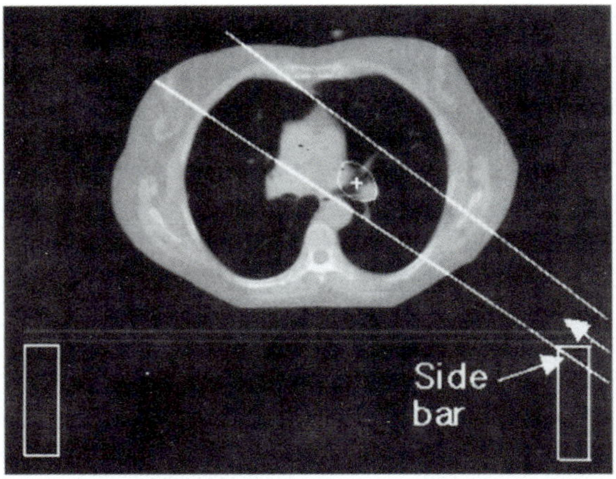

A

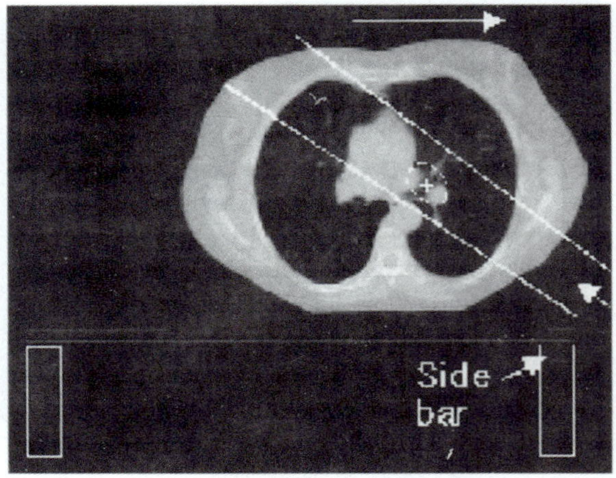

B

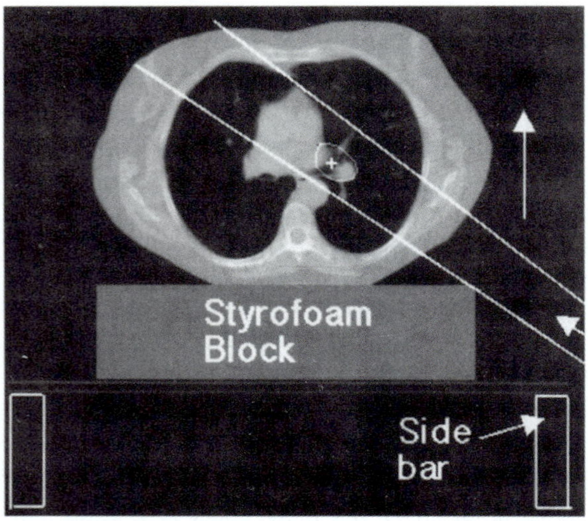

C

Fig. 3-8 Collimator/couch collisions and beam interception by the side bars in posterior oblique fields (*A*) may be eliminated by moving the patient to the side on the couch (*B*) or by elevation off the treatment couch (*C*). In both situations, the isocenter *and* the patient are shifted relative to the side bars.

IMMOBILIZATION DEVICES

Many types of positioning and immobilization devices are available to aid in patient repositioning and to help the patient *maintain* the position during each treatment. A positioning aid can be as simple as a bed pillow under the knees or as complex as a total-body mold. A range of devices are described, site by site, in the following chapters of this book.

SIMPLE DEVICES

A host of different positioning pillows and supports that can be used to make the patients more comfortable are available, many of them in every radiation therapy department. For example, a bed pillow under the head that is not thick enough can be boosted by adding a second pillow or a Styrofoam block under the pillow. Almost every patient feels more comfortable when the head is raised to a natural

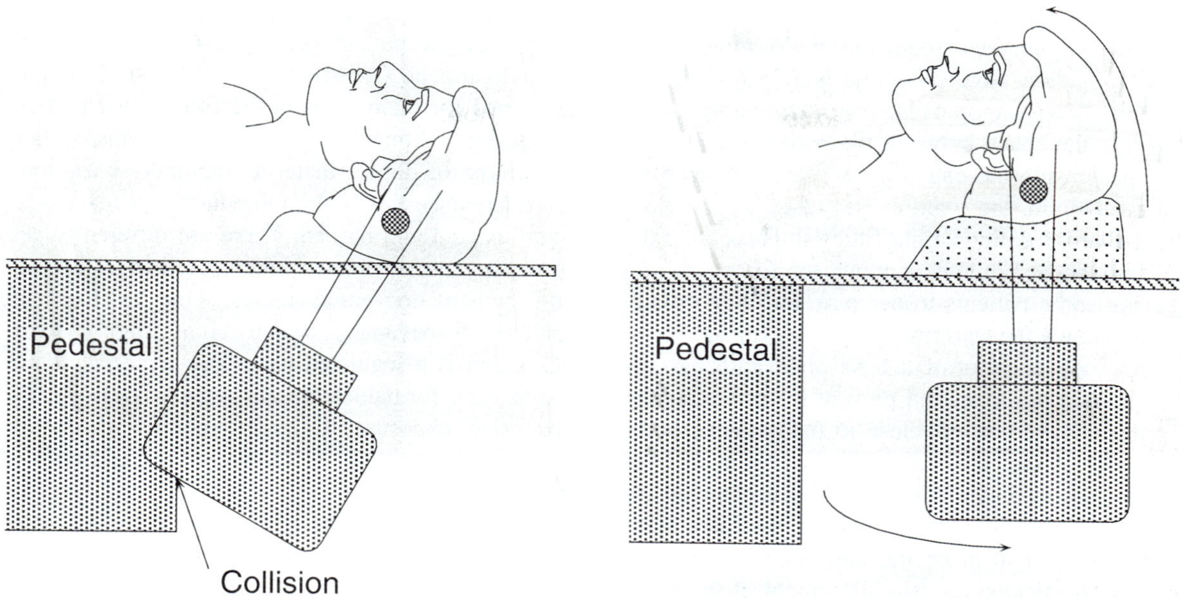

Fig. 3-9 When a brain or head and neck tumor is treated via a posterior/caudal field, the couch is often turned 90° and the gantry is rotated to the appropriate angle. The gantry angle is often limited by the risks of a gantry/pedestal collision (*A*). To facilitate such a posterior/caudal field, the patient's head can instead be flexed (*B*).

position. A bed pillow under the bent knees tends to relax the lower back when the patient is lying on a hard treatment couch. In many cases, the width of the treatment couch is not sufficient to support the patient's arms. Removable Plexiglas supports on each side can be used during most treatments but may interfere with treatments to the upper torso. For patients treated in the decubitus position, adding a small pillow or folded towel between their knees and/or feet usually improves comfort. To reproduce the foot separation for a supine/prone patient position, a Styrofoam block, where a section for each foot is removed, can be padded and used during each treatment.

Many simple devices are commercially available. Some of these are site-specific and may have restraining straps to achieve immobilization. Although these devices and the pillows and supports described above may assist in the daily alignment and immobilization of the patient, they do not permanently register the patient's initial treatment position for subsequent treatments. In a large number of treatments, such registration is not essential (e.g., whole-brain treatment, irradiation of bone metastases, some palliative lung treatments).

POSITIONING MOLDS

In head and neck and brain irradiation, facial masks are often used. These are described in detail in Chap. 4. Positioning molds used for various other treatment sites include the Alpha Cradle®,* Vac-Lok®,† and Aqua-Plast®.‡

*Smithers Medical Products, Inc., North Canton, Ohio.
†MED-TEC, Inc., Orange City, Iowa.
‡WFR/AQUAPLAST Corporation, Wyckoff, New Jersey.

Alpha Cradle. An Alpha Cradle is made by pouring polyurethane foam into a Styrofoam shell placed inside a large polyvinyl bag before the patient lies down on top of the bag. The foam expands and fills the space between the patient's body and the shell inside the bag (Fig. 3-10). After approximately 10 min, the foam ceases to expand and becomes hard, forming a tight-fitting impression of the patient's body. While expanding, the form is warm, causing some patients to perspire, but they usually seem to enjoy the warmth.

The shell consists of a base plate with barriers that contain the foam and prevent it from escaping. By placing the barriers close to the patient's body, the walls of the finished mold are prevented from becoming too thick. When the barriers are placed immediately adjacent to the patient, the foam tends to expand and displace the barriers, forming adequate wall thicknesses. The placement of the barriers also serves as a guide to the amount of foam needed. In general, when there is more space between the patient and the barriers, a larger volume of foam is needed. When more foam is used, the walls become thicker and the size of the mold increases, possibly leading to the collision problems discussed above. It may also be problematic with fitting the patient into diagnostic scanners [e.g., CT or magnetic resonance imaging (MRI)]. Thick walls may also cause excessive skin erythema when the radiation beam traverses the mold. On the contrary, the mold needs to be strong to withstand the stress caused by the patient getting in and out of it for every treatment. Construction of an Alpha Cradle is described for many sites in the following chapters.

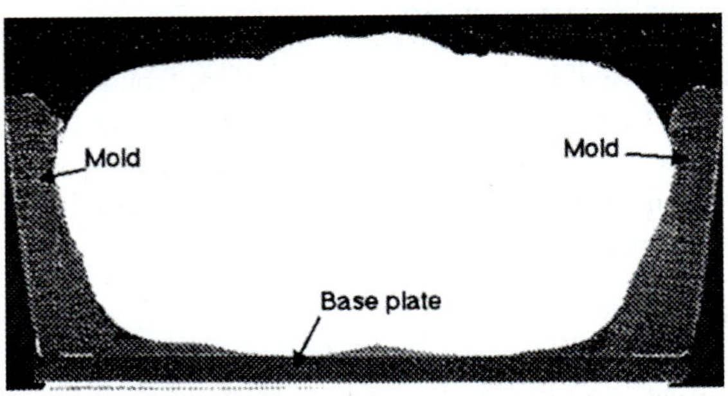

Fig. 3-10 A positioning mold should fit tightly to the patient's external contour.

Toxicity. Almost all polyurethane foams contain some type of diisocyanate, a potentially hazardous material, since this is the ingredient that makes the foam expand and harden. There are different types of diisocyanates, many of them used in industrial- and construction-grade foams. One of these is toluene diisocyanate, which emits highly toxic gases and is a regulated hazardous material. Some foams emit formaldehyde gas, which is also toxic. Extensive exposure to large amounts of certain types of diisocyanates is known to have caused respiratory disease.*

The foam used in the *Alpha Cradle* product *does not* contain these hazardous types of gases. In it, the ingredient used to make the foam expand and harden is diphenylmethane diisocyanate. The personal exposure level (PEL) set by the Occupational Safety and Health Administration (OSHA) for this material is 0.02 parts per million (ppm). When this material was tested, it registered 0.004 ppm, which is well below the standard set by OSHA. No adverse health effects should result from the proper use of this material. Other brands of foam used for making immobilization molds may not have been tested for toxic gases. It is important that each user obtain toxicology information for the particular brand being used.

Effect on Dose. The effects of foam molds on the depth dose are generally small relative to other heterogeneities that are often ignored in routine clinical practice (irregular external contour, air cavities, lung and bone density). The effect on the surface dose, however, should be considered, especially if lower beam energies (≤4 MV) are used and the beam traverses a large thickness of foam (5 to 7

*Further information can be obtained from National Institute for Occupational Safety and Health, 4676 Columbia Pkwy., Cincinnati, Ohio 45226 (Tel: 1-800-356-4674; or e-mail: pubstaft@niosdt1.em.cdc.gov).

cm). The doses in the buildup regions under different thicknesses of expanded foam were measured and compared to an open field. Measurements were made using a commercial scanning system* with a photon diode on a linear accelerator† using a 6-MV photon beam (10 × 10 cm field). The dose was measured at 1.5 mm of depth and extrapolated surface doses were 46, 65, and 75% for 2-, 5-, and 7-cm foam, respectively. The extrapolated surface dose for an open field was 35%. When there are concerns with respect to skin dose, the thickness of the foam within the radiation fields can be trimmed. The plastic bag should be secured over the trimmed areas to prevent direct contact with the foam.

In our more than 20 years of experience in using the Alpha Cradle at Duke University Medical Center, we have rarely seen any harmful effects from the interception of treatment fields by the molds. One moderately large patient with lung cancer received 73.6 Gy through a combination of opposed anterior/posterior and oblique fields using 6-MV photon beams. The posterior fields traversed the mold and a 1.2-cm-thick Plexiglas insert on the couch. Following completion of radiation therapy, she had a small area of moist desquamation on the posterior surface of her chest, where all fields overlapped. It is possible that this reaction was, in part, caused by the presence of the Plexiglas insert. Skin erythema was observed in the lateral fields of one moderate-sized patient irradiated for prostate cancer. The foam was 6 to 8 cm thick, and a dose of ~66 Gy was delivered via a four-field plan using 6-MV photons. Increased erythema has been seen in some patients treated using 6-MV photons and where the beams traversed a foam thickness in excess of ~7 cm.

Storage and Disposal. Concerns regarding storage and disposal of foam molds are sometimes expressed. At Duke University Medical Center, approximately 30 to 35 molds are stored vertically inside cabinets in each treatment room (Fig. 3-11*A*). The vertical storage appears to cause the molds to warp; however, the patients' weight usually flattens the molds on the treatment couch during treatment. When space inside the cabinets is insufficient, some molds are stored on "baker's racks" (Fig. 3-11*B*). Disposal has been through the customary discard system within the hospital. Recently, a business firm that recycles foam packaging, with more than 180 collection sites in the United States, has offered to recycle foam molds.‡

Vac-Lok System. Another system that can be used to form an immobilization mold consists of a urethane bag filled with small polystyrene beads. The patient is placed on top of the bag and, while the bag is semideflated, it is molded around the patient's body (Fig. 3-12). The mold becomes rigid when air is evacuated by a vacuum compressor, connected via a valve in the bag. Any cut or tear in the bag caused by handling or storing during the treatment course or by a patient's or staff member's jewelry, nails, or other sharp object causes air to enter, and the mold loses its shape. When the mold is remade, it is unlikely that the patient's position will be reproduced and that the setup marks on the device will be in precisely the same position. Therefore, the simulation procedure would also need to be repeated. When three-dimensional treatment-planning/(3DTP) techniques are used, the CT scanning and treatment-planning process would also need to be repeated, an obvious drawback. When a bag is damaged, it is returned to the manufacturer for repair or is replaced.

The effects of Vac-Lock molds on the depth dose are generally small relative to other heterogeneities that are often ignored in routine clinical practice. The surface dose, however, should be considered. With a 2-cm-thick mold, using a 6-MV photon beam (15 × 15 cm field), the surface dose is approximately 60%, versus 43% for an open field.

*Wellhöfer Dosimetrie, Schwarzenbrück, Germany.

†Varian 6/100, Varian Oncology Systems, Palo Alto, California.

‡Smithers Medical Products, Inc., North Canton, Ohio, can be contacted for information.

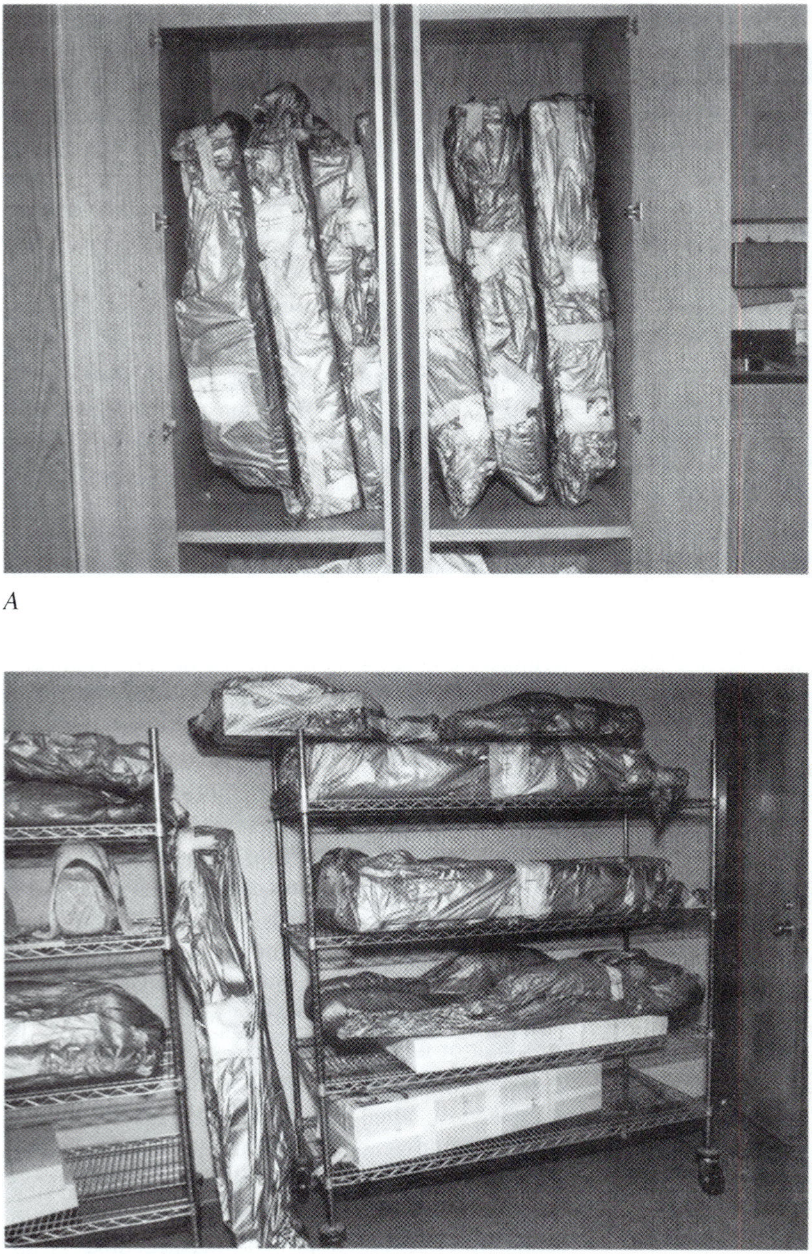

A

B

Fig. 3-11 Cabinet for vertical storage of positioning molds (*A*) and "baker's rack" for horizontal storage (*B*).

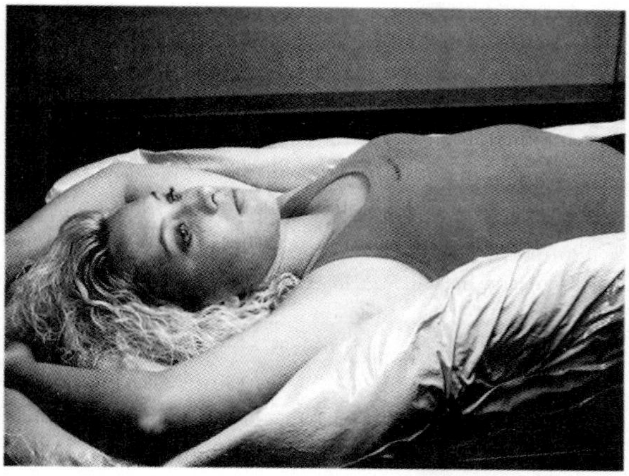

Fig. 3-12 A vacuum bag, molded to the patient's external contour, is often used for patient positioning. (Courtesy of MED-TEC, Inc., Orange City, Iowa.)

Since the urethane bags are reusable, they require cleaning and removal of setup marks between patients. Bags are available in many sizes and shapes; some have a "window" to prevent buildup in the treatment area, and others have "belly-board-type" openings.

Aqua-Plast. The most common use of thermoplastic materials is probably in head and neck or brain radiation therapy (Chaps. 4 and 5). Thermoplastic molds are also used for pelvic and breast immobilization.[6-8] The thermoplastic material is softened in a warm-water bath and is molded to conform to the patient's external contour. The mold is secured to a base plate on each side and, for pelvic molds, also between the patient's legs (Chap. 9). When the thermoplastic material cools, it forms a rigid mask or mold of the patient's body.

EFFICACY OF IMMOBILIZATION

The effectiveness of an immobilization device depends on the care with which it is conceived, fabricated, and used. Construction of an effective immobilization device requires a thorough understanding of anatomy and physiology as well as experience in working with various materials. If not designed carefully, an immobilization device may become a detriment to patient repositioning (e.g., a sharp edge on the device may cause patients not to reposition themselves correctly).

A patient who understands the importance of the immobilization and is willing and able to cooperate is more likely to remain motionless during the therapy and to get into awkward positions willingly. At Duke University Medical Center, the purpose of the immobilization device is explained to patients prior to the mold/mask making. The patients are instructed to think about how the position/mold feels when the fabrication is completed so that they do reproduce the position when they return for treatment. Instructions regarding how to enter the mold for each treatment are also given—e.g., they first sit straight in the mold and then recline to facilitate consistent positioning.

The effectiveness of an immobilization device is often determined by comparing simulation and portal films of the treatment fields. It is important to recognize, however, that many other factors play an important role in the accuracy of the patient-beam alignment observed on portal films: for example, fit of the immobilization device (clothing, gowns, and sheets under the patient must be avoided), mobile skin marks, thickness of setup lines, precision of alignment systems, couch sag in the simulation/CT and treatment rooms, and—perhaps the most important variable—the patience and meticulousness of the treating technologists in setting up treatments.

REFERENCES

1. Bentel GC, Marks LB, Sherouse GW, et al: The effectiveness of immobilization during prostate irradiation. *Int J Radiat Oncol Biol Phys* 31:143–148, 1995.
2. Bentel GC, Marks LB, Hendren K, Brizel DM: Comparison of two head and neck immobilization systems. *Int J Radiat Oncol Biol Phys* 38:867–873, 1997.
3. Bentel GC, Marks LB, Krishnamurthy R, Prosnitz LR: Comparison of two repositioning devices used during radiation therapy for Hodgkin's disease. *Int J Radiat Oncol Biol Phys* 39:791–795, 1997.

4. Bentel GC, Marks LB, Krishnamurthy R: Impact of cradle immobilization on setup reproducibility during external beam radiation therapy for lung cancer. *Int J Radiat Oncol Biol Phys* 38:527–531, 1997.
5. Rosenthal SA, Roach M III, Goldsmith BJ, et al: Immobilization improves the reproducibility of patient positioning during six-field conformal radiation therapy for prostate carcinoma. *Int J Radiat Oncol Biol Phys* 27:921, 1993.
6. Creutzberg AL, Althof VG, Huizenga H, Visser AG: Quality assurance using portal imaging: The accuracy of patient positioning in irradiation of breast cancer. *Int J Radiat Oncol Biol Phys* 25:529–539, 1993.
7. Leibel SA, Heiman R, Kutcher GJ, et al: Three dimensional conformal radiation therapy in locally advanced carcinoma of the prostate: Preliminary results of a Phase I dose-escalation study. *Int J Radiat Oncol Biol Phys* 28: 55–65, 1993.
8. Zierhut D, Flentje M, Frank C, et al: Conservative treatment of breast cancer: Modified irradiation technique for women with large breasts. *Radiother Oncol* 31:256–261, 1994.

PROBLEMS

3-1 When target margins are small, patient immobilization is
- (*a*) not necessary because the patients are told to hold still during the treatment
- (*b*) more important than when margins are generous, because small target margins are more vulnerable to misalignments
- (*c*) the same as when margins are generous because the patients are told to not move during the treatment
- (*d*) not necessary because it does not improve setup accuracy

3-2 In repositioning a patient for treatment, it is
- (*a*) necessary to position the patient straight on the couch regardless of how he or she was positioned during the simulation/CT procedure
- (*b*) necessary to position the patient so that he or she is comfortable and not necessarily the same as during the simulation/CT procedure
- (*c*) most important that the patient is comfortable
- (*d*) necessary to position the patient in the same position as during the simulation/CT procedure

3-3 In treating spinal fields
- (*a*) it is necessary to undress the patient above the waist and move skirts or pants below the hips
- (*b*) clothing need be removed only so that the field marks can be visualized
- (*c*) clothing and bed sheet should remain under the patient
- (*d*) the patient can remain on the stretcher during the treatment, as it may be painful to move him or her onto the treatment couch

3-4 Patients receiving treatment via multiple fields
- (*a*) may be moved between treatment fields
- (*b*) preferably should remain in the same position for all fields
- (*c*) should be encouraged to move between fields
- (*d*) should be treated to only one field per day

3-5 To avoid having posterior oblique lung fields intercepted by side bars on the couch, the
- (*a*) patient can be moved on the couch closer to the gantry
- (*b*) patient can be elevated off the couch
- (*c*) attenuation by the side bars should be disregarded
- (*d*) patient should be treated on another machine

3-6 For an immobilization device to be effective,
(*a*) it should fix the patient's body rigidly at least 10 in. on each side of the treated area
(*b*) it should be made of a softly padded cushion so that the patient will be comfortable and remain still during treatment
(*c*) it should rigidly fix at least the nearest joint on each side of the treatment area
(*d*) it should immobilize the feet and chest

3-7 To facilitate maximum space in which to maneuver the patient/couch, a treatment machine should have
(*a*) a short distance from the x-ray source (target) to the collimator
(*b*) a short distance from the collimator to the isocenter
(*c*) a long collimator-to-isocenter distance
(*d*) large outer dimensions of the distal part of the collimator

3-8 The purpose of an immobilization device is to
(*a*) make the patient's position comfortable
(*b*) facilitate reproducing and maintaining the position
(*c*) prevent the patient from falling off the couch
(*d*) help the therapist set up the treatment faster

3-9 Foams used in making positioning molds
(*a*) contain some sort of diisocyanate, since this is what causes the foam to expand and harden
(*b*) are different and should be tested for toxicity before being used to make immobilization devices
(*c*) and labeled Alpha Cradle brand have been tested for toxic levels by OSHA and found to be well within its standards
(*d*) *a*, *b*, and *c* are true
(*e*) *a*, *b*, and *c* are false

3-10 In comparing simulation and port films to detect misalignments,
(*a*) only the effect of the immobilization device is measured
(*b*) the combined effects of all uncertainties are measured
(*c*) the effect of the immobilization device is not measurable
(*d*) only misalignments $\geq$5 mm are visible

CHAPTER

4

Head and Neck

INTRODUCTION

The ability to position the patient accurately and reproducibly during a course of radiation is fundamental to fractionated radiation therapy. This is particularly true when the target is located adjacent to radiosensitive structures or when the margins surrounding the target are small. This situation is frequently encountered when the head and neck area is irradiated. The risks of inadvertently irradiating nontarget tissues must be minimized and every effort should be made to accurately irradiate the target.

In earlier years, radiation therapy was often delivered using cobalt-60 machines, some without isocentric rotation capabilities.[1] Treatment fields were shaped by loosely stacking (not fastening) lead blocks onto a tray fixed to the collimator, thus precluding machine angulation. The machine was therefore stationary with the beam pointing toward the floor while the patient's position was adjusted to achieve the desired beam/patient relationship. Patients receiving radiation therapy for head and neck or brain tumors were thus often treated while lying on their sides,[2] with a tape stretched across the head to prevent motion (Fig. 4-1). When opposed

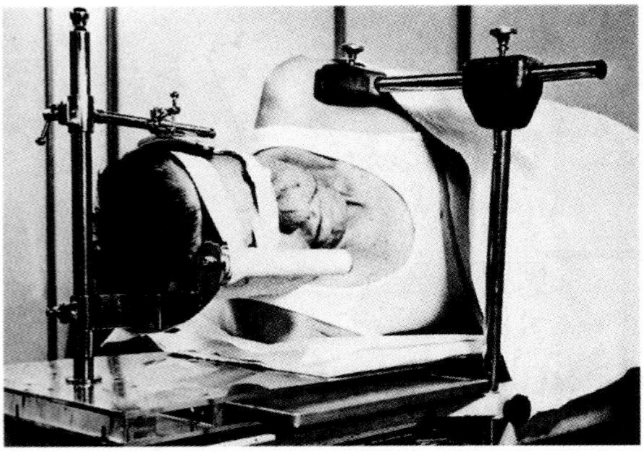

Fig. 4-1 Positioning device used in earlier years to treat patients in the lateral (decubitus) position. (From Fletcher GH: *Textbook of Radiotherapy,* 3d ed. Philadelphia: Lea & Febiger, 1980. Reproduced with permission of Williams & Wilkins, Baltimore.)

lateral fields were used, the patients would alternate lying on the right or left side. If an anterior lower neck/supraclavicular field was also used, the patient would be in the supine position for this field. The treatment would thus be delivered with the patient in three different positions, with obvious field-matching difficulties. It was also common to treat only one of the opposing fields during each treatment session. The position was not comfortable or reproducible, and, in patients with a short neck, the beam would exit in the shoulder on which the patient was resting.

As treatment machines have become more sophisticated during the last 15 to 20 years and beam-shaping blocks are *fastened* onto a tray, all fields can be treated with the patient in one position while the machine is turned to the appropriate angle.

The need for accuracy in field matching and concern for normal tissue damage has led to many sophisticated positioning and immobilization techniques in the head and neck area. The proximity of the eyes, optic chiasm, spinal cord, and brain requires precise reproducibility of the setup, particularly when the target dose exceeds the tolerance of the neighboring normal tissues. The need for a reproducible yet comfortable patient position and the use of restraining devices has become evident; as a result, many positioning aids and immobilization devices are currently available.

TREATMENT POSITION

SUPINE, PRONE, OR DECUBITUS

In the majority of head and neck and brain treatments, the patient's position is supine and rarely is the prone position desirable. In addition to being more comfortable, the supine position has been shown to be superior to the lateral position.[2] Marks and Haus found 16% of setup errors in unimmobilized patients treated in the lateral position, while there was only 1% of setup errors in patients immobilized using a bite-block system and treated in the supine position ($p < 0.001$). The supine position also allows the patient to visualize the staff during the setup. For a child or an anxious patient, the ability to see the staff during the setup can have a calming effect and be important for the successful day-to-day repositioning. The supine position also allows the staff better visualization of the patient and often also of the treatment fields.

Consideration should be given to the patient's condition when the position is chosen. For example, for an anesthetized child, it may be necessary to place a rolled up towel under the neck in order to facilitate easier breathing. A patient who is short of breath may need to be treated in a semirecumbent position, and a claustrophobic patient may not tolerate any type of restraining device. The patient's ability to maintain the position for the duration of the treatment should also be considered when the position is chosen.

HEAD POSITION

Neutral. The neutral head position is one in which the forehead and chin lie on a nearly horizontal plane (Fig. 4-2*A*). The head elevation required to achieve this position is variable but is largely determined by the size of the patient's torso (Fig. 4-2*B*). In a larger (thicker) patient, the midcoronal plane of the torso is elevated more above the couch than it is

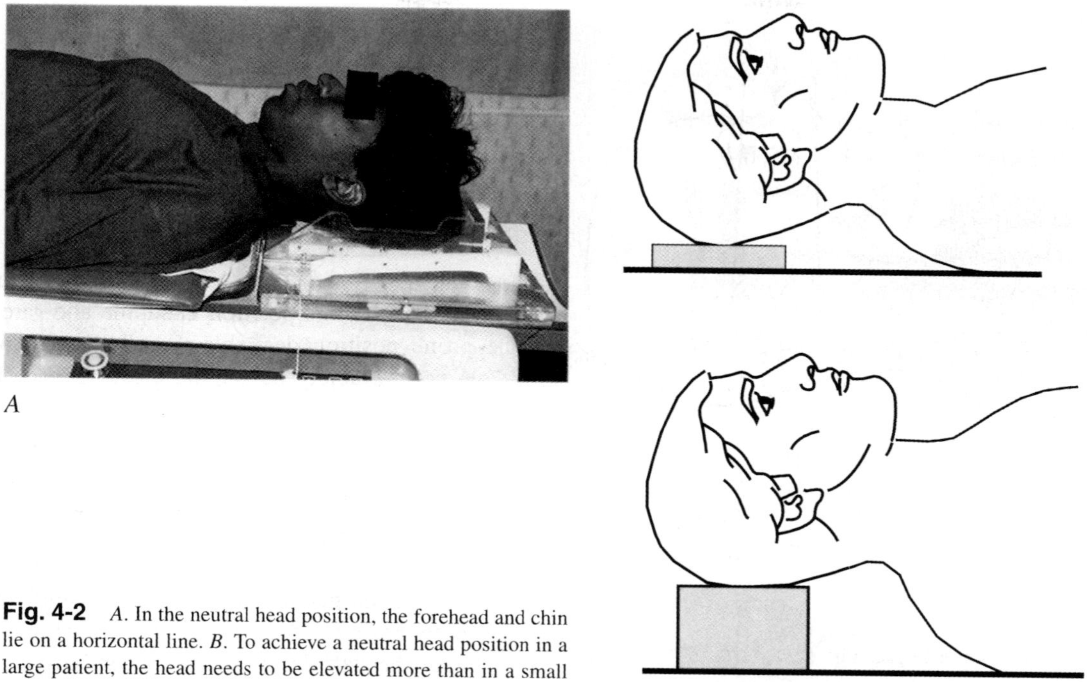

A

B

Fig. 4-2 *A*. In the neutral head position, the forehead and chin lie on a horizontal line. *B*. To achieve a neutral head position in a large patient, the head needs to be elevated more than in a small patient.

in a smaller (thinner) patient, while the heads of the two patients are of approximately the same size. To elevate the head in the supine patient so that it is in the neutral position, a thicker head support is thus required for the larger patient (Fig. 4-2*B*). In small children, where the head is large relative to the body, it may be necessary to elevate the torso to achieve a neutral head position.

Extended. In treating certain tumors in the head and neck region, it may be necessary to elevate the patient's chin. For example, an anterior field, frequently used in the treatment of tumors in the maxillary antrum, may include a large portion of the eye if the head is in a neutral position (Fig. 4-3*A*). By extending the chin, the apex of the maxillary antrum (which extends cephalad and posterior to the eye) can be included while reducing the amount of the eye in the beam (Fig. 4-3*B*). The same patient/beam arrangement can be achieved by turning the couch 90° and rotating the gantry to the appropriate angle while the patient is in the neutral head position (Fig. 4-3*C*). One disadvantage of this position (Fig. 4-3*B* and *C*) is that the volume of brain within the anterior field is increased. In situations where the eye cannot be spared (e.g., tumor invasion of the orbit), elevation of the chin may not be necessary. Many patients are uncomfortable with the chin extended, especially if it is hyperextended. Elevating the patient's shoulders by placing a thick pad under the chest often increases the chin elevation and may reduce the strain and discomfort of extending the chin (Fig. 4-4).

Flexed. A flexed head position may be desired when a frontal or vertex field is used in treating pituitary or brain lesions (Chap. 5). Alternatively, the head position could be neutral and the appropriate beam angles achieved by rotating the gantry, couch, and collimator. This is difficult unless three-dimensional treatment planning (3DTP) capabilities are available.

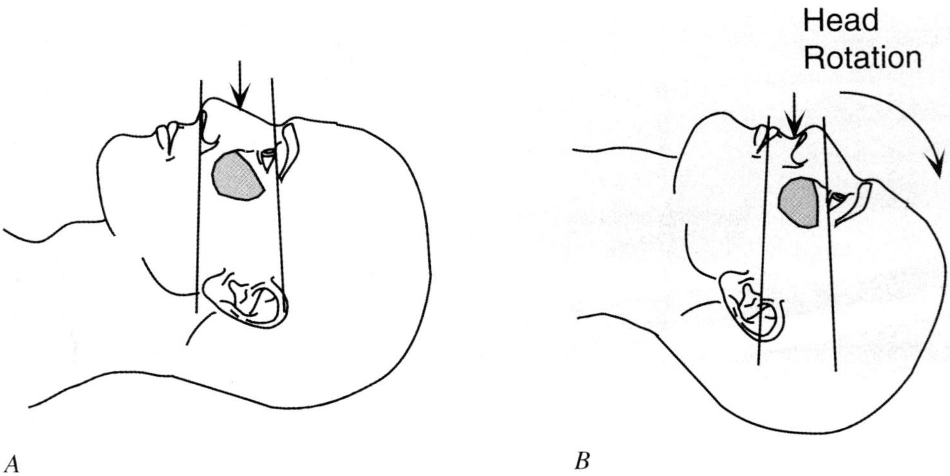

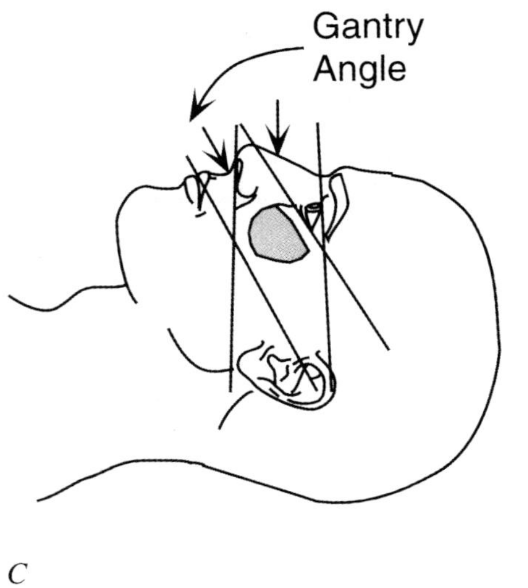

Fig. 4-3 *A*. In treating a lesion of the maxillary antrum with the patient's head in the neutral position, the eye may also be included. *B*. By extending the chin, the apex of the maxillary antrum can be included while avoiding the eye. *C*. With the patient's head position neutral, the same patient/beam arrangement can be achieved by turning the couch 90° and rotating the gantry.

In the era of 3DTP, where the selection of beam orientations is practically unlimited, the patient's head can remain in a neutral position (i.e., the forehead and chin lie on a horizontal plane), and the beams are then arranged on the desired plane by turning the gantry, couch, and collimator (Fig. 4-3*C*).

IMMOBILIZATION AND RESTRAINING

The ability to reproduce the patient's position from treatment to treatment may be compromised in the absence of positioning aids. The possibility of some involuntary motion associated with swallowing or coughing during a treatment is always present. Moreover, patients placed in an uncomfortable (unnatural) position are generally more likely to move involuntarily during the treatment. Immobilization and restraining devices may be helpful in reproducing the position from treatment to treatment *and* in maintaining the position during each treatment.

Uncooperative patients may also require restraining of arms and trunk to the treatment couch. Such rigorous immobilization should be used judiciously, since the risks associated with the patient's inability

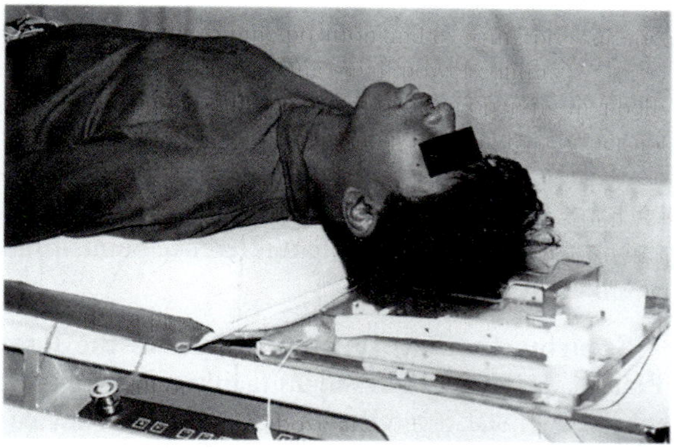

Fig. 4-4 To increase the chin extension, the patient's shoulders can be elevated.

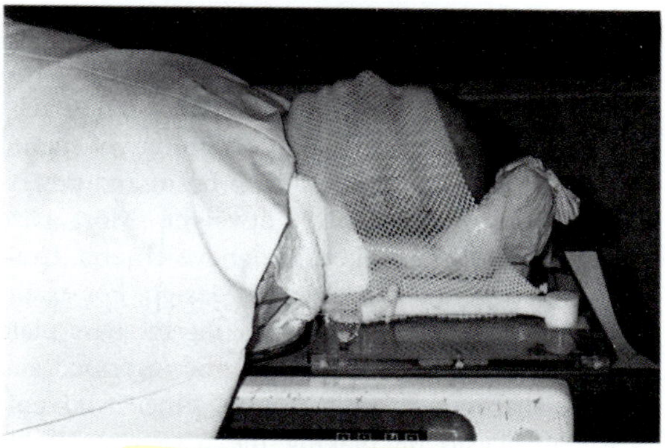

Fig. 4-5 Head and neck immobilization device consisting of a customized head support and a facial mask attached to a base plate that is secured to the treatment couch.

to release the restraints in emergencies (vomiting, seizures, etc.) can be serious.

There are a large number of head immobilization systems available and it would be impossible to describe them all in this text, but an overview of the basic components is given. Additional head immobilization devices are described in Chap. 5.

IMMOBILIZATION DEVICES: FACIAL MASK-BASED

A modern head immobilization device usually consists of a support under the head and a facial fixation mask, both attached to a base plate on top of the couch (Fig. 4-5). Such a system appears most effective when the base plate is reproducibly secured to the treatment couch.[3] Rigid immobilization devices should be designed with a patient-controlled quick-release mechanism for emergency situations.

The type of immobilization device used should be carefully considered for each patient. Some patients may not tolerate a facial mask that covers the eyes. For many claustrophobic patients and children, it may be necessary to remove parts of the mask over the eyes, mouth, or nares. In patients whose face masks have been weakened by such openings (or by stretching during molding) and in uncooperative patients, the setup reproducibility may be compromised. This uncertainty should be reflected in the selection/design of the treatment fields.

There are many issues that need to be considered when a head immobilization device is designed. The efficacy of the device is of main concern, but the patient's comfort, ease of using it, fixation to the couch, beam attenuation, loss of skin sparing, and the ability to rotate the treatment machine around the patient and the device without a collision should also be considered. Many commercial systems have been designed with these considerations in mind, and some clinics have designed their own devices.

The purpose of a facial fixation device is to reproduce and securely maintain the head position during the treatment. It is possible for the rounded posterior surface of the head to fit comfortably into the bowl-shaped support even when the head is turned slightly to either side (e.g., ball in socket). This rotation may be prevented by the facial fixation mask. Facial fixation masks can either cover the entire face or be made from two or three strips (approximately 1 in. wide) that are molded to the chin and forehead. The more extensive facial mask can be made using a perforated or solid thermoplastic sheet* or a solid plastic sheet. The common feature of these materials is that they can be molded to the patient's external surface when softened and that they harden within a few minutes.

*AquaPlast™, WFR Aquaplast Corp., Wyckoff, New Jersey.

BASE PLATE

Design. The plate onto which the head immobilization system is fastened is usually referred to as a *base plate.* Its material should be strong yet should minimally attenuate the radiation beam and preferably be transparent and lightweight. Most base plates are acrylic and meet the above criteria. Concession may be made in terms of design. For example, if emphasis is placed on making the base plate strong, the beam attenuation may be increased and the skin sparing reduced. If, on the other hand, emphasis is placed on making the base plate lightweight to minimize beam attenuation, the strength of the base plate may be reduced and it could possibly break if it were accidentally dropped on the floor.

Dimensions and Securing the Base Plate to the Couch. The dimensions of the base plate should be as small as possible to minimize the possibilities of gantry collision and beam interception and also to reduce its weight. The precise dimensions depend on how it is to be fastened to the treatment couch. It is important that the base plate be secured to the treatment couch such that it will not shift during setup or treatment.[3] In many designs, the width is customized to facilitate fixation to the couch via a "lip" that fits snugly over each side of the treatment couch, preventing rotation on a horizontal plane above the couch ("skewing") (Fig. 4-6). These lips also center the base plate on the couch. Since the couch designs vary from machine to machine [computed tomography (CT), simulator, treatment], one base plate, customized to the particular treatment couch, is usually needed for each room. A small peg inserted through a hole in the base plate and extending into the treatment couch can prevent the base plate from sliding along the couch. Since drilling a hole into the treatment couch may not be feasible, other options to secure the base plate to the couch are use of a C-clamp or strips of Velcro.* In one design, the base plate is sized to fit snugly into the opening in the couch, intended for the "tennis racket" insert. Usually, CT and simulation couches are designed without such an opening; therefore other means of securing the base plate must be used. One treatment couch has been developed that facilitates fastening of immobilization devices to the couch.† Each immobilization device is designed to be locked onto the couch in exactly the same position, thus providing consistent reference points from treatment to treatment.

Securing the Face Fixation Mask to the Base Plate. The base plate should facilitate fastening of the facial mask (or other head-restraining device) and provide a centering mechanism for the head. These two requirements are combined by the addition of a three-sided box centered on the base plate with a locking mechanism for the facial mask (Figs. 4-6 and 4-7*A*). This box is approximately 20 cm long, 14 cm wide, and 5 cm high. To reduce the risk of any sharp corners touching the patient, the height of the sides should be tapered toward the patient's shoulders and the surfaces should be smooth.

In the head-immobilization device used at Duke University Medical Center, the facial mask is secured to the base plate by three protrusions on each side of the box onto which the thermoplastic material is fastened. An arm that has holes corresponding to the protrusions is then locked into place over the protrusions, clamping the softened thermoplastic material securely to the base plate (Fig. 4-7B). The arm, which is attached to the base plate, is designed with a double joint, allowing it to be moved into place without otherwise interfering with the softened thermoplastic material. A hole in the base plate adjacent to the locking arm allows an acrylic peg to be placed such that it prevents the arm from inadvertently releasing the mask (Fig. 4-7*C*). Removal of this peg and loosening of the locking arm allows the patient to release the mask quickly in case of an emergency.

The width of the box, which is important for the effectiveness of the mask, should be about the same as the width of a patient's head (14 to 16 cm). This allows the mask, after being draped over the patient's face, to be pulled straight down (posteriorly)

*Velcro USA, Manchester, New Hampshire.

†Exact™, Varian Associates, Inc., Palo Alto, California.

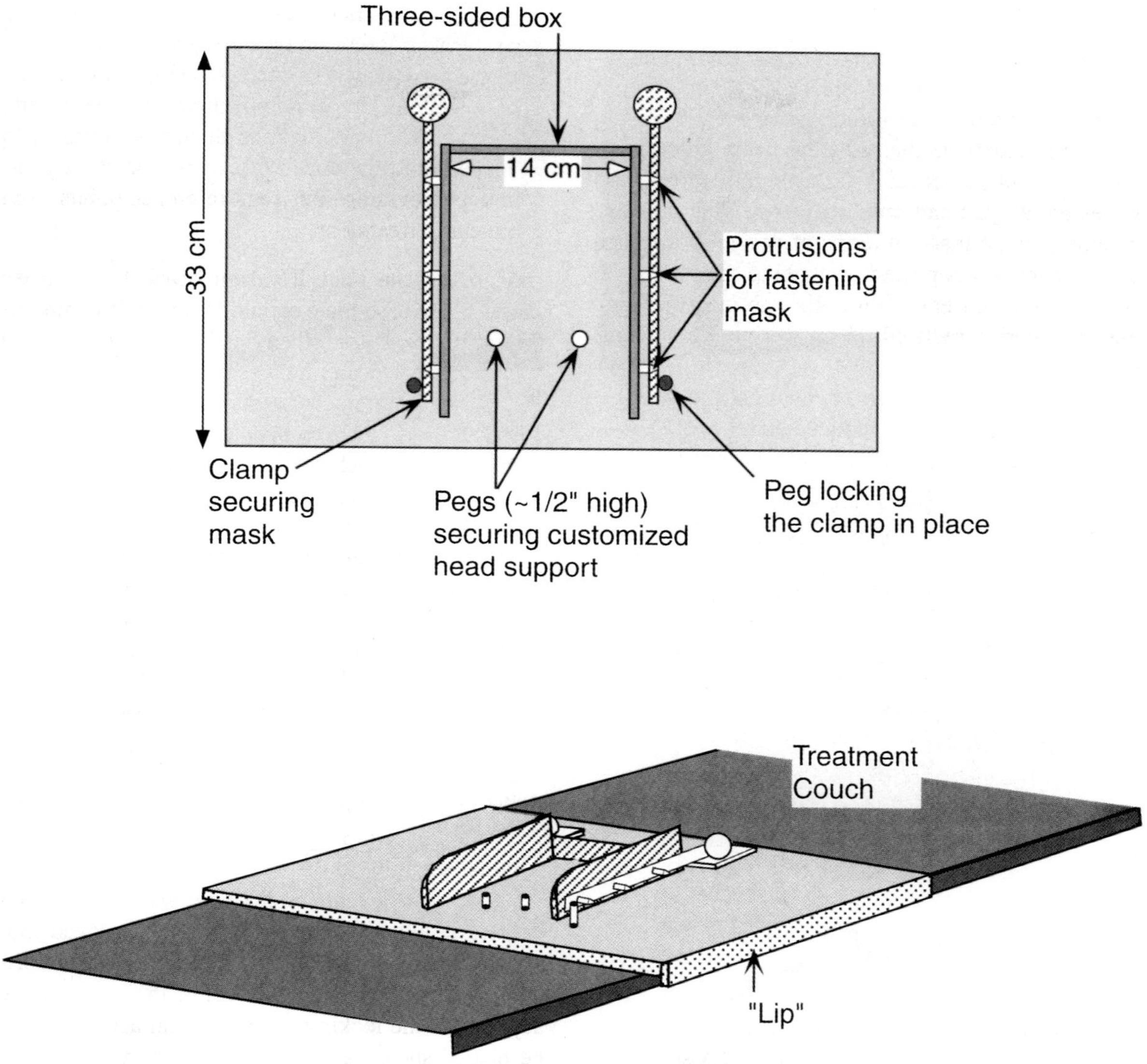

Fig. 4-6 A base plate designed with "lips" that fit over the width of the treatment couch to prevent skewing. The head support is secured inside the three-sided box in the center and the face mask is secured by a clamp on each side of the head support.

to the anchor points on the base plate and to follow the sides of the patient's head as closely as possible. If the anchor points are placed too far from the patient's head, the mask must be pulled away from the head in order to be fastened, and thus it will be less effective (Fig. 4-8).

Special Devices. Treatment techniques utilizing unconventional beam orientations and beam-modifying accessories, attached to the collimator, may not be implementable due to gantry-couch collisions. An extension of the treatment couch, wide enough to accommodate the patient's head, can be

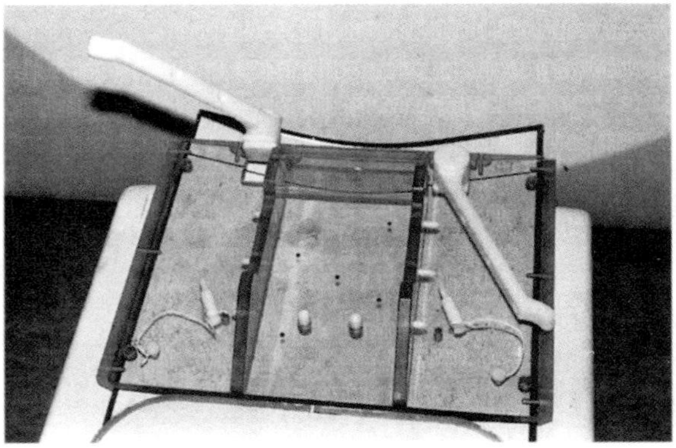

A

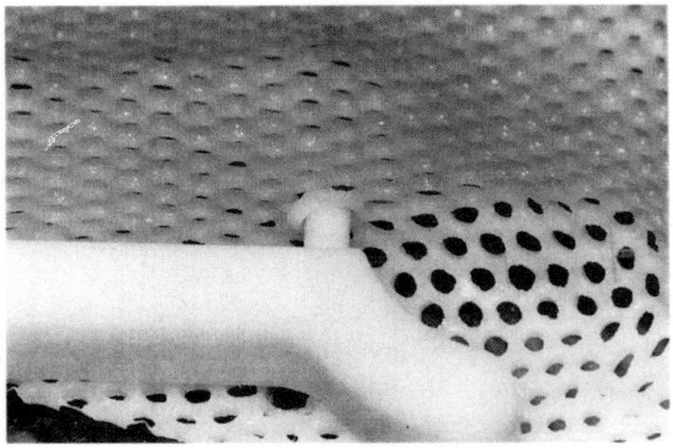

B

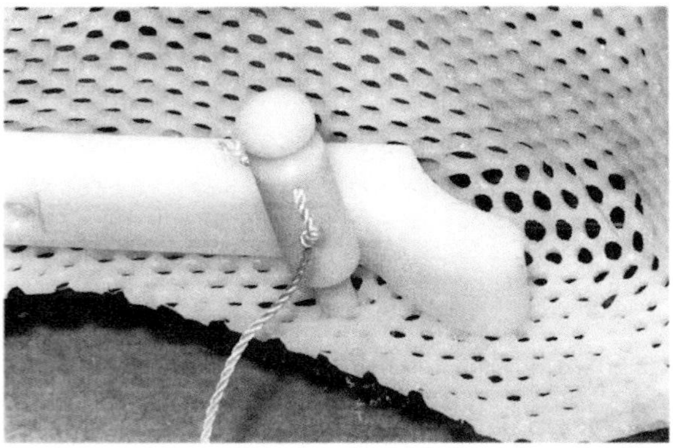

C

Fig. 4-7 *A*. Base plate, diagrammed in Fig. 4-6, secured via lips over the CT couch. *B*. Closeup of the mask fastened over one protrusion on the three-sided box and clamp being pushed over it to lock the mask in place. *C*. An acrylic peg is placed to prevent inadvertent release of the mask.

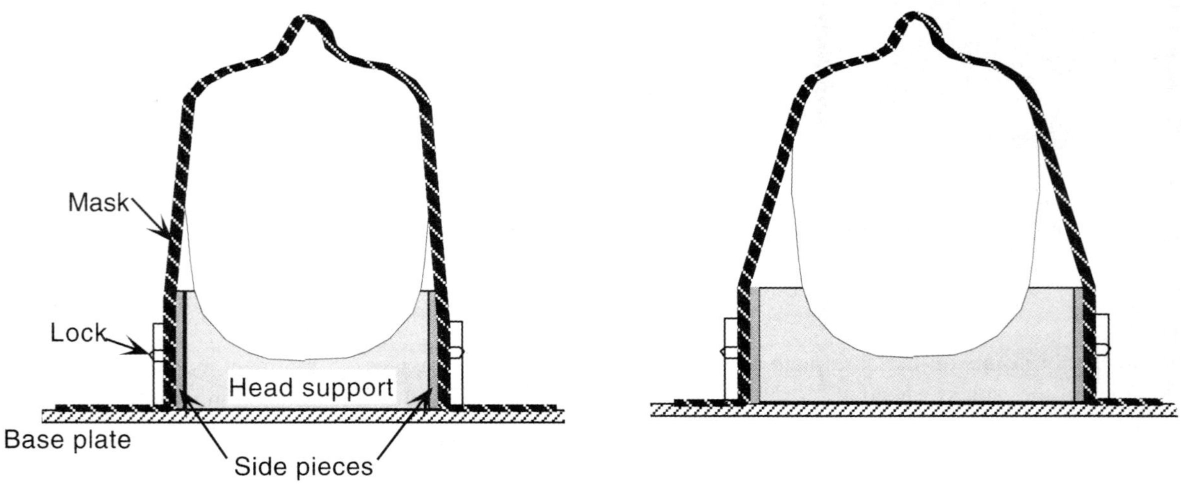

Fig. 4-8 The mask should be pulled straight down and follow the sides of the patient's head (*left*). When the anchor points are too far from the head, the mask is less effective (*right*).

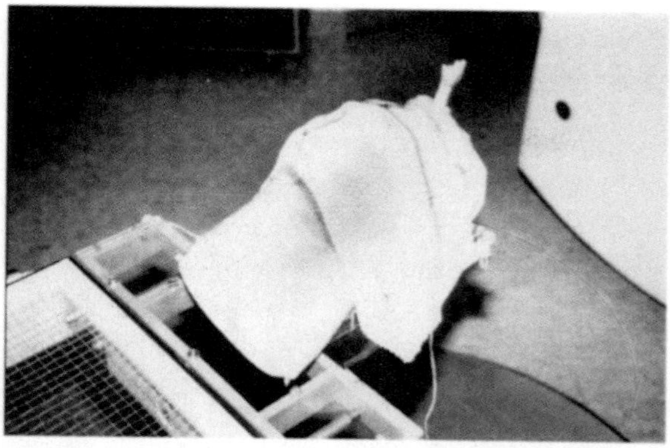

Fig. 4-9 To minimize the risks of collimator/couch collisions, an extension, approximately 6 in. wide and 8 to 10 in. long, can be added to the treatment couch for head and neck treatments. A base plate that fits over the extensions is used for these treatments.

attached at the end of the couch to minimize the risk of collisions (Fig. 4-9).

Some base plates are designed such that the central portion, on which the patient's head rests, can be angled (up to about 45°) to achieve the flexed head position (Fig. 4-10*A*). In some designs, the base plate is built with a small opening or a thin sheet of acrylic under the head to facilitate a posterior field without loss of skin sparing. Base plates for prone head immobilization are also available (Fig. 4-10*B*). These are sometimes used when a vertex field is required for treatment of pituitary or certain brain tumors.

HEAD SUPPORTS

Standard Head Supports. A support under the patient's head is necessary to achieve the desired elevation above the treatment couch. The most commonly used standard head supports are available in sets of six, offering a variety of sizes and shapes. These are made of molded polyurethane foam and their shapes are intended to follow the posterior surface of a patient's head and neck (Fig. 4-11*A*). Since these supports have different shapes and are of different heights, the beam attenuation varies both *within* and *among* the supports.

A similar head support system is hollow and is made of transparent plastic (Fig. 4-11*B*) that allows visualization of the posterior surface of the head, e.g., to determine the source–surface distance

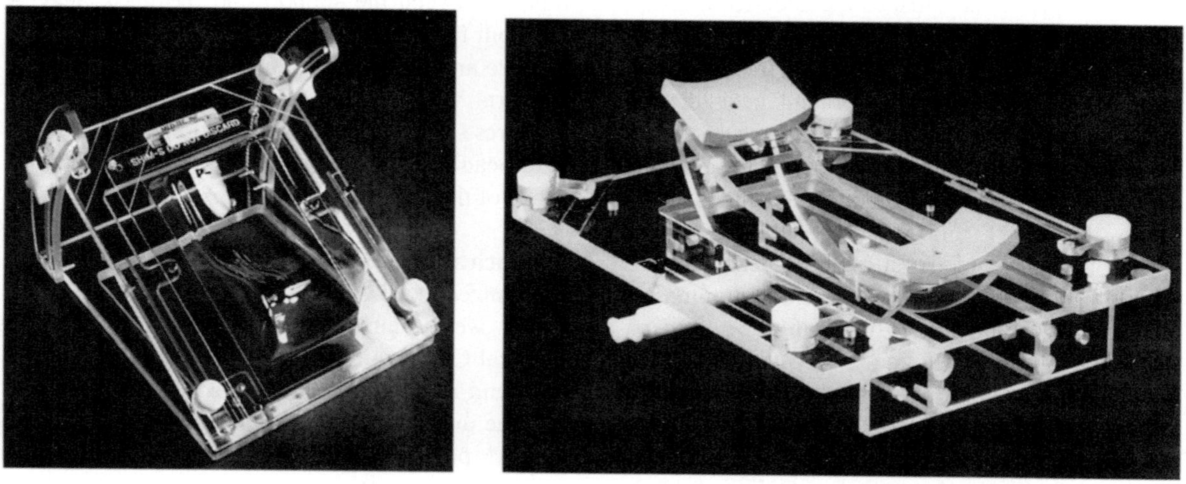

A *B*

Fig. 4-10 *A*. A head positioning system that can be angled may be used to achieve a flexed head position. *B*. A prone head position system with adjustable angulation. (Courtesy of MED-TEC, Inc., Orange City, Iowa.)

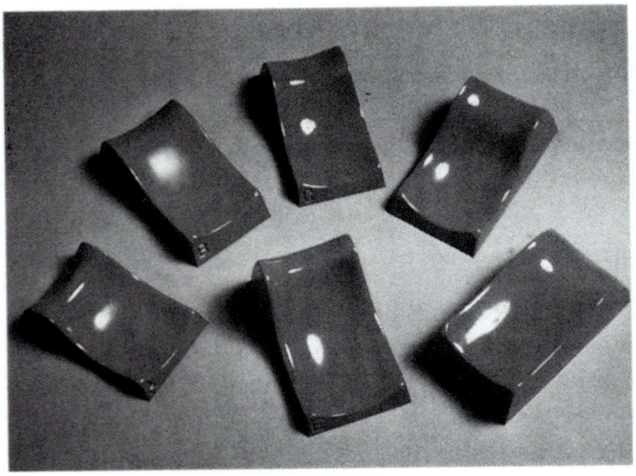

A

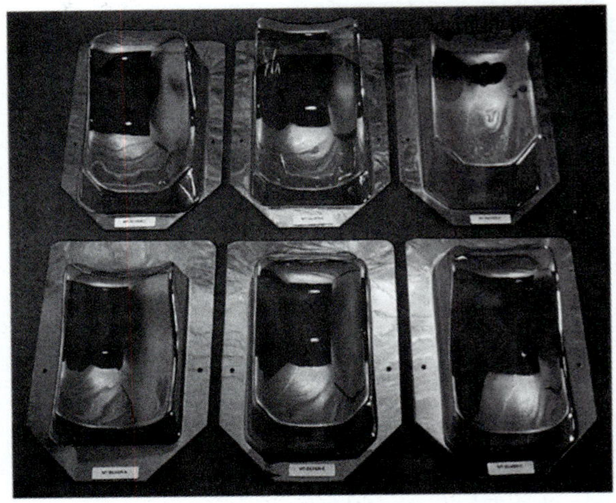

B

Fig. 4-11 *A*. A set of standard polyurethane head supports. *B*. A set of standard transparent head supports. (Courtesy of MED-TEC, Inc., Orange City, Iowa.)

(SSD) of posterior or posterior oblique fields. It also attenuates the beam less than the polyurethane supports. Neither of these supports can be tailored to a particular patient's head and neck, and they may therefore be uncomfortable, particularly in extreme situations, as when the chin is hyperextended. To find one support that satisfies the need for a certain head position while also providing a comfortable support for the head and neck can be problematic.

In patients with a short and/or thick neck, the portion of the head rest intended for the neck is too high and the bowl-shaped portion intended for the head is too low.[4] Thus the patient's head is not resting in the bowl (Fig. 4.12). When a space is present between the support and the head, it leaves room for motion even when a facial fixation mask is used. This position is also uncomfortable, and patients must strain to maintain the position. In selecting the most appropriate head support, consideration should be given to the desired head position, the height of the head support, and the shape and length of the patient's neck. Repositioning of the head on the support is also important for treatment accuracy (Fig. 4-13).

Customized Head Supports. Fabricating a customized head support for each patient is an alternative that reduces the difficulties described. A customized support usually facilitates better reproducibility of the head position and is more comfortable than the standard support. The head fits tightly between the support and the mask, leaving no room for motion. In one study, the variability of the size and shape of the customized posterior head supports was found to exceed that of "standard" head rests, verifying the impression that the standard head rests, in many patients, do not match the shape of the posterior head and neck.[4]

Fabrication of Customized Head Supports. A customized head support and thermoplastic facial mask were implemented at Duke University Medical Center during 1991 in an effort to improve head and neck immobilization as 3DTP capabilities became available. The support is made of foaming agents* poured into a small plastic bag, which is

*Polyurethane, Smithers Medical Products, Inc., North Canton, Ohio.

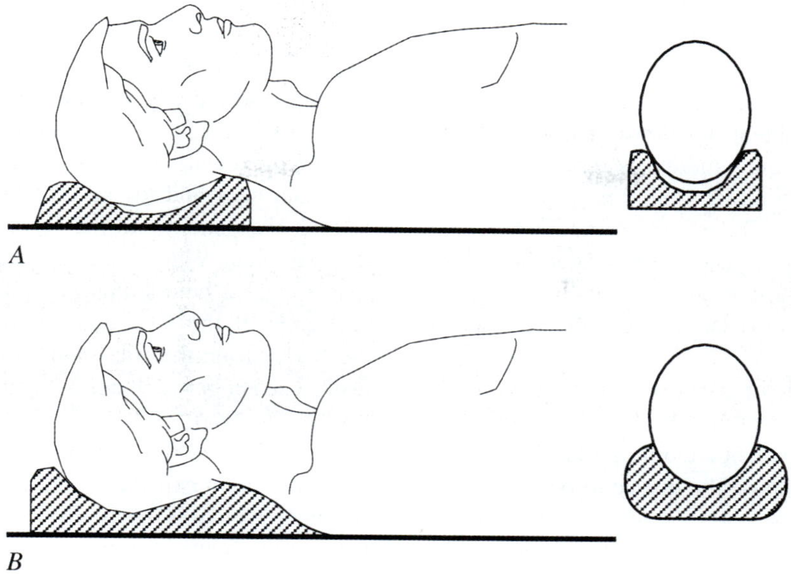

Fig. 4-12 *A*. Standard head supports frequently do not follow the patient's posterior head and neck, thus leaving room for motion. *B*. A comfortable support, tailored to the patient's posterior head, neck, and upper shoulders, leaves no room for motion.

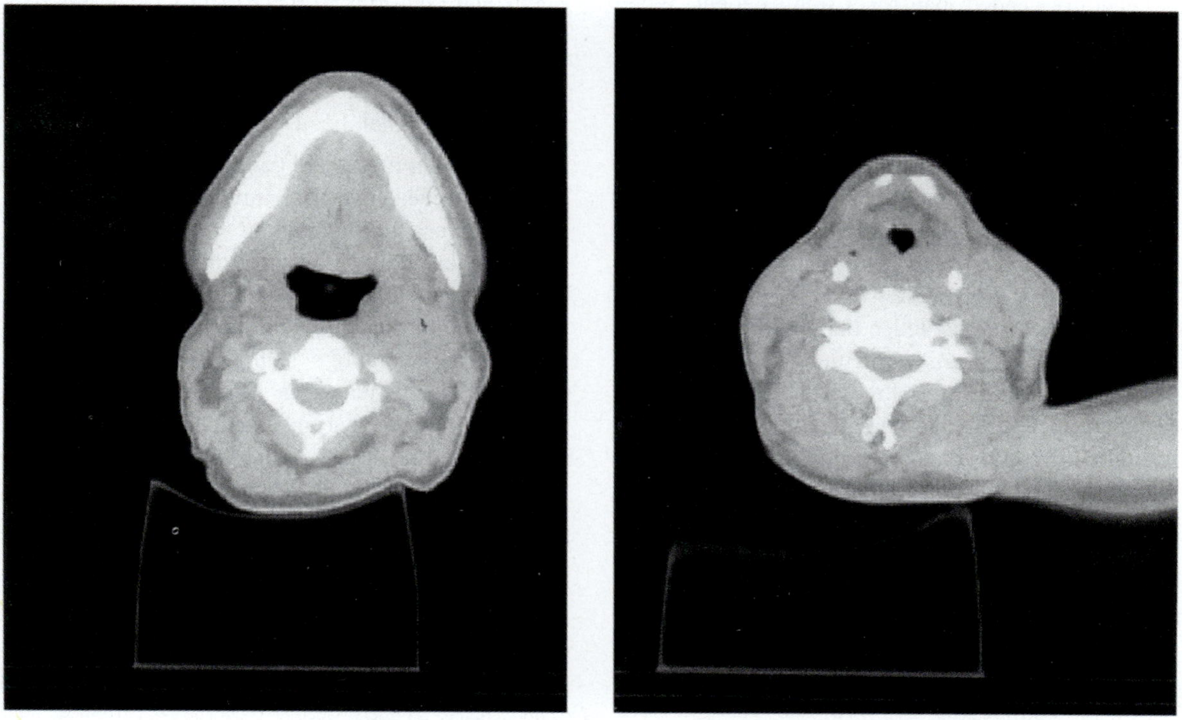

Fig. 4-13 Careless positioning of the patient's head on the support may be uncomfortable and can lead to setup difficulties.

placed in the three-sided box centered on the base plate before the patient lies down. The foam (same as used in positioning molds used in other sites) swells and forms a mold contoured to the patient's posterior surface. There are certain steps and considerations that are necessary in order to make a customized head support meet the requirements of a particular situation. These are described in the following sections.

The patient's clothing above the waist should be removed prior to making the head support, since variations in the patient's clothing during the treatment course may cause the device to be too tight or too loose.

The desired head position (neutral, extended, or flexed) is decided first, and the head elevation (above the couch) needed to achieve this position is accomplished by placing Styrofoam* spacers under the head (Fig. 4-14*A*). To achieve the neutral head position in a large patient, a larger (thicker) spacer is generally needed than for a small patient. When the extended chin position is required for a large patient, where the torso is elevated more above the couch than with a small patient, the Styrofoam spacers may be omitted or be of minimal height (Fig. 4-14*B*). For a small patient, the torso may need to be elevated in order to achieve the desired chin extension (Fig. 4-15*A*). When the flexed head position is required, a larger (thicker) head support is needed. Such a support may be of a triangular shape and may also extend under the shoulders, causing the patient to be in a semirecumbent position (Fig. 4-15*B*). (Also, see Fig. 6-4 in Chap. 6.)

When the appropriate head position has been determined, the Styrofoam spacers are taped together and placed inside a plastic bag approximately 10 in. wide and 18 in. long. This bag is placed in the three-sided box on the base plate with the opening toward the top of the head and the bag itself extending under the neck and upper shoulders. Approximately 100 mL of the foaming agent is mixed and poured into the plastic bag. Air is squeezed out of the bag, and the bag is sealed to prevent the foam from leaking. The patient resumes the position and the foam expands and fills the spaces between the head and neck and the base plate, thus conforming to both the patient and the repositioning guides of the base plate. While the foam is expanding, the patient's head is held straight by placing one hand on each side of the head and simultaneously guiding the foam up on the sides and around the top of the head. The support will conform to the posterior contour of the head, neck, and shoulders and will also form an elevated ridge around the head (Fig. 4-16). Since the foam expands in the direction of least resistance, which is away from the patient's head, guiding the foam up around the head is very important. It is also important that the plastic bag be wide enough to provide adequate space for the foam to expand.

Another custom-made head support consists of a water-cured pad that, when soaked in water, expands and conforms to the patient's head and neck within 4 to 5 min.†

FACIAL FIXATION

Facial fixation masks are commonly used during irradiation of head and neck tumors. Such masks provide excellent immobilization and facilitate making setup marks on the rigid mask rather than the mobile skin, possibly an advantage in terms of reproducibility, and unsightly skin marks are thus eliminated. A *disadvantage* is the inability to directly visualize the patient—an important consideration when setting field margins intended to include scars, palpable lymph nodes, superficial lesions, and so on, or irradiating fields near the eyes. Alternatively, lead markers can be placed on these features during the simulation. However, visualization during the treatment setup may still be desired.

The effectiveness of a head immobilization system may, in part, be related to the rigidity and size of the facial fixation device. As a minimum, a facial

*Dow Chemical, Midland, Michigan.

†Quick-Form™, MED-TEC, Inc., Orange City, Iowa.

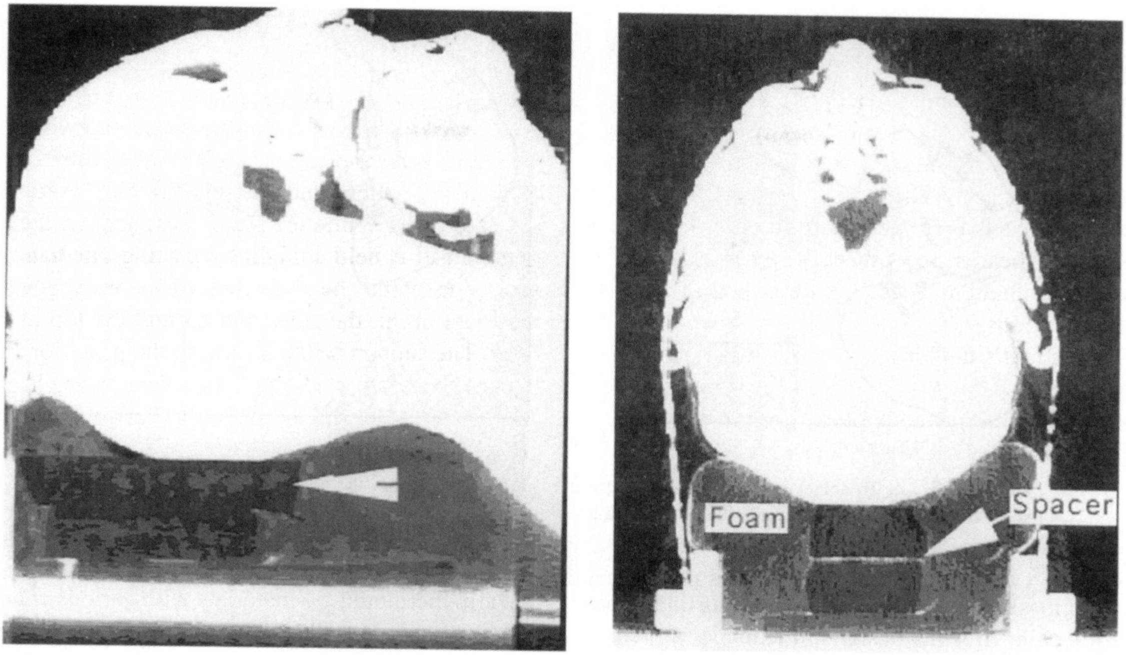

A

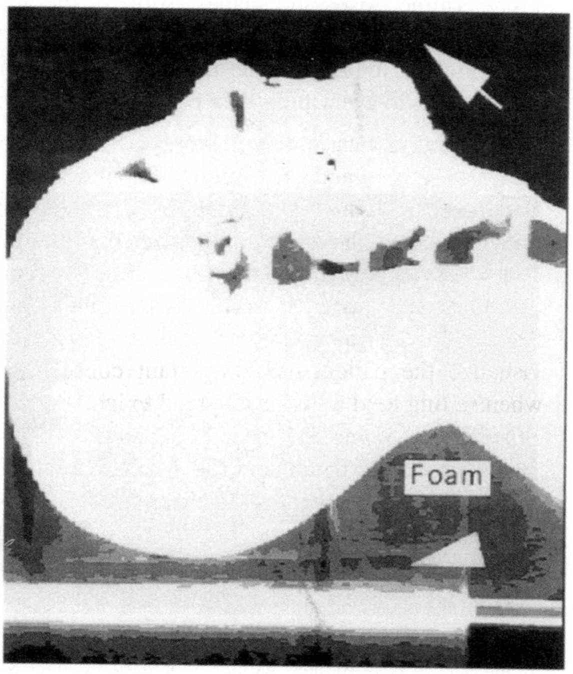

B

Fig. 4-14 The required head elevation can be achieved by varying the thickness of spacers under the head. *A*. To achieve a neutral head position, two pieces of 1-in. Styrofoam were needed in this patient. *B*. For the extended position, no Styrofoam spacers were used and the head is resting on the base plate.

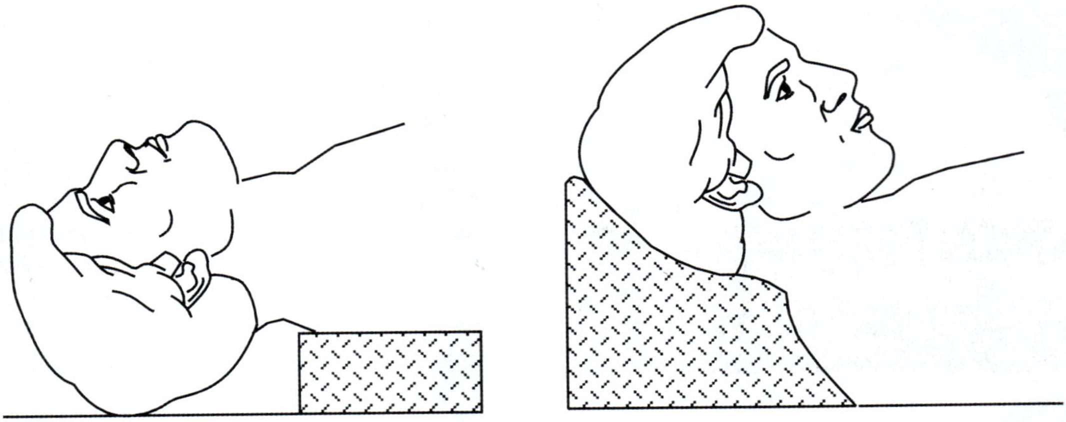

Fig. 4-15 *A*. To achieve the extended chin position in a small patient, the chest can be elevated on a sheet of Styrofoam. *B*. To achieve the flexed head position, a larger head and shoulder support is needed.

fixation mask should extend from the hairline to below the chin. In some designs, it extends to include the top of the head, facilitating additional field marks in this area (Fig. 4-17). Extending the mask to include the shoulders may improve the accuracy of field matching between opposed lateral and an anterior lower neck/supraclavicular field (Fig. 4-18).

Face-Mask Materials. A commonly used head immobilization material is a thermoplastic sheet that is softened in hot water (to approximately 160°F) and molded to the patient's facial contour.[3-13] Several thermoplastic materials with various characteristics and designs are available either as solid sheets or with perforations and in different thicknesses and colors. They can also be purchased in predetermined sizes and shapes. Some of the materials have a soft surface to make the mask more comfortable. Some are easier to handle because they do not stick to everything they come in contact with

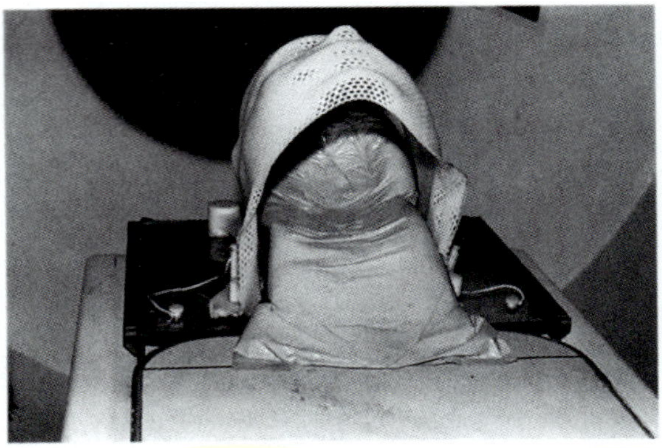

Fig. 4-16 A head support, molded to the posterior contour of the head, neck, and upper shoulders, leaves no room for motion when used with a tight-fitting facial mask.

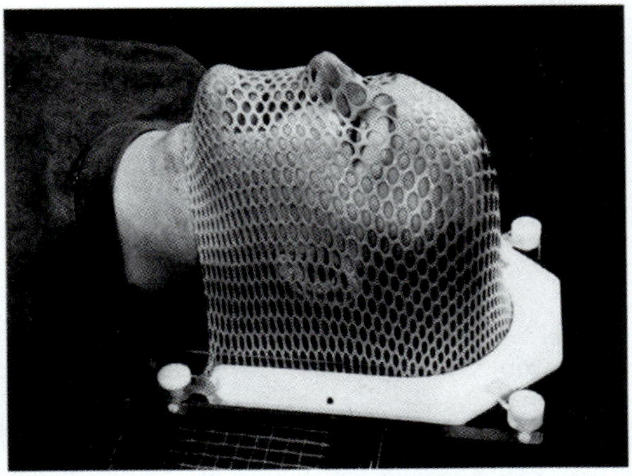

Fig. 4-17 The facial mask can be extended to include the top of the head so as to facilitate marking of brain fields on the mask. A larger piece of thermoplastic material is needed when the mask is extended beyond the face, as stretching the material reduces the firmness. (Courtesy of MED-TEC, Inc., Orange City, Iowa.)

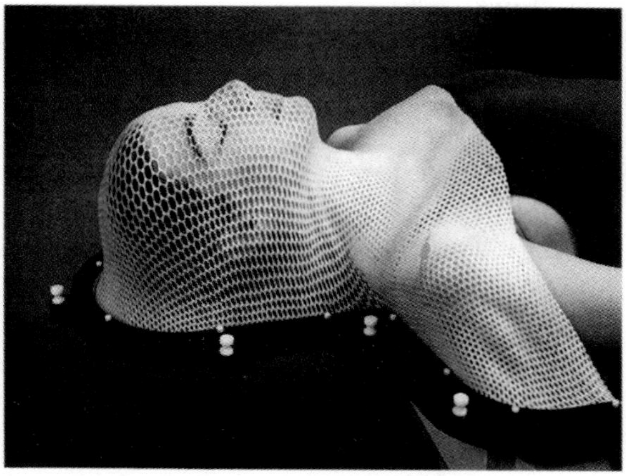

Fig. 4-18 The facial mask, extended to include the shoulders, may improve reproducibility of the head/shoulder position and thus reduce uncertainties of field matching. (Courtesy of MED-TEC, Inc., Orange City, Iowa.)

(hot-water pan, hands, latex gloves, the base plate, and so on).

A few other facial fixation materials are available. For example, relatively inexpensive glass-fiber bandages have been used.[14] Another alternative is a resin-impregnated casting adhesive* that becomes rigid a few minutes after being submerged in warm water.

Choosing Face-Mask Materials. The primary selection criteria for mask material should be the effect on skin sparing and the strength of the finished mask. A thinner material would more likely afford better skin sparing than a thicker material. On the other hand, the thicker material may produce a stronger immobilization mask. One should remember that if the thermoplastic material is stretched as it is draped over the patient, it becomes thinner and therefore weaker. In one design, the thermoplastic material is fastened in a horseshoe-shaped frame that fits to the base plate above and on each side of the patient's head (Fig. 4-17).† In this design, the thermoplastic material, which is approximately 15 × 15 cm, must be stretched until it covers the patient's face and reaches down to the base plate on each side of the patient. In patients with greater head elevation, the material is stretched more, simply because the distance over which it has to be stretched is increased.

Fabrication of a Thermoplastic Facial Fixation Mask. Prior to making a face mask, it is important to determine if the patient wears dentures or bridges that need to be removed during treatment. Likewise, one must decide whether a bite block or other similar devices (wax to prevent secondary scatter from fillings, lead shields when electron beams are used, and so on)[15–22] are needed during the treatments. Lead markers to indicate, for example, the eyes, incisions, and so on should also be placed prior to making the mask. If such devices or markers are added after the face mask is made, the mask may not fit and will have to be remade.

Facial masks used at Duke University Medical Center consist of a 3-mm-thick, perforated thermoplastic sheet that is approximately 20 × 45 cm. The thermoplastic sheet is softened in hot water and, after the excess water is shaken off, is draped over and molded to the face before it becomes rigid (3 to 5 min). The softened sheet is draped over the patient's face from the hairline to below the chin and is fastened onto the base plate on each side of the head. Immediately, while the thermoplastic is still soft, it is gently molded to the forehead, bridge of the nose, and chin. It is particularly important that the mask conform well to the bridge of the nose, where the soft tissues are thin, as well as to the bony prominences. These areas are reliable reference points for the mask.

While the mask should be shaped to conform closely to the facial features, it should not be so tight that it distorts the soft tissues. Pressure points formed during the molding of the mask may prove prohibitive during future use of the mask. As some of these materials harden, some shrinkage may occur, making the mask too tight when the patient returns for treatment. It is therefore important to gently mold the mask to the face.

Other Facial Fixation Devices. Three strips of resin-impregnated casting adhesive placed across the patient's head and attached to the base

*Scotchcast™, 3M Corp., St. Paul, Minnesota.

†Uniframe™, MED-TEC, Inc., Orange City, Iowa.

plate can offer good reproducibility. One strip is formed around the chin and is fastened to a post, which in turn is secured to the base plate above (cephalad of) the patient's head to maintain chin position. Another strip is formed around the chin and is fastened to the cephalad portion of the base plate on each side of the head. The third strip is placed across the forehead and is fastened to the base plate near the shoulders. These three strips overlap and adhere to one another on each side of the patient's head, thus forming a partial face mask (Fig. 4-19).

A more elaborate facial mask system consists of a thin transparent plastic formed to the face through a process requiring a plaster model of the patient's head and a vacuum machine. In this process, an impression is made of the patient's head and then the impression is filled, usually with plaster of paris, to form a model of the patient. This hard model is placed inside a vacuum machine and a softened plastic sheet is draped over the model. The vacuum forces the plastic sheet to conform tightly to the head model. Within a few seconds, the mask becomes solid and is removed.

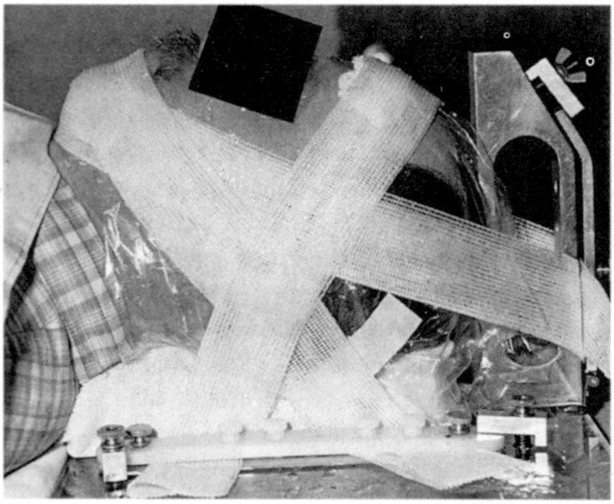

Fig. 4-19 Head immobilization masks can also be made from resin-impregnated casting strips. Three strips placed across the patient's head and fastened to a base plate may offer adequate reproducibility.

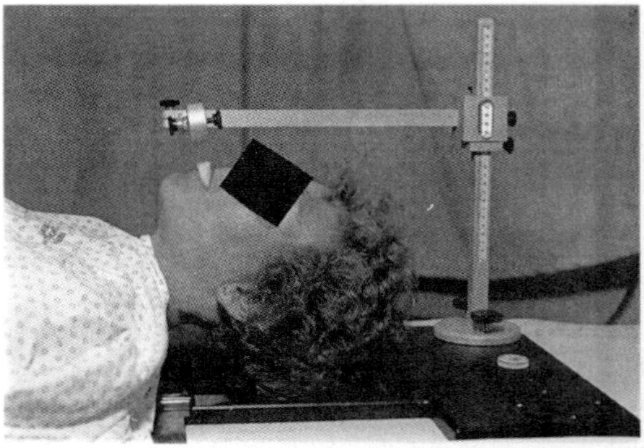

Fig. 4-20 A bite-block type of head immobilization device with a reference system. The bite block is molded to the patient's teeth and is attached to the reference system, which is secured to a base plate.

IMMOBILIZATION DEVICES: DENTAL FIXATION

Another type of head and neck immobilization device relies on dental fixation and consists of a bite block molded to the patient's teeth.[23] The bite block is made by having the patient bite into a softened impression material, which hardens within a few minutes. A tube may also be inserted within the bite block to make breathing easier. The bite block attaches to an external reference system fixed to the base plate (Fig. 4-20). This type of bite block should not be confused with the bite blocks (described below) sometimes used in radiation therapy for the purpose of keeping the patient's mouth open during treatment. In this context, the bite block is made for the purpose of immobilizing the patient's head. There might be situations in which a bite block would be used for both immobilizing the head and keeping the mouth open.

IMMOBILIZATION OF SMALL CHILDREN

Small children requiring irradiation of head and neck tumors present a special problem in that they almost always need general anesthesia. Another problem is the head size of infants, since their heads may be too small for a mask-based immobilization system to be effective. Treatment fields in children irradiated for retinoblastoma are set clinically each day by direct visualization of the eye. Because of the very small distance between the target and the lens of the eye and the need for a fixed gaze, these children are always treated while under general anesthesia. In these children, use of a facial immobilization mask may not be possible because it would interfere with both the anesthesia mask or intubation and the ability to see the radiation field relative to the eye.

An alternative immobilization method consists of making an anterior plaster cast of the child's torso and head, leaving the eyes, mouth, and nose uncovered to facilitate anesthesia and visualization of the eyes (Fig. 4-21). An opening is also made over the upper abdomen to facilitate visualization of respiratory motion from outside the room during the "beam-on" period. In cases where a facial immobilization mask *is* possible, the anesthesia equipment (mask or tube) can be included in the immobilization mask. The same anesthesia equipment must then be used for each treatment or it will not fit to the mask. An opening can be made in the immobilization mask to facilitate visualization of the eye during the setup.

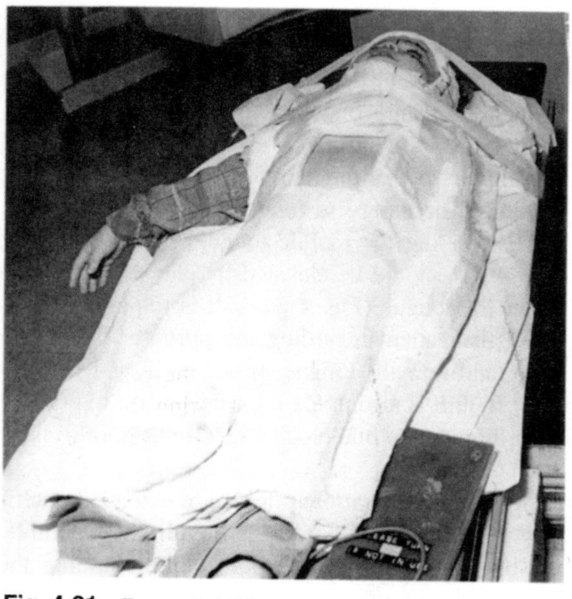

Fig. 4-21 For small children treated for retinoblastoma and requiring general anesthesia, an anterior plaster cast may be a better alternative than a facial mask. An opening is left for the eyes, mouth, and nose to facilitate anesthesia and visualization of the eyes. An opening is also made over the upper abdomen to facilitate visualization of respiratory motion during "beam-on" time.

OTHER IMMOBILIZATION AIDS

BITE BLOCKS

Bite blocks are sometimes used to reduce the volume of oral mucosa within the radiation field by keeping the patient's mouth open during treatment. Bite blocks can be made from impressionable dental materials molded to the teeth and then hardened. One such material is Silicone Tray Material, Type III.* This consists of a base that has a paste-like consistency and, when mixed with an accelerator, attains a hard-rubber consistency within 3 to 5 min. Another bite block material is Impression Compound Type 1†, which becomes soft when left in hot water (about 160°F) for a few minutes. Approximately 5 min after removal from the hot water, the material becomes hard and sometimes brittle.

While the impression material is soft, a tongue blade and some type of airway can be molded into it; the device is then inserted into the widely opened mouth (Fig. 4-22). The tongue blade is used to press down or elevate the tongue and can also be used as a handle when inserting and removing the bite block. An airway is often necessary, as some patients may have difficulty breathing through the nose. (An airway for a patient with a tracheostomy is, of course, superfluous.) The patient is asked to bite lightly into the material to make an impression of the teeth (or gums in an edentulous patient), but with the mouth open. If the patient bites down hard, the mouth is no

*Coe Laboratories, Inc., Chicago, Illinois.
†Kerr USA, Romulus, Michigan.

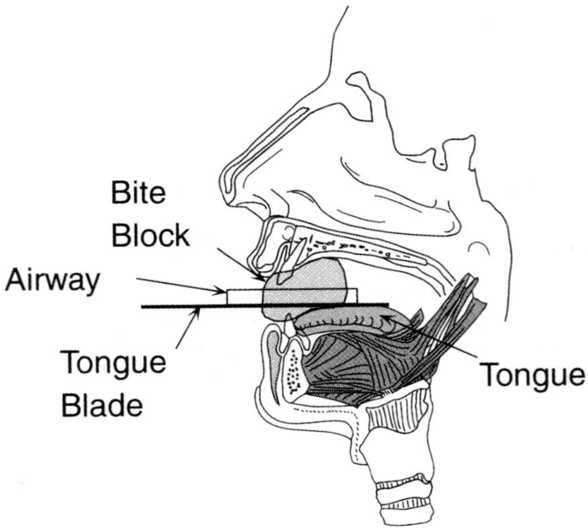

Fig. 4-22 A bite block used to keep the patient's mouth open and press the tongue down.

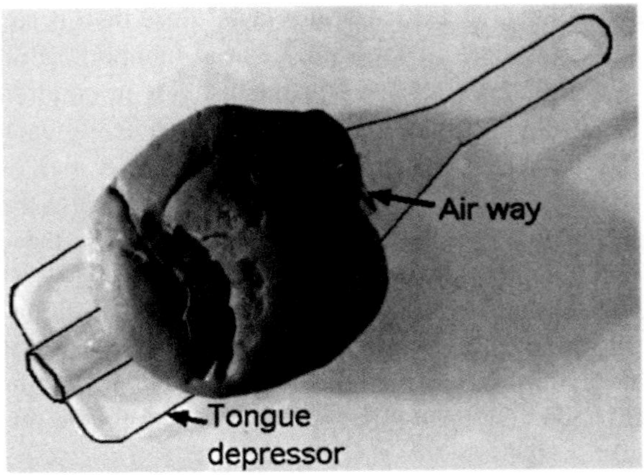

Fig. 4-23 An acrylic tongue depressor/airway device with a dental impression material, when inserted properly, keeps the mouth open and the tongue depressed, facilitating easy breathing. Repositioning of the device is aided by the impression of the teeth in the mold.

longer open, defeating the purpose of the bite block. After approximately 5 min, the material becomes hard and the device can be removed. The impression of the teeth assures that the patient's mouth remains opened to the same degree for each treatment. The airway can be the barrel of a syringe or some other hard tube of adequate caliber. A combination tongue depressor/airway,* made of Plexiglas, is available on the market (Fig. 4-23) but can also be made in most radiation therapy clinics. One disadvantage of using a wooden tongue depressor is that it frequently becomes wet from the impression material. When it dries, it tends to warp; thus, as it changes shape, it may break the brittle bite block.

When a bite block/tongue blade is constructed, it is very important that the staff *and* the patient understand its purpose. For example, the placement of the tongue blade with respect to the impression material depends on how the device is to be used. When a tumor in the maxillary antrum is treated, the purpose of the bite block/tongue blade arrangement is to keep the mouth open and the mobile tongue/mandible pressed down, away from the radiation fields, thus reducing incidental irradiation to these structures (Fig. 4-22*A*). It is important for the patient to understand that in this situation, the tongue needs to be held *under* the tongue blade. When the tongue needs to be treated, the same bite block/tongue blade arrangement is desired; now, however, for the purpose of sparing the roof of the mouth. In yet other situations, it may be necessary to treat the floor of the mouth while avoiding the mobile tongue. In this situation, the tongue should be elevated by placing the device *under* the tongue (Fig. 4-24*A*). It is important to instruct the patient regarding the purpose of the bite block and how the tongue should be placed with respect to it. It is also prudent for the patient to practice repositioning the bite block a few times prior to initiation of treatment.

Some lateral treatment fields are extended anteriorly to include the floor of the mouth, the mandible, the buccal mucosa, and so on, while avoiding the lips. A roll of gauze can be inserted between the front teeth and the lips such that the lips are pushed farther anterior and away from the radiation field. A more reproducible lip position may be achieved by adding a piece of the dental material to a bite block such that it fits between the front teeth and the lips (Fig. 4-24*B*).

*Van Arsdale Innovative Products, Inc., Pensacola, Florida.

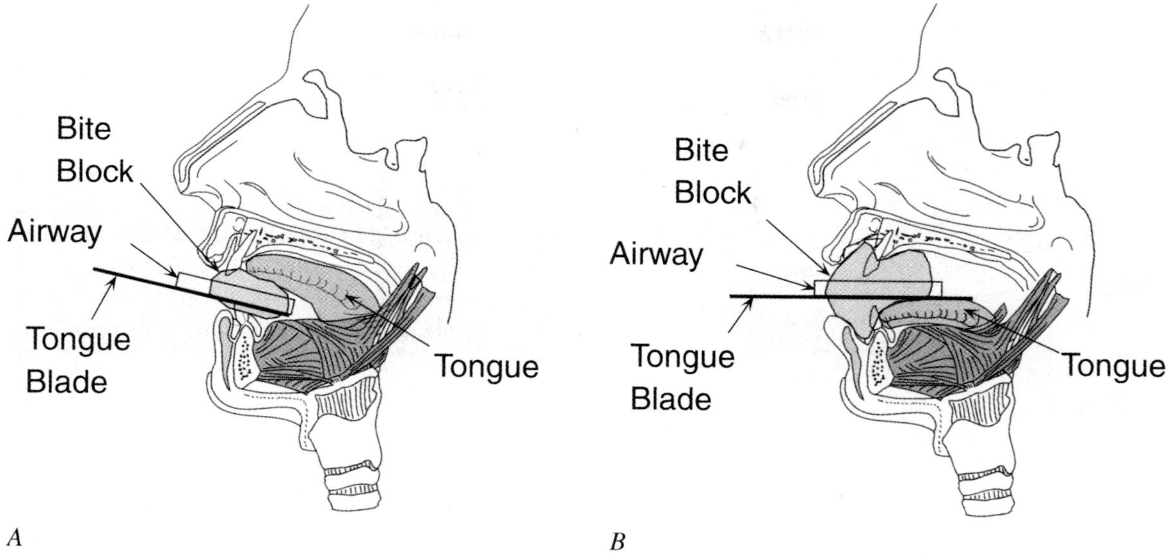

Fig. 4-24 *A*. When a floor-of-mouth lesion is treated, the tongue may have to be elevated; thus the bite block should be placed under the tongue. *B*. The lips can be pushed anteriorly by placing a small amount of impression material (or a dental roll) between the front teeth and the lips.

DENTAL SHIELDS

Radiation therapy fields used to treat head and neck tumors frequently include portions of the oral cavity. During the irradiation, metallic dental materials (e.g., cavity fillings) emit secondary electrons, thus increasing the dose in their vicinity. A high radiation dose can occur on the lingual and buccal mucosa adjacent to dental crowns and fillings, increasing the mucositis.[15-22,24,25] The secondary scatter can be sufficiently reduced by placing a 2- to 4-mm tissue-equivalent absorber over the teeth. Such an absorber can be made from wax softened and molded to the shape of the patient's teeth.* Other materials, such as acrylic resin and silicone, have been described.[26-28]

CHIN STRAPS

In irradiating tumors in the lower neck or upper mediastinum through opposed anterior and posterior fields (modified mantle fields, lymphoma, thymoma), it is often necessary to extend the patient's chin. Due to the beam divergence, it is most important to extend the chin while the posterior field is being treated. A patient may think that since the machine is rotated to his or her back, it is no longer necessary to extend the chin, or the patient may forget and gradually move the chin down to a more comfortable position. A chin strap can then be used to reproduce the chin extension and also to serve as a reminder for the patient (Fig. 4-25).

SHOULDER RETRACTION

In the patient with a short neck or one where opposed lateral fields are used to treat the neck, the shoulders sometimes need to be retracted caudally to avoid entrance and exit doses in the shoulders. Elastic straps, equipped with handles and attached to each side of the treatment couch, can be used for the patient to pull on.† The length of these straps should be adjustable to facilitate appropriate tension

*Smithers Medical Products, Inc., North Canton, Ohio.

†MED-TEC, Inc., Orange City, Iowa.

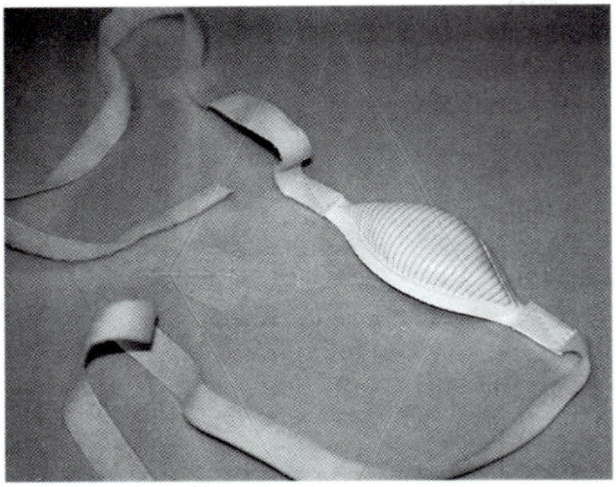

Fig. 4-25 A chin strap used to maintain correct chin position. (Courtesy of Smithers Medical Products, Inc., North Canton, Ohio.)

(Fig. 4-26). In the absence of such straps, the patient can pull on each end of an elastic bandage or other strap placed below his or her feet or around the foot end of the treatment couch. Another method, sometimes used to avoid inclusion of the shoulder on the entrance side of the beam, is to turn the foot end of the couch 5 to 10° away from the collimator. This causes a larger volume of the opposite shoulder to be in the exit beam. Field matching would be a difficult problem when this technique is used.

INTRAORAL CONE FIXATION

Intraoral cones are occasionally used with orthovoltage or electron beams to treat small, fixed lesions (< 3 cm) in the floor of the mouth.[29] When such treatment is delivered *following* external beam irradiation, the oral mucosa may be quite sore, causing difficulty in positioning the cone. Due to the discomfort, the patient may have difficulty remaining motionless during the treatment. An acrylic appliance, made from an impression to fit over the cone and the patient's teeth (or gums in an edentulous patient), will help in repositioning and holding the cone in place during the treatment. The impression of the teeth and cone must be made with the cone in the precise position; the acrylic is then formed to the impression (the negative) (Fig. 4-27). Daily confirmation of the placement is necessary. A detachable telescopic mirror or fiberoptic scope inserted through the cone can be used for direct visualization of the lesion at the end of the cone.

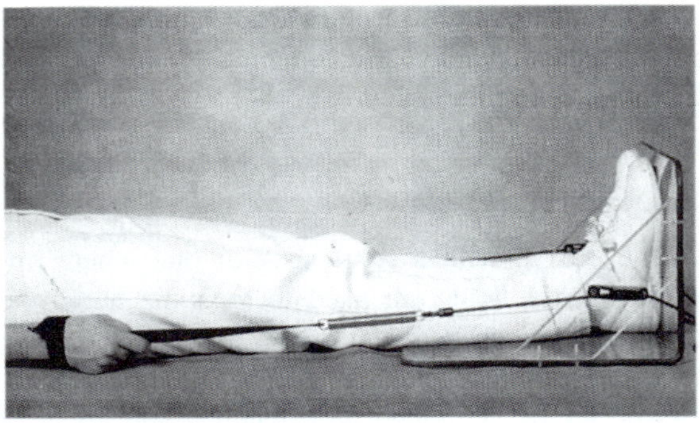

Fig. 4-26 The shoulders can be retracted by having the patient pull on an elastic strap placed under the feet. This device, with a platform under the feet, may also be used to prevent the patient from sliding down on the couch when he or she is placed in a semirecumbent position. (Courtesy of Van Arsdale Innovative Products, Inc., Pensacola, Florida.)

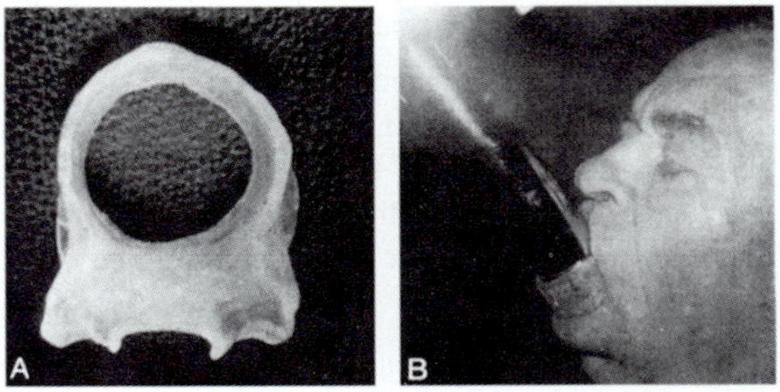

Fig. 4-27 An acrylic appliance (*A*) molded to the patient's teeth and an intraoral cone (*B*) may be used to reproduce and stabilize the position of the intraoral cone. Visual confirmation of cone placement is necessary prior to each treatment. (From Perez C, Brady L: *Principles and Practice of Radiation Oncology.* Philadelphia: Lippincott, 1987. Reproduced with permission of Lippincott-Raven Publishers, Philadelphia.)

TREATMENT CHAIR FOR HEAD AND NECK IRRADIATION

There are a variety of clinical situations in which a conventional recumbent position is not possible. Shortness of breath is sometimes exaggerated when the patient is in a recumbent position; the treatment must therefore be delivered with the patient in an upright position. Patients whose weight exceeds the tolerance of the treatment couch may also require a sitting treatment position. The repositioning of a patient in the sitting position poses a special challenge, and special devices may be needed to facilitate treatment of a sitting patient.[30–34]

Most modern radiation therapy machines are capable of a 360° rotation with the axis of rotation (isocenter) fixed in space. Repositioning the sitting patient correctly with respect to the isocenter requires that the chair be flexible and meet several requirements. For example, it needs to be usable with both a simulator and an isocentrically mounted linear accelerator. The chair should allow vertical and horizontal motion and isocentric rotation about a vertical axis. The chair should also allow an adequate range of vertical travel. Since the height of the isocenter is fixed, one must be able to elevate or lower the patient to the appropriate level. Another important requirement of a treatment chair is that it allow treatment from a variety of directions, including anterior and posterior, opposed laterals, as well as multiple oblique fields.[33]

One treatment chair features an adjustable back support consisting of a carbon-fiber grid panel facilitating a window for posterior fields (Fig. 4-28).* This chair is also equipped with adjustable arm supports and hand grips, facilitating a raised-arm position. One model facilitates the use of a head immobilization system consisting of a standard head support and a thermoplastic facial mask.

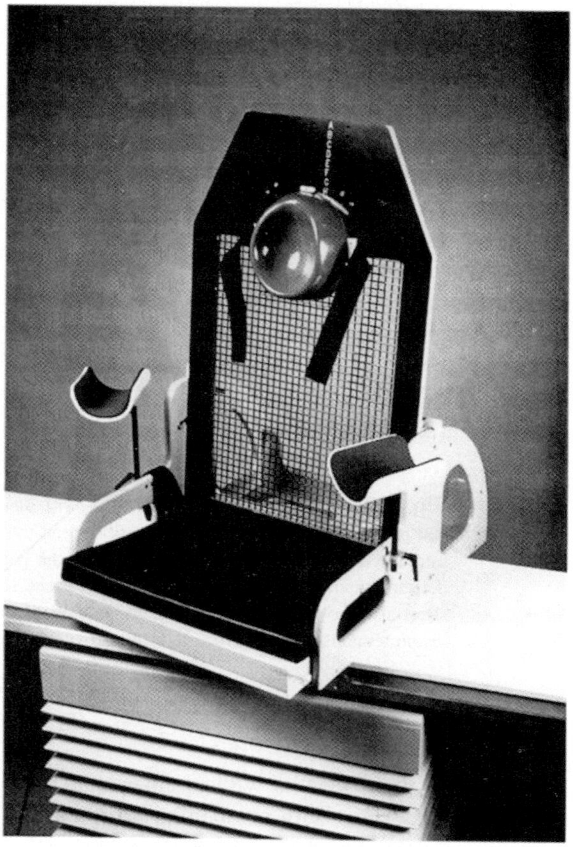

Fig. 4-28 A treatment chair that can be used for head and neck and thoracic irradiation. A thermoplastic mask can be used for head immobilization and the carbon-fiber back panel facilitates a posterior chest field. (Courtesy of MED-TEC, Inc., Orange City, Iowa.)

STABILIZATION AND SHIELDING DURING IRRADIATION OF SUPERFICIAL LESIONS

When superficial lesions are irradiated, it is usually necessary to visualize the skin or palpate the area to ensure proper margins around the target. Facial masks often negate this, so that other methods of restraining the patient's head must be utilized. For example, the patient's head can be stabilized by using a standard head support and Velcro straps across the forehead. Skin lesions are often treated using an electron beam or a superficial x-ray beam. In both of these setups, a treatment cone extending from the head of the machine to the patient's skin surface is usually utilized. The treatment cone, which is in direct contact with the skin surface, also helps to maintain the head position.

*MED-TEC, Inc., Orange City, Iowa.

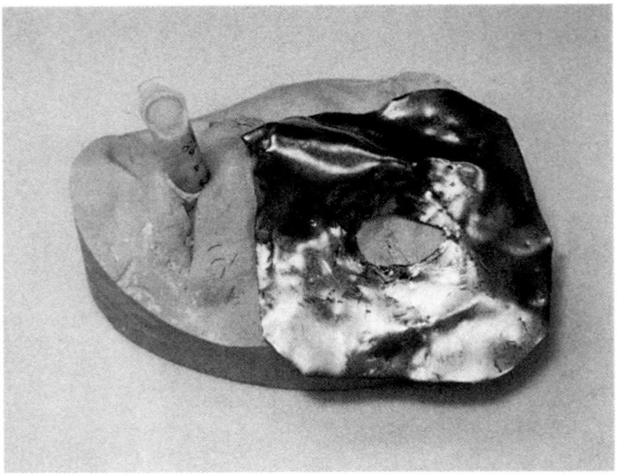

A

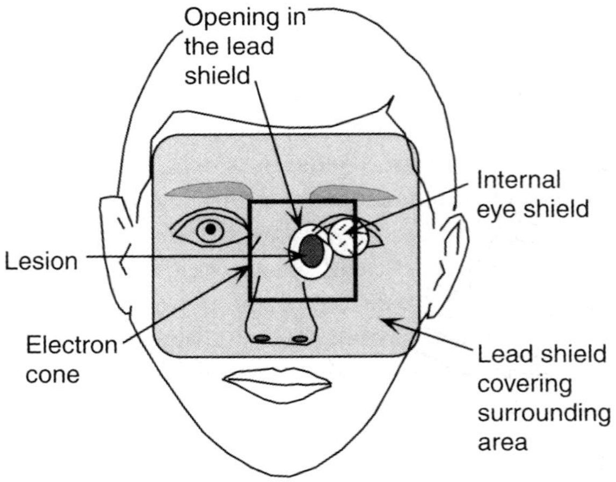

B

Fig. 4-29 *A*. A protective lead sheet—with an opening for the treatment area, molded to the patient's facial prominences—should extend well beyond the treated area to prevent normal tissues from being moved into the (stationary) radiation field in case the patient moves. *B*. A protective lead sheet with an opening defining the radiation field is fixed to the patient. If the patient moves, the target and the opening in the lead sheet also move. Thus, the treatment cone needs to be larger than the opening in the lead sheet, so that the lesion remains within the beam if the patient moves.

In treating these lesions with a superficial x-ray machine, a lead sheet with an opening for the lesion (plus margins) is placed over the patient's face (Fig. 4-29*A*). If the lead sheet is formed so that it conforms to the irregular surface of the patient's face, it will aid in achieving precise repositioning and may prevent shifts during treatment. Making the protective lead shield conform to the facial prominences usually requires that a model of the patient's face be made from dental stone or some other hard material that can withstand the process of hammering out the lead sheet.

The size of the treatment cone should be 1 to 2 cm larger than the opening in the lead sheet, so that even with small patient movements, the target remains within the beam. The protective lead sheet should cover the patient well beyond the treatment cone so that if the patient moves, the radiation beam remains over the shielded areas (Fig. 4-29*B*). It is important to recognize that the radiation beam (cone) is fixed in space while the patient with the protective lead shield may move.

When skin lesions on the eyelids or near the eyes are treated, it may be necessary to place an internal tungsten eye shield over the globe of the eye and under the eyelids (Fig. 4-30). Internal eye shields are available in different sizes (Fig. 4-31). Eye shields are sometimes coated with an acrylic to reduce secondary scatter.

When lip lesions are irradiated using a nonpenetrating beam, an internal shield can be placed immediately behind the lip to shield the buccogingival sulcus (Fig. 4-32). Such a shield can be secured by embedding it in a thin (stretched) layer of thermoplastic material extending over and formed to the patient's exterior surface. Similarly, when a lesion on the helix of the ear is irradiated, a lead shield can be placed behind the ear to protect the brain from the exit dose (Fig. 4-33). When an external skin lesion on the nose is irradiated, a lead shield can be inserted into the nostril to protect the underlying mucosa (Fig. 4-34). A string attached to such nostril shield and taped to the external skin surface will secure the shield and prevent the patient from accidentally inhaling it.

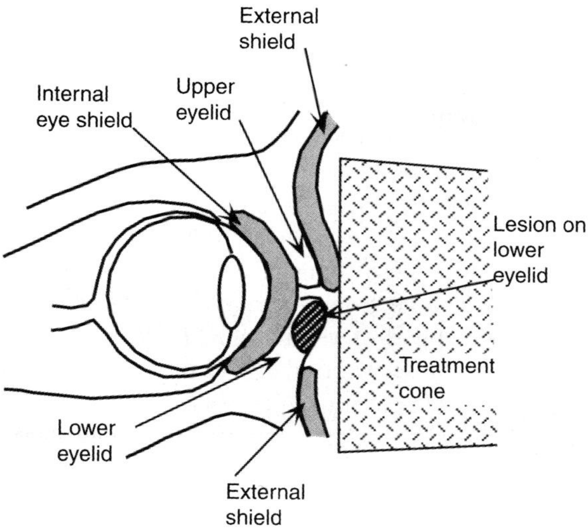

Fig. 4-30 Internal eye shields can be placed over the globe of the eye under the eyelids when lesions on or near the eyelids are treated using low-energy irradiation.

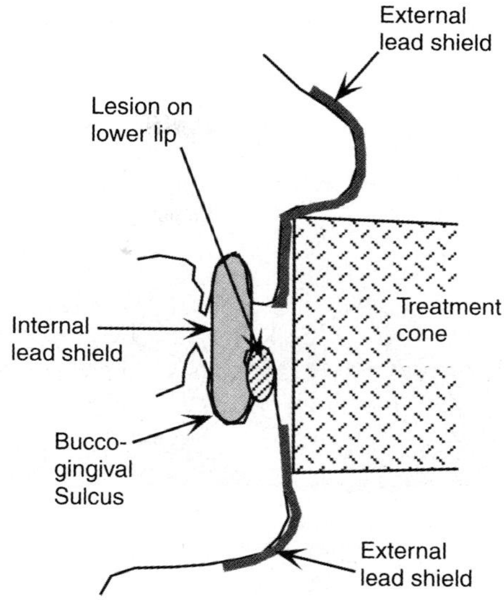

Fig. 4-32 When a lip lesion is treated, a lead shield can be placed in the buccogingival sulcus to protect oral mucosa from the exit beam.

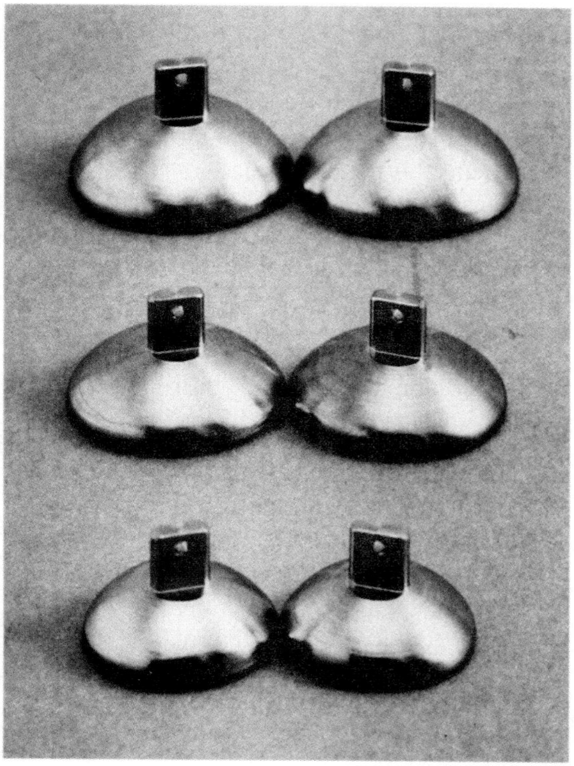

Fig. 4-31 Internal eye shields are available in different sizes. (Courtesy of MED-TEC, Inc., Orange City, Iowa.)

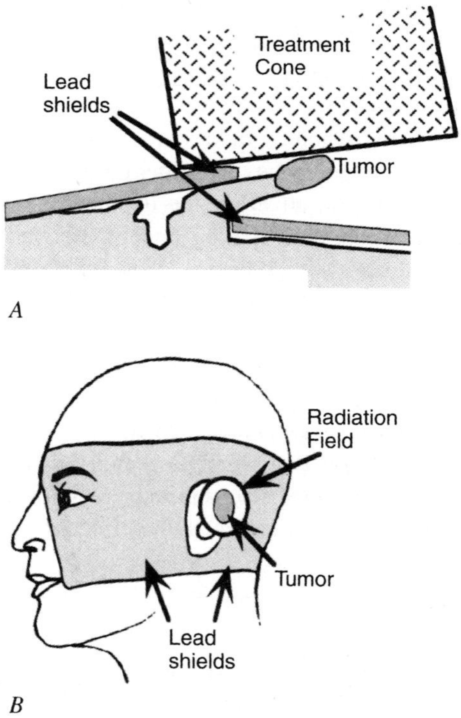

Fig. 4-33 A lead sheet can be placed behind the helix of the ear to protect the scalp and brain from the exit beam. *A*. Transverse view of a lead shield anterior to the ear and another behind the ear. *B*. Placement of anterior and posterior lead shields in treating a tumor on the helix of the ear.

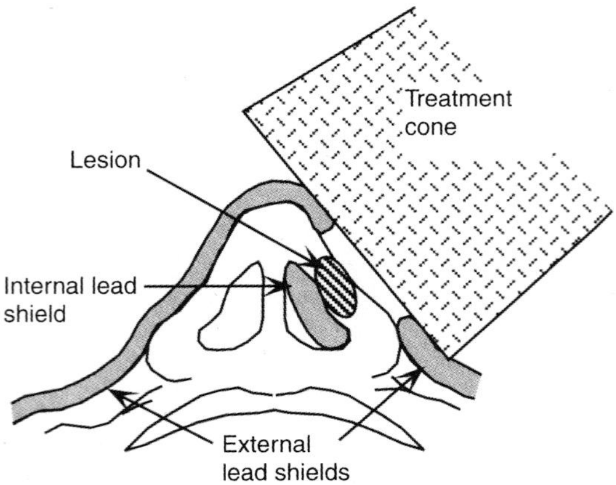

Fig. 4-34 A lead shield attached to a string can be placed inside the nostril when irradiating a lesion on the ala nasi. Such a field may flash over the nose and include the contralateral face and eye. A large protective lead shield is advocated in such treatment.

EFFECT OF IMMOBILIZATION DEVICES ON THE RADIATION DOSE

In treatments where a radiation beam traverses an immobilization device, consideration should be given to both the effect on the depth dose and the reduction of the skin-sparing benefits derived from the use of megavoltage beams. Most radiation fields used in head and neck treatment originate from the lateral or anterior direction, eliminating the problems associated with treating through the posterior head support, base plate, couch top, and so on. The effect of these materials on the depth and surface dose depends on their thickness and density, and, for the surface dose, also the distance between the material and the surface; thus, the effect varies with each setup.

DEPTH DOSE

The effects of immobilization devices on the depth dose are generally small relative to other heterogeneities that are often ignored in routine clinical practice (irregular external contour, air cavities, lung and bone density, and so on). When the entire radiation field is intercepted by an attenuator of uniform thickness and density, the effect on the depth dose is uniform within the field. This attenuation can be compensated by increasing the number of monitor units. However, when the thickness or density of the material varies within the field, the problem becomes more complex. For example, a posterior head and neck field may traverse a base plate and head support of varying thickness and density, causing the dose within the field to vary. This presents a dilemma of how to compensate for the dose changes; increasing the number of monitor units will increase the dose, but the heterogeneity still remains. Depending on the magnitude of the dose variation within the field, the size of the area affected, and the tissues being irradiated, the attenuation may be disregarded or an average attenuation factor applied. Caution should be used in increasing the number of monitor units to compensate for attenuation in situations where only a portion of the treatment field is intercepted by attenuating material. By increasing the number of monitor units, the depth dose in the *unattenuated* portion of the field increases, possibly causing adverse effects. In such a situation, it might be preferable to accept a lower dose in the attenuated portion of the field.

The effect of the thermoplastic materials used in facial masks on the depth dose percentage is negligible; however, the point of maximum ionization is shifted a few millimeters toward the surface.[10]

SURFACE DOSE

Immobilization facial masks and strips are the main cause of reduction of the skin-sparing benefits derived from the use of megavoltage beams. Special attention should be paid to immobilization materials when they lie in the path of the beam, as they may significantly increase the dose in the first few millimeters of tissue. The increase in skin dose caused by such immobilization devices varies with their thickness and density. The effect on the skin dose caused by perforated thermoplastic material, which is commonly used for facial masks, is probably less than that of a solid sheet (nonperforated) of the same thickness. Fiorino et al. investigated the effect of three commercially available thermoplastics

(Orfit Raycast,* Posicast,† and Optimold‡) on the skin dose using a 6-MV photon beam.[7,11] Surface-dose measurements of 2.4-mm Optimold, 2-mm Orfit, and 2.5-mm Posicast showed no large differences between the three materials; surface doses ranged from 55 to 65% of D_{max} dose for a 10 × 10 cm field. A significant difference in the skin dose between 3.2-mm Orfit and Optimold was found, with Optimold showing better skin sparing. This was attributed to the difference in perforation of the two materials. These measurements were made using flat, unstretched sheets of the thermoplastic materials.

Fontenla et al. made similar measurements of solid and perforated thermoplastic material (Aquaplast§) and of plaster (about 3 mm thick) using 6- and 15-MV photon beams.[10] With a 6-MV photon beam and a 12 × 12 cm field, the surface dose under 3 mm of solid thermoplastic material increased from 24% without to about 80% of D_{max} dose with the material present, an increase of about 56 percentage points. For a 15-MV beam, the 3-mm solid thermoplastic material increased the surface dose from 19 to 58% of D_{max} dose. For the perforated thermoplastic material, the surface dose increased by 33 and 21% for 6 MV and 15 MV, respectively. For the plaster, the surface dose increased by 43 and 30% of the open-field D_{max} dose using 6- and 15-MV photons, respectively. The effect of the plaster on the buildup dose is more noticeable than that of the perforated form of thermoplastic material but not as significant as that of the thicker, solid form of thermoplastic material.

The skin dose measured on molded masks is invariably less than the skin dose measured with the unmolded material. This is because of the stretching that inevitably occurs when the mask is molded to the patient's face. It is extremely difficult to determine the true skin dose caused by finished facial masks because of a large variability in thickness and perforation within and between masks. Measurements of surface dose have been made for molded masks using 2-mm Orfit and 3.2-mm Optimold. The surface dose with molded Orfit masks ranged from 40 to 50% of D_{max} dose (mean, 45%) and from 30 to 50% of D_{max} dose (mean, 38%) with Optimold masks using a 10 × 10 cm field.[7,11]

*Luxilon Industries, Vijnegem, Belgium.
†Sinmed, Reenwijk, Holland.
‡WFR Aquaplast Corp., Wyckoff, New Jersey.
§AquaPlast™, WFR Aquaplast Corp., Wyckoff, New Jersey.

TREATMENT ACCURACY

Increased accuracy of daily setup provides an opportunity to improve the therapeutic ratio, both by increased likelihood of tumor control and by decreased risk of complications in normal tissue. Reproducing the setup in the head and neck area is particularly important due to the proximity of many critical organs (eye, optic chiasm, brain, spinal cord, and so on), which often limits the field margins. Assessing the effectiveness of an immobilization device is therefore important and the result should be considered when field margins are designed, with respect both to the target and to normal tissues. Thus, the frequency and magnitude of treatment field misalignments during irradiation of head and neck malignancies has been extensively studied.[2,3,12–14,35–45]

Portal imaging is an important quality assurance procedure for monitoring the reproducibility of setup geometry in radiation therapy. The role of portal imaging has become more critical in recent years due to the increased use of three-dimensional treatment planning technology, facilitating high-precision conformal therapy with relatively small margins. The most common methods are visual comparison of simulation film (prescription) and port film (treated), computer-based comparison of films, and, more recently, electronic portal imaging.

Traditional methods of acquiring weekly port films interpreted by visual comparison of a prescription image suffer from deficiencies[46]; these fuel speculation that some setup errors go undetected and others persist for a clinically significant portion of the prescribed dose.[42] For example, a field-shaping block omitted or inserted in the wrong orientation during a treatment delivered between port-filming days would not be detected. Likewise, misinterpretation of setup marks leading to setup errors could go undetected for several days. Significant improvements in both the accuracy and the efficiency of detecting and correcting setup errors can, in principle, be achieved by using electronic portal imaging devices where the setup is verified prior to each treatment and in some situations also during the treatment.[47]

Visual comparison of simulation and port films is clinically practical but cannot readily determine if a misalignment is due to isocenter placement (translational error) or a rotation of the patient's head (rotational error). Since it is difficult to determine the cause of the misalignment, a translational correction is usually made (i.e., shifting the isocenter). By placing wax molds with metal markers into the outer ear[48] or metal markers injected into the cranium,[49] one can more readily determine the cause of the misalignment, since these markers are fixed to the patient's anatomy.

In evaluating the effectiveness of an immobilization device, it is important to recognize that systematic errors frequently occur in the transfer of information from the simulation to the treatment unit.[12,13,36,41,44,50–52] Such errors can be due to discrepancies between the couch top, the laser alignment system, crosshair alignment, and so on. The couch top in the simulation or CT unit is often solid, whereas in the treatment room there are "windows" in the couch to facilitate posterior fields. Such windows may be covered by a tennis racket–type mesh that may sag under the patient's weight. Although verification of laser alignment systems and field congruence on each machine is frequently made, discrepancies may be present, causing misalignments when the treatment setup is transferred from the simulation to the treatment unit.

It is difficult to determine whether a misalignment is due to failure to reposition the patient relative to the positioning mold or to inaccuracies in field placement relative to the positioning mold (gantry or couch angles, thickness of alignment lines, mobility of skin marks, and so on). Patients who are incorrectly repositioned within a tight-fitting immobilization device are likely to be uncomfortable and therefore to require a position adjustment. Precise patient repositioning in an immobilization device requires that the patient understand the importance of repositioning and that the staff take the time to make sure that the patient is returned to the device correctly. Dunscombe et al. used a computer-based method to resolve field placement errors into those due to patient motion within the immobilization shell and those due to incorrect beam position, orientation, and shape.[36] Their study suggests that the patients' motion within the immobilization shell is greater than field placement errors.

Hess et al. studied the accuracy of field alignment in 95 head and neck patients immobilized with facial masks.[12] Measurements were made from identifiable anatomic landmarks to the field edges on simulation and portal films to determine setup variability. All measured deviations were normally distributed, with mean values of 0 to 3 mm and standard deviations of 3 to 5 mm. Of the absolute deviations, 50 and 90% were within 3 and 9 mm, respectively, and about 20% of the absolute deviations exceeded 5 mm. These figures representing the accuracy of field alignment in clinical routine are similar to those reported by other authors[40,53] and may therefore be predictive of the expected accuracy of field alignment in head and neck treatment.

Halverson et al. used an on-line radiotherapy imaging system to study treatment setup variability.[38] Daily digital portal images of 17 patients undergoing head and neck irradiation were acquired and variations in the daily setup were quantified using a cumulative verification image-analysis method. Isofrequency distributions, or contours of the treated fields, were calculated and examined with respect to the prescription treatment area defined by the simulator film. The frequency with which the prescription area was treated was also determined. At best, approximately 95% of the prescribed area was treated 100% of the time during the entire course of radiation therapy, and, in the worst case, approximately 70% of the prescribed area was treated 100% of the time. These results indicate that despite patient immobilization, large setup variations can occur.

Recalculation of dose distributions, including daily setup variation, is helpful to illustrate the dosimetric consequences of setup errors. Frazier et al. compared the dosimetry measured in a solid water phantom using multileaf collimators and custom blocks with the dose distribution resulting from the same field but including daily setup variations.[37] Sequential port films obtained during the course of radiation therapy were aligned with the prescription film and setup errors were calculated for each patient. The measured and composite dose distributions, including daily setup variations, were compared in the beam's-eye view. The field's penumbra width was calculated (20/80% isodose lines), and the ratio of areas covered by the 90 and 20% (90/20% isodose lines) was determined. With and without daily setup variation, the use of custom blocks was more favorable than that of multileaf collimators in terms of field penumbra width and 90/20 ratio. In the absence of daily setup variation, the multileaf collimator's penumbra width was on the average 1.3 mm larger than that of the custom blocks and 0.9 mm larger in the presence of daily setup variations. For both the custom blocks and the multileaf collimator, daily setup variability produced a significant increase in the field's penumbra width—2.3 mm for the custom blocks and 1.9 mm for the multileaf collimator—and a decrease in the 90/20 ratio—0.06 and 0.05, respectively. The impact of setup variations on "effective" penumbra is far greater than the penumbra difference between the custom blocks and the multileaf collimator. Thus, in practical terms, there is no clinical difference between the custom blocks and multileaf collimators.

Michalski et al. performed a similar study exploring the impact of geometric treatment variations on the dose. They used an on-line radiotherapy imaging system to capture the daily beam positions in 12 patients treated for head and neck, thoracic, and pelvic malignancies.[54] Each daily portal image was aligned with the prescription image using a template of anatomic structures. The outline of the actual block position was then superimposed on the prescription image. Daily block positions were summed to give a summary image represented by the "block overlap isofrequency distribution." These summary data were used to analyze the geometric variation relative to the prescription boundary on a histogram distribution plot. Dose distributions were recalculated considering daily setup variations. The results were expressed in isofrequency distributions where the 100% isofrequency curve represented areas covered throughout the treatment course and the 0% curve represented the extreme limits of variation; i.e., areas outside this curve were never within the primary beam. Head and neck sites had the least random variation, with an average 0 to 100% block overlap isofrequency distribution width of 7 mm, compared with 12 mm for thoracic and 14 mm for pelvic sites.

In some of the studies quoted above, the immobilization device is not described in detail. In other studies, where facial masks were used, the authors report a repositioning ability varying from <1 to about 5 mm.[3,5,6,13,41] When the reproducibility is presented in terms of distance (millimeters), it implies that the discrepancy represents translational errors only. In other studies, the reproducibility is described in distance and number of degrees, indicating an ability to separate translational from rotational errors. It is important to consider not only the maximum, minimum, and average accuracy, but also the *frequency* with which setup errors occur. The latter would require daily port films, which would be impractical and costly. Using rapidly growing electronic portal imaging techniques, these questions may be addressed more satisfactorily in the future.[42,47,48,55–59] One of the major advantages of electronic portal imaging systems is that patient-positioning and field-shaping errors can be detected and corrected before the daily radiation has been delivered.[57,60–63]

Using the frequency of physician-requested isocenter shifts as an indicator of the accuracy of patient repositioning is a clinically practical but not precise measure of the magnitude of setup errors. In our own experience, isocenter shifts are usually requested in 0.5-cm increments, since it is difficult to make smaller shifts in the treatment room. For example, the setup marks on the mask (or on the patient) and the laser alignment lines are often a few millimeters thick; it would be impossible to set up each treatment to precisely the same portion of such a line. Small variations may also exist between how different technologists would set up the same treatment from one treatment to another.

Interpretation of the data illustrating setup accuracy is difficult due to many variables. For example, is it the strength of the immobilization device or the technologists' compulsiveness that is the true source of the result? Are some patients more cooperative than others, causing the results to vary? Are there variables in interpretation of the portal images? These questions cannot be answered; it is therefore important that each user evaluate his or her own immobilization technique and decide if it is acceptable or if improvements need to be made.

REFERENCES

1. Bentel GC: *Radiation Therapy Planning*, 2d ed., New York, McGraw-Hill, 1996.
2. Marks JE, Haus AG: The effect of immobilization on localization error in the radiotherapy of head and neck cancer. *Clin Radiol* 27:175, 1976.
3. Bentel GC, Marks LB, Hendren K, Brizel DM: Comparison of two head and neck immobilization systems. *Int J Radiat Oncol Biol Phys* 38:867–873, 1997.
4. Bentel GC, Marks LB, Sherouse GW, Spencer DP: A customized head and neck support system. *Int J Radiat Oncol Biol Phys* 32:245–248, 1995.
5. Thornton AF, Ten Haken RK, Weeks KJ, et al: A head immobilization system for radiation simulation, CT, MRI, and PET imaging. *Med Dosim* 16:51–56, 1991.
6. Thornton AF, Ten Haken RK, Gerhardsson A, Correll M: Three-dimensional motion analysis of an improved head immobilization system for simulation, CT, MRI, and PET imaging. *Radiother Oncol* 20:224, 1991.
7. Fiorino C, Cattaneo GM, Del Vecchio A, et al: Skin-sparing reduction effects of thermoplastics used for patient immobilization in head and neck radiotherapy. *Radiother Oncol* 30:267–270, 1994.
8. Niewald M, Lehmann W, Uhlmann U, et al: Experience in the use of face masks for radiotherapy of head and neck tumors. *Strahlentherapie* 161:681–684, 1985.
9. Niewald M, Lehmann W, Scharding B, et al: Face masks for radiotherapy of head and neck tumors: Comparative tests of different materials. *Strahlenther Onkol* 162: 448–454, 1986.
10. Fontenla DP, Napoli JJ, Hunt M, et al: Effects of beam modifiers and immobilization devices on the dose in the build-up region. *Int J Radiat Oncol Biol Phys* 30: 211–219, 1994.
11. Fiorino C, Cattaneo GM, Del Vecchio A, et al: Skin dose measurements for head and neck radiotherapy. *Med Phys* 19:1263–1266, 1992.
12. Hess CF, Kortmann RD, Jany R, et al: Accuracy of field alignment in radiotherapy of head and neck cancer utilizing individualized face mask immobilization: A retrospective analysis of clinical practice. *Radiother Oncol* 34:69–72, 1995.
13. Mitine C, Dutreix A, van der Schueren E: Black and white in accuracy assessment of megavoltage images: The medical decision is often grey. *Radiother Oncol* 28:31–36, 1993.
14. Rubio AM, Ferrer E, Algara M, et al: Dosimetry and use of an immobilization system for head and neck radiotherapy treatments. *Med Dosim* 16:163–167, 1991.
15. Gagnon WF, Cundiff JH: Dose enhancement from backscattered radiation at tissue-metal interfaces irradiated with high energy electrons. *Br J Radiol* 53:466, 1980.
16. Gibbs FA, Palos B, Goffinet DR: The metal/tissue interface effect in irradiation of the oral cavity. *Radiology* 119:705, 1976.
17. Khan FM, Moore VC, Levitt SH: Field shaping in electron beam therapy. *Br J Radiol* 49:833, 1976.
18. Klevenhagen SC, Lambert GD, Arbari A: Backscattering in electron beam therapy for energies between 3 and 35 MeV. *Phys Med Biol* 27:363, 1982.
19. Saunders JE, Peters BG: Back-scattering from metals in superficial therapy with high energy electrons. *Br J Radiol* 47:467, 1974.
20. Thambi V, Murthy AK, Alder G, Kartha PK: Dose perturbation resulting from gold fillings in patients with head and neck cancer. *Int J Radiat Oncol Biol Phys* 5:581, 1979.
21. Thilmann C, Adamietz IA, Rahn R, et al: The in-vivo determination of dosage intensification due to dental alloys in the therapeutic irradiation of the oral cavity. *Strahlenther Onkol* 171:468–472, 1995.
22. Weidlich GA, Nuesch CE, Fuery JJ: Added aluminum shielding to attenuate back scatter electrons from intraoral lead shields. *Med Dosim* 21:165–167, 1996.
23. Nelson TJ, Lindberg RD: Biteblock-head immobilizer system. *Med Dosim* 14:147–151, 1989.
24. Farahani M, Eichmiller FC, McLaughlin WL: Measurement of absorbed dose near metal and dental material interfaces irradiated by x- and gamma-ray therapy beams. *Phys Med Biol* 35:369–385, 1990.
25. Niroomand-Rad A, Razavi R, Thobejane S, Harter KW: Radiation dose perturbation at tissue-titanium dental interfaces in head and neck cancer patients. *Int J Radiat Oncol Biol Phys* 34:475–480, 1996.
26. Cheng VST, Oral K, Aramy MA: The use of acrylic resin oral prosthesis in radiation therapy of the oral cavity. *Int J Radiat Oncol Biol Phys* 8:1245, 1982.
27. Schratter-Sehn AU, Schmidt FW, Kielhauser R, et al: Prävention lokaler Schleimhautläsionen während Oropharynxbestrahlung durch einen Plombenschutz. *Strahlenther Onkol* 168:35, 1992.

28. Thilmann C, Adamietz IA, Ramm U, et al: In vivo dose increase in the presence of dental alloys during ^{60}Co-gamma-ray therapy of the oral cavity. *Med Dosim* 21: 149–154, 1996.
29. Fayos JV, Lampe I: Peroral irradiation of carcinoma of the oral tongue. *Radiology* 93:387–394, 1969.
30. Allain YM, Schlienger M, Houy JC: Artifice de technique dans l'irradiation au betatron. *J Radiol d'Electrol* 52: 189–192, 1971.
31. Boag JW, Hodt HJ: Adjustable chair for radiotherapy of head and neck cancer. *Br J Radiol* 44:316–317, 1983.
32. Karzmark CJ, Bagshaw MA, Huisman PA, Lawson J: A versatile radiotherapy treatment chair. *Br J Radiol* 53:1190–1194, 1980.
33. Miller RW, Raubitschek AA, Harrington FS, et al: An isocentric chair for the simulation and treatment of radiation therapy patients. *Int J Radiat Oncol Biol Phys* 21:469–473, 1991.
34. Wiernik G: A new radiotherapy treatment chair. *Br J Radiol* 34:676–678, 1961.
35. Byhardt RW, Cox JD, Hornburg A, Liermann G: Weekly localization films and detection of field placement errors. *Int J Radiat Oncol Biol Phys* 4:881, 1978.
36. Dunscombe PB, Fox K, Loose S, Leszczynski K: The investigation and rectification of field placement errors in the delivery of complex head and neck fields. *Int J Radiat Oncol Biol Phys* 26:155–161, 1993.
37. Frazier A, Yan D, Du M, et al: Effects of treatment setup variation on beam's eye view dosimetry for radiation therapy using the multileaf collimator vs. the cerrobend block. *Int J Radiat Oncol Biol Phys* 33:1247–1256, 1995.
38. Halverson KJ, Leung TC, Pellet JB, et al: Study of treatment variation in the radiotherapy of head and neck tumors using a fiber-optic on-line radiotherapy imaging system. *Int J Radiat Oncol Biol Phys* 21:1327–1336, 1991.
39. Huizenga H, Levendag PC, DePorre PMZR: Accuracy in radiation field alignment in head and neck cancers: A prospective study. *Radiother Oncol* 11:181, 1988.
40. Mitine C, Leunens G, Verstatete J, et al: Is it necessary to repeat quality control procedures for head and neck patients? *Radiother Oncol* 21:201, 1991.
41. Rabinowitz I, Broomberg J, Goitein M, et al: Accuracy of radiation field alignment in clinical practice. *Int J Radiat Oncol Biol Phys* 11:1857, 1985.
42. Valicenti RK, Michalski JM, Bosch WR, et al: Is weekly port filming adequate for verifying patient position in modern radiation therapy? *Int J Radiat Oncol Biol Phys* 30:431–438, 1994.
43. Verhey LJ, Goitein M, McNulty P, et al: Precise positioning of patients for radiation therapy. *Int J Radiat Oncol Biol Phys* 2:289–294, 1982.
44. Hunt MA, Kutcher GJ, Burman C, et al: The effect of setup uncertainties on the treatment of nasopharynx cancer. *Int J Radiat Oncol Biol Phys* 27:437–447, 1993.
45. Weiser JC, Gur D, Cano ER, et al: Verification of electron beam therapy with storage phosphor images: Precision of field placement. *Radiology* 175:257–259, 1990.
46. Rosenman J, Roe CA, Cromartie R, et al: Portal film enhancement: Technique and clinical utility. *Int J Radiat Oncol Biol Phys* 25:333, 1993.
47. Fritsch DS, Chaney EL, Boxwala A, et al: Core-based portal image registration for automatic radiotherapy treatment verification. *Int J Radiat Oncol Biol Phys* 33:1287–1300, 1995.
48. Bel A, Keus R, Vijlbrief RE, Lebesque JV: Setup deviations in wedged pair irradiation of parotid gland and tonsillar tumors, measured with an electronic portal imaging device. *Radiother Oncol* 37:153–159, 1995.
49. Lam KL, Ten Haken RK, McShan DL, Thornton AF: Automated determination of patient setup errors in radiation therapy using spherical radio-opaque markers. *Med Phys* 20:1145–1152, 1993.
50. McCullough EC, McCullough KP: Improving agreement between radiation-delineated field edges on simulation and portal films: The edge tolerance test tool. *Med Phys* 20:375, 1993.
51. Gildersleve J, Dearnaley DP, Evans PM, Swindell W: Reproducibility of patient positioning during routine radiotherapy, as assessed by an integrated megavoltage imaging system. *Radiother Oncol* 35:151–160, 1995.
52. Lirette A, Pouliot J, Aubin M, Larochelle M: The role of electronic portal imaging in tangential breast irradiation: A prospective study. *Radiother Oncol* 37:241–245, 1995.
53. Lebesque JV, Bel A, Bijhold J, Hart AA: Detection of systematic patient setup errors by portal film analysis. *Radiother Oncol* 23:198, 1992.
54. Michalski JM, Wong JW, Gerber RL, et al: The use of online image verification to estimate the variation in radiation therapy dose delivery. *Int J Radiat Oncol Biol Phys* 27:707–716, 1993.
55. Boyer AL, Antonuk L, Fenster A, et al: A review of electronic portal imaging devices (EPIDs). *Med Phys* 19:1, 1992.
56. Creutzberg AL, Althof VG, Huizenga H, Visser AG: Quality assurance using portal imaging: The accuracy of patient positioning in irradiation of breast cancer. *Int J Radiat Oncol Biol Phys* 25:529–539, 1993.
57. Michalski JM, Graham MV, Bosch WR, et al: Prospective clinical evaluation of an electronic portal imaging device. *Int J Radiat Oncol Biol Phys* 34:943–951, 1996.
58. Bissett R, Leszczynski K, Loose S, et al: Quantitative vs. subjective portal verification using digital portal images. *Int J Radiat Oncol Biol Phys* 34:489–495, 1996.
59. Yin FF, Rubin P, Schell MC, et al: An observer study for direct comparison of clinical efficacy of electronic to film portal images. *Int J Radiat Oncol Biol Phys* 35:985–991, 1996.
60. Balter JM, Chen GT, Pelizzari CA, et al: Online reposi-

tioning during treatment of the prostate: A study of potential limits and gains. *Int J Radiat Oncol Biol Phys* 27:137–143, 1993.

61. DeNeve W, Van den Heuvel F, DeBeukeleer N, et al: Routine clinical on-line portal imaging followed by immediate field adjustment using a telecontrolled patient couch. *Radiother Oncol* 24:45, 1992.
62. DeNeve W, Van den Heuvel F, Coghe M, et al: Interactive use of on-line portal imaging in pelvic radiation. *Int J Radiat Oncol Biol Phys* 22:517–524, 1993.
63. Ezz A, Munro P, Porter AT, et al: Daily monitoring and correction of radiation field placement using a video-based portal imaging system: A pilot study. *Int J Radiat Oncol Biol Phys* 22:159–165, 1992.

PROBLEMS

4-1 In head and neck treatment, the most reproducible position appears to be
(*a*) prone with a facial support
(*b*) supine without immobilization
(*c*) decubitus with a tape across the forehead
(*d*) supine with a facial mask

4-2 A neutral head position is one in which
(*a*) the forehead and chin lie on a horizontal line
(*b*) the forehead and the tip of the nose lie on a horizontal line
(*c*) the head is elevated 2 in. off the top of the treatment couch
(*d*) the shoulders are elevated about 4 in.

4-3 To achieve a neutral head position in a large patient (large chest)
(*a*) a sheet of Styrofoam is usually needed under the chest
(*b*) no head elevation above the couch is needed
(*c*) the head elevation required is usually thicker than for a thin patient
(*d*) the head elevation required is usually thinner than for a thin patient

4-4 To achieve an extended head position in a thin patient, it may be necessary to
(*a*) elevate the chest and not use any head elevation
(*b*) place a very large support under the head and shoulders
(*c*) use a head support that is much thicker than that needed for a large patient
(*d*) elevate both the head and the shoulders until the forehead and chin lie on a horizontal plane

4-5 In designing a head immobilization system, consideration should be given to
(*a*) weight, strength, and ease to use
(*b*) weight, strength, effect on the dose, and ease of quick release
(*c*) weight and size
(*d*) weight, size, and effect on the dose

4-6 Head and neck immobilization devices are more effective when
(*a*) the base plate is sized to the specific treatment couch
(*b*) the face mask is secured to the base plate
(*c*) the face mask is secured to the base plate and the base plate is fixed to the treatment couch
(*d*) the fixation of the face mask and the base plate makes no difference

4-7 Customized head supports are likely to be more comfortable for the patient because they
(*a*) conform to the sides and top of the head and do not cause neck pain
(*b*) are soft and pliable
(*c*) are transparent and permit visualization of posterior fields
(*d*) conform to the patient's head and neck

4-8 Stretching of thermoplastic face-mask materials
(*a*) is always recommended since it reduces the effect of the mask on the skin dose
(*b*) should be avoided because it makes the mask weak and thus less effective
(*c*) is often necessary in order for the mask to reach across the patient's face and be attached to the base plate on each side of the head
(*d*) all of the above

4-9 Bite blocks are sometimes used in head and neck irradiation for the purpose of
(*a*) opening the patient's mouth
(*b*) protecting the oral mucosa from secondary scatter off fillings in the teeth
(*c*) facilitating easier breathing
(*d*) reducing the volume of oral mucosa within the beams

4-10 In treating a tumor in the maxillary antrum, the purpose of a bite block is to
(*a*) move the tongue and mandible away from the radiation fields
(*b*) move the tongue into and the mandible away from the radiation fields
(*c*) keep the mouth open to facilitate easier breathing
(*d*) move the mandible into and the tongue away from the radiation fields

4-11 When superficial lesions are irradiated
(*a*) protective lead sheets with an opening for the radiation field need to extend only 1 cm from the lesion as long as they conform to the surface of the adjacent structures
(*b*) the smallest cone available should always be used
(*c*) protective lead sheets with an opening for the radiation field should conform to adjacent structures and be generous in size
(*d*) the size of the treatment cone is always irrelevant

4-12 The effect of thermoplastic mask immobilization devices on the skin dose
(*a*) depends on the beam energy only
(*b*) depends on the beam energy used and the thickness of the face mask
(*c*) depends on the thickness of the face mask only
(*d*) the skin dose is not affected by the mask

CHAPTER

5

Central Nervous System

INTRODUCTION

Although positioning and immobilization for patients with brain tumors is similar to that for patients with head and neck tumors (Chap. 4), there are some differences, which are discussed in this chapter.

BRAIN

PATIENT POSITION

Patients receiving radiation therapy for brain tumors are usually positioned supine. Whether the patient's head is extended, flexed, or in neutral position is partly determined by the anticipated field arrangement. The extended head position, described in Chap. 4, is rarely needed when brain tumors are treated with the patient supine. This is because in the neutral position, the base of the skull lies at approximately a 20° angle in the anterior-to-posterior direction (Fig. 5-1). Thus, the head needs to be flexed, not extended, in order to treat an anterior field without including the face.

Patients should be positioned such that the degree of beam attenuation by the "thick" portions of the immobilization device is minimized, thereby reducing loss of skin sparing. Skin reactions in the posterior region of the head may prove prohibitive during future use of a tight-fitting facial mask. Therefore, in a patient with a posterior lesion being treated by opposed lateral fields in the typical immobilization device used at Duke University (described in Chap. 4), the loss of skin sparing due to the acrylic will be reduced by elevating the head (Fig. 5-2).

For some tumors, an anterior field may be used to spare tissues on the right or left side of the tumor (Fig. 5-3*A*). For tumors near the skull base, an anterior field may include the face when the head is in the neutral position (Fig. 5-3*B*). With this situation, the patient's

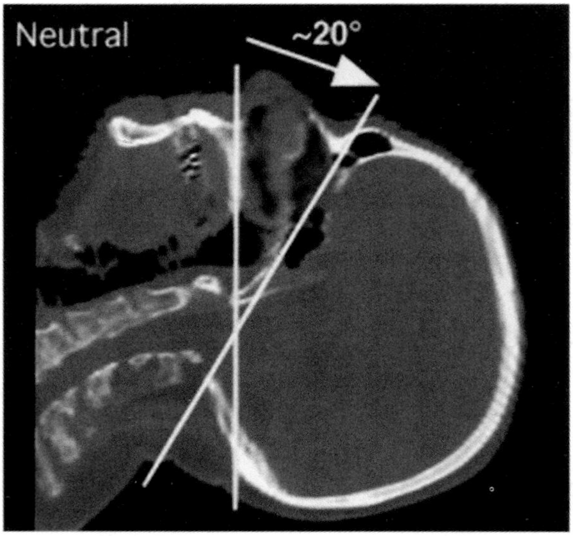

Fig. 5-1 The base of the skull lies at approximately 20° in the anterior-to-posterior direction when the patient's head is in the neutral position.

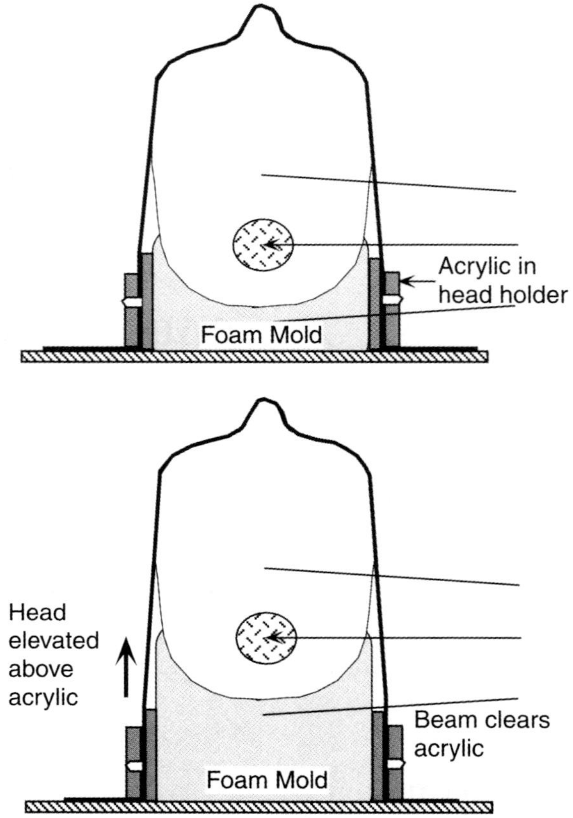

Fig. 5-2 Beam attenuation caused by head immobilization devices can be reduced by adjusting the head position. In this situation, a small head elevation prevents the lateral field from traversing the acrylic walls of the immobilization device.

head needs to be flexed (forward) until the anterior/vertex field projects superior/posterior of the eyes (Fig. 5-3*C*) or a couch and gantry angle can be used (Fig. 5-3*D*). A patient unable to flex his or her head sufficiently can have the chest elevated to a semirecumbent position to achieve the same result (Fig. 5-4). Patients may have difficulties maintaining this position and tend to slide down. A support or brace below the feet may alleviate this problem (Figs. 5-5 and 4-26). Alternatively, the patient can be placed in the prone position with the head and chest raised to facilitate a vertex field (Fig. 5-6). The exit beam from this vertex arrangement might include the mouth.

With the patient's head in the neutral and more comfortable and reproducible position, the preferred technique to treat a third field is to rotate the couch 90° and the gantry to the desired orientation. In this manner, the orientation of the vertex field is selected based on anatomic considerations rather than on the patient's ability to flex (in prone position, extend) the neck. This approach enables one to be less concerned with the head position, since the beam orientation can be adjusted by turning the gantry. Nevertheless, even when this approach is used, the orientation of the head does affect the exit path of the vertex field into the neck.[1] Three-dimensional treatment planning (3DTP) tools are very useful to help shape and direct these vertex fields (Fig. 5-7). When 3DTP tools are available, the patient's head can remain in the neutral position and the beam direction is achieved by turning the gantry, couch, and collimator (Fig. 5-3*D*). Such tools provide great flexibility to design treatment beams limited only by risks of gantry/couch collision.

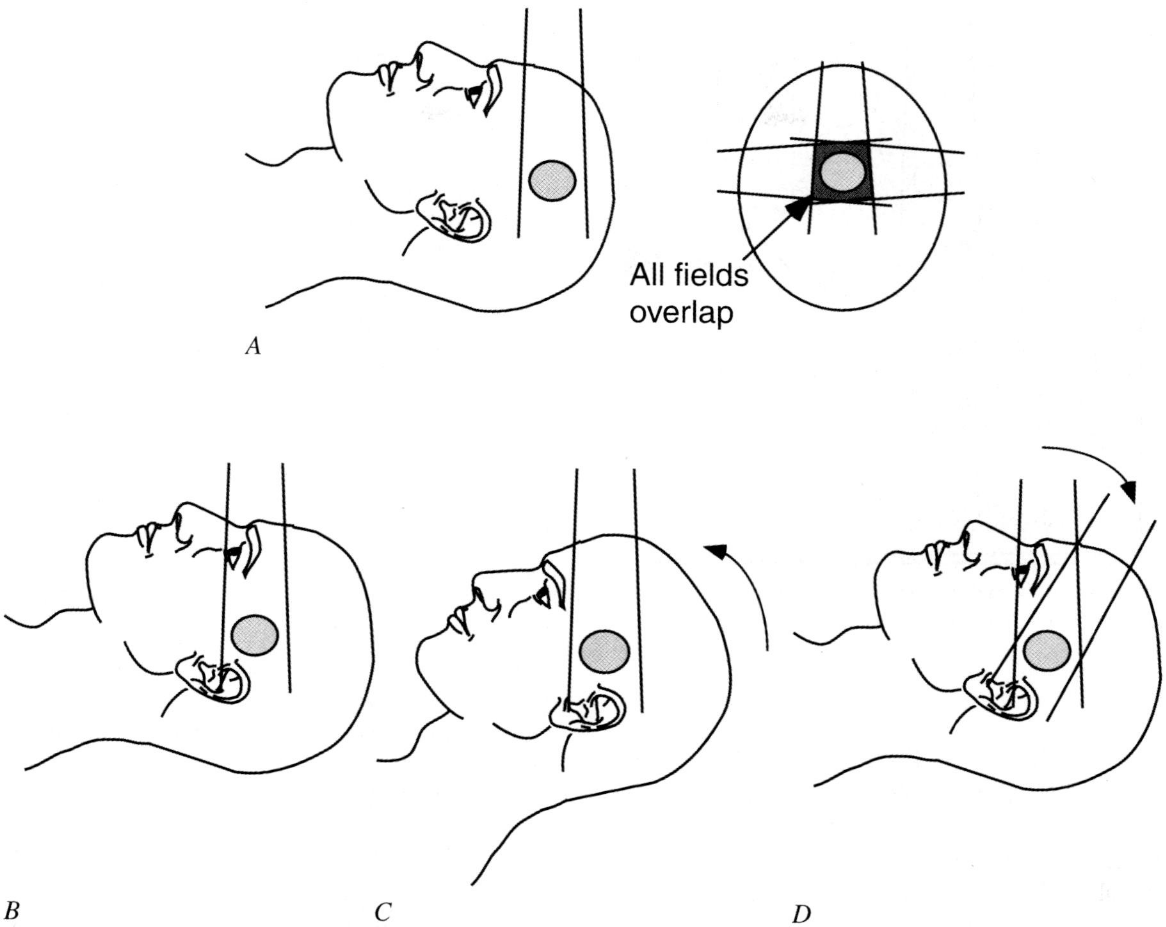

Fig. 5-3 *A*. An anterior field is sometimes used to treat brain tumors in order to reduce the dose in the surrounding brain tissue. The maximum dose is delivered where all three fields overlap (*shaded area on the right*). *B*. When the tumor lies close to the skull base, an anterior field would include the face when the head position is neutral. *C*. The patient's head needs to be flexed until the caudal margin of the anterior/vertex field lies superior/posterior of the eyes (approximately 20°). *D*. The same patient/beam arrangement can be achieved by turning the couch 90° and the gantry to the appropriate angle.

DEFINING CLINICAL CONTINUUM OF CARE

Organ motion is a major issue for extracranial sites but is not generally considered during brain irradiation, since the brain is relatively confined within the skull. The skin overlying the head is also less mobile than that elsewhere on the body, making skin marks somewhat more reliable in this area. Nevertheless, the scalp and facial skin *are* mobile; therefore reliance on skin marks alone is *not* recommended. Furthermore, marks on the scalp are difficult to make and to visualize and they tend to smear, particularly in patients with oily hair.

There are many ways to immobilize the head, with variable accuracy, invasiveness, and logistic limitations. The selection depends upon the type of treat-

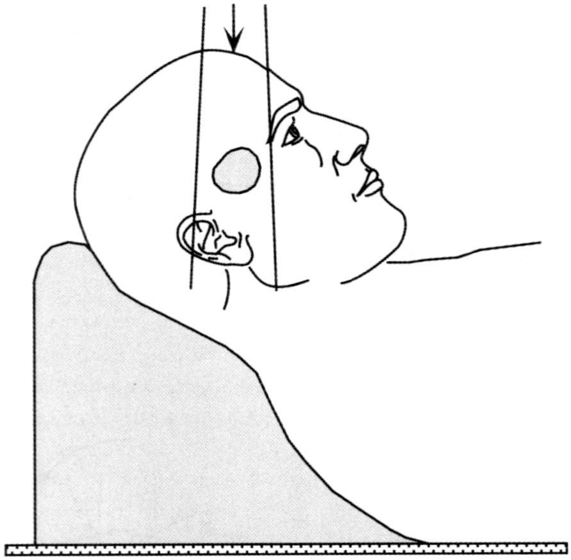

Fig. 5-4 In patients unable to flex the head sufficiently, a support can be built to elevate the head and chest to a semirecumbent position.

ment desired. The most accurate are generally the most invasive and are typically used during highly conformal and short (single-fraction) high-dose therapy termed *radiosurgery*. For such treatments, since normal brain tissue does not tolerate large single fractions of radiation therapy, extreme care is taken (typically with rigid fixation to the skull) to be as accurate as possible. Several authors have studied the accuracy and precision requirements for stereotactic radiosurgery.[2–8] As immobilization becomes less rigid and the possibilities for motion increase, the target margins are generally increased to avoid a geometric miss. As the target margins increase, a larger volume of normal tissue is irradiated; therefore, the fraction size is often lower to reduce the risk of injury to the normal brain tissues.

The term *stereotactic radiosurgery* (SRS) generally refers to a technique in which a high dose (~12 to 15 Gy) of radiation is delivered to a small (4 to 50 mm in diameter) target volume in a single fraction. In SRS techniques, unlike conventional radiation therapy, no attempt is made to spare normal tissues *within* the irradiated volume by fractionating the radiation dose. An extension of stereotactic radiosurgery techniques is frequently used in which normal cells within the treatment volume are spared by *fractionating* the dose in hopes of improving the therapeutic ratio. This fractionated radiosurgery technique is termed *stereotactic radiotherapy* (SRT) or fractionated conformal radiation therapy.

Fractionated conformal radiation therapy is different from single-fraction SRS in terms of fraction size and generally also margins; however, there is a continuum. The size of the margins is related to the accuracy of the target localization and patient immobilization. The fraction size is related to the volume of normal tissues within the treatment volume. In SRS, the entire therapeutic dose is delivered in *one* fraction and generally with *no* target margins; it

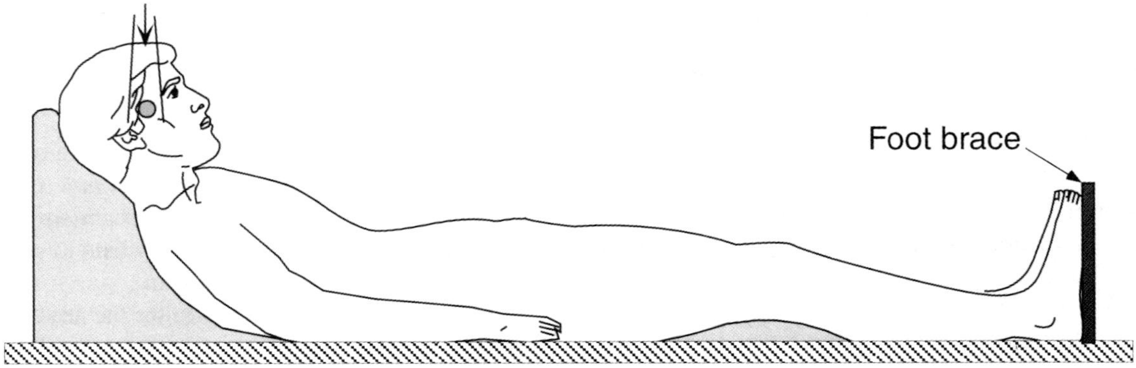

Fig. 5-5 A brace or support below the patient's feet may prevent the patient from sliding down on the couch.

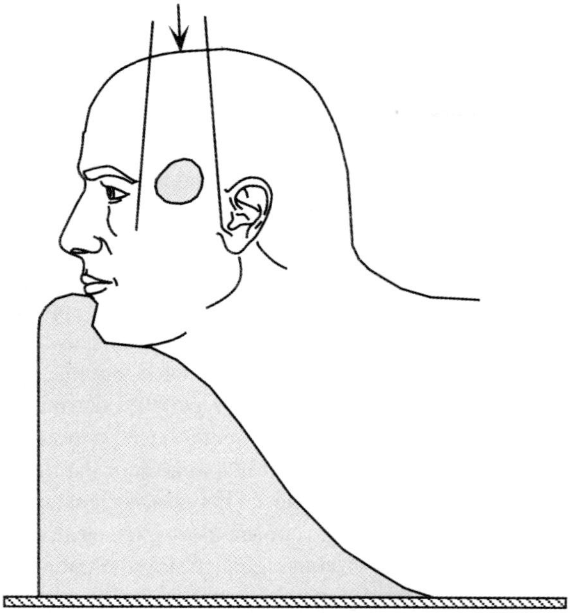

Fig. 5-6 Prone position used to achieve a vertex field.

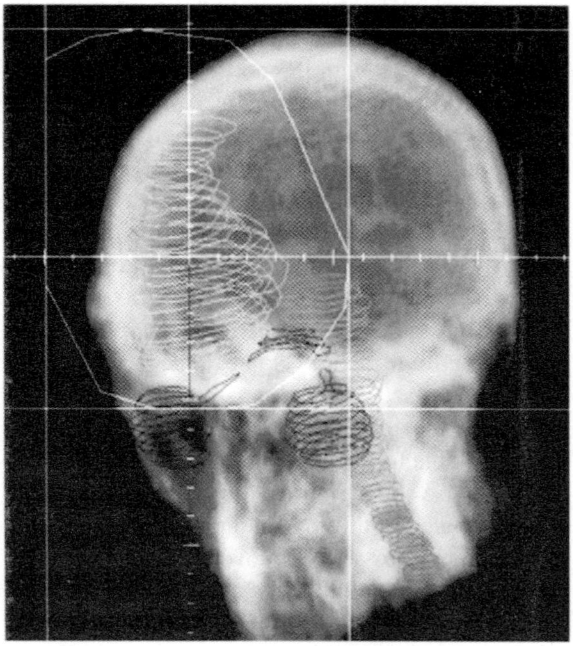

Fig. 5-7 Utilizing three-dimensional treatment-planning tools to determine the optimal direction and shape of a vertex field is very useful. This "vertex" field, angled to avoid brainstem, spinal cord, and as much as possible of the optics, would not be possible without three-dimensional treatment-planning capabilities.

therefore requires *very* accurate methods (< 1 mm). In conformal SRT, the dose is fractionated and thus some margin around the target is often used. However, if very accurate repositioning is performed, fractionated treatment with minimal or no margin can be delivered.

The goal of precision brain irradiation is to *conform* the therapeutic dose volume tightly around the target in three dimensions. A steep dose gradient at the target edge provides excellent sparing of surrounding normal tissues. This can be accomplished by using several conformally fixed, shaped fields, multiple linear accelerator (linac)-based arcs,[9–12] or a Gamma Knife.*[13–15] The Gamma Knife consists of a large lead sphere that holds 201 well-collimated cobalt-60 sources where the radiation from all sources converges at a single point. During the treatment, the patient's head is placed inside this lead sphere such that the point where the radiation converges lies in the target. The isodose distribution can be shaped to conform to the target by selectively blocking some of these sources or by moving the location of the point where the radiation converges to multiple locations (multiple isocenters). A linac-based system provides comparable isodose distributions via multiple arcs converging at the isocenter of the linear accelerator and by using multiple isocenters.

In these precision radiation therapy techniques, the patient's position is sometimes arbitrary, since the beam orientation relative to the patient is accomplished by gantry and couch rotations. However, there are some practical physical limitations. For example, in posterior lesions irradiated using posterior fields, the head may need to be elevated or flexed to avoid gantry/floor stand collisions.

PATIENT IMMOBILIZATION

Single-Fraction Radiation Therapy. Stereotactic radiosurgery was developed in Sweden by Dr. Lars Leksell[16,17] for the purpose of treating inaccessible intracranial targets in a single treatment in lieu

*Electa Instrument AB, Stockholm, Sweden.

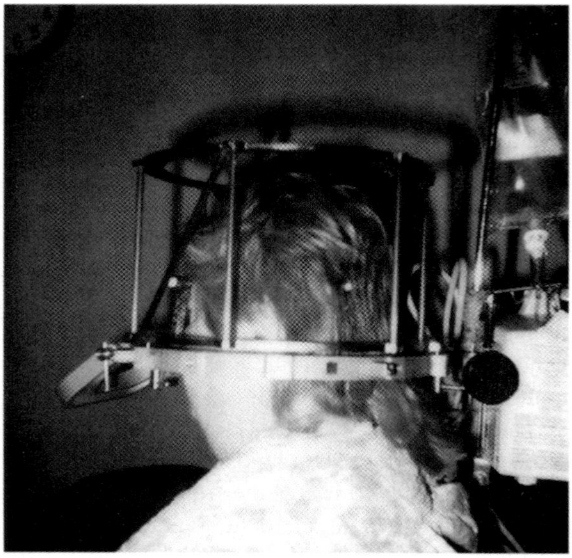

Fig. 5-8 A stereotactic head frame is rigidly attached to the patient's head by four screws in the cranium.

of invasive surgery. The technique was first established to treat functional disorders. It was later used to treat other "nonmalignant" diseases such as arteriovenous malformation (AVM), "benign" tumors such as acoustic neuromas, and, more recently, a wide variety of benign and malignant conditions.[12,18–21]

In SRS, a head ring such as the Brown-Roberts-Wells (BRW)* is attached to the patient's skull by screws, where it remains during target localization and treatment delivery (Fig. 5-8). A series of removable devices, rigidly attached to the head ring, define the stereotactic coordinate space, thus quantitatively linking the diagnostic imaging data to the treatment.[22] Provided that the ring remains rigidly fixed to the patient, the stereotactic coordinates of any point of the intracranial anatomy are also fixed.[9] During treatment delivery, the BRW frame is rigidly docked with the stereotactic accessories on the linear accelerator, thus fixing the beam/skull relationship.

A frameless radiosurgical treatment system, referred to as a Cyberknife†, is currently appearing on the horizon.[23–25] In this system, two orthogonal real-time x-ray cameras are coupled to a robotically manipulated linear accelerator, thus guiding the therapy beam to the treatment site within the patient's cranium. These cameras observe the position and orientation of the patient's head in the treatment system coordinate frame. An image registration algorithm compares the two real-time radiographs to a corresponding pair of digitally synthesized radiographs derived from a computed tomography (CT) study of the patient. The algorithm determines the difference between the patient's head position in the CT coordinate space and its position in the treatment room coordinate space. This allows translation of treatment planning coordinates into treatment room coordinates without rigidly fixing the patient's head position during image acquisition or treatment delivery.

Fractionated Conformal Radiation Therapy. Fractionated SRT, often used to treat relatively localized tumors, combines the advantages of conformal dose delivery with the potential radiobiological advantages of fractionation. In traditional conventional fractionated external beam irradiation, significant volumes of normal tissues are often intentionally included, thus limiting the dose that can safely be delivered. In fractionated conformal radiation therapy, the therapeutic dose volume is "conformed" in three-dimensional space to the target volume, thus allowing larger fraction sizes (e.g., 16 to 20 Gy in four fractions) to be delivered.[26]

The stereotactic head ring, intended for use in single-fraction irradiation techniques, is somewhat uncomfortable for the patient, thus essentially eliminating its use for a protracted course of irradiation. In fractionated conformal radiation therapy, where the treatments are delivered over several days, relocatable head immobilization devices are more frequently used. There is no rule as to what type of localization and immobilization system should be used for single- or multiple-fraction therapy. Thus,

*Radionics Inc., Burlington, Massachusetts.

†Cyberknife™, Accuray, Inc., Sunnyvale, California.

relocatable systems may be used for single-fraction therapy and stereotactic halo-ring systems for multiple-fraction therapy.[27]

INVASIVE HEAD IMMOBILIZATION DEVICES FOR FRACTIONATED THERAPY

A technique has been described in which a stereotactic frame is invasively attached to the patient's cranium for target localization and the first treatment.[28–30] Following the first treatment, coordinates of the target center are marked on the patient's skin with tattoos and the stereotactic frame is removed. For subsequent treatments, another device (a standard neurosurgical halo ring) is attached to the patient's skull and used for setup and immobilization during the remainder of the treatment course. For these treatments, the repositioning of the patient is made by aligning the tattoos with the laser alignment system designating the linear accelerator's isocenter.

This halo-based fractionated treatment approach proved somewhat cumbersome with regard to patient repositioning. There was also some concern about the shifting of skin tattoos due to tissue swelling as a result of frame placement and removal. In the belief that the most reliable approach would be to treat all fractions with the use of only one stereotactic frame, a stereotactic frame built in house, attached to the cranium and used during target localization and throughout the treatment course (usually 12 days), was used.[31] The coordinates of the target center are determined using a target localization box that contains fiducial markers and a target localization grid. This box is used during target localization and treatment but is removed between treatments.

NONINVASIVE RELOCATABLE HEAD IMMOBILIZATION DEVICES

Several noninvasive and possibly more comfortable relocatable head immobilization devices intended for use in fractionated radiation therapy have been designed.[9,32–45] Many of these noninvasive systems are designed and built in house. The design is often based on using dentition combined with a cranial mask or cast for patient fixation.

1. The Latinen relocatable system* consists of a lightweight frame fixed to the patient by means of earplugs and a nose bridge (Fig. 5-9). A millimeter scale on the frame is used in repositioning of the frame and for realigning the patient with the radiation beam. A high degree of reproducibility with little patient discomfort has been demonstrated using this system for stereotactic fractionated radiotherapy.[33,37,41]

2. A device designed for repeated attachment to the head in precisely the same position consists of dental and occipital impressions and a strap that forces these impressions against the head (Fig. 5-10). The original device, referred to as the Gill-Thomas (GT) frame,†[32,35,40] consists of an aluminum alloy base ring that is compatible with the BRW stereotactic frame. The dental appliance is individually constructed for each patient from an impression of the upper and lower teeth. It is firmly attached to the base ring; thus the ring is fixed relative to the cranium. The patient's head is supported by an occipital tray constructed from a malleable vinyl polysiloxane. The frame is fixed to the patient's head by three quick-release nylon straps.

3. Several modifications to the original Gill-Thomas device have been described by Kooy et al.[39]; these were developed in an attempt to improve relocatability and also to make the device usable in children requiring anesthesia. The modifications include an improved strapping system, construction of the oral appliance at the in-house dental clinic, and construction of a depth-confirmation helmet to confirm the position of the frame rapidly on a daily basis.

The original nylon strapping system was replaced by a Velcro‡ head strap, which attaches to the occipital support plate, and two lateral anterior hooks. The occipital support was modified so that it mounts

*Sandström Trade & Technology, Inc., Welland, Ontario, Canada.
†Radionics, Inc., Burlington, Massachusetts.
‡Velcro USA, Manchester, New Hampshire.

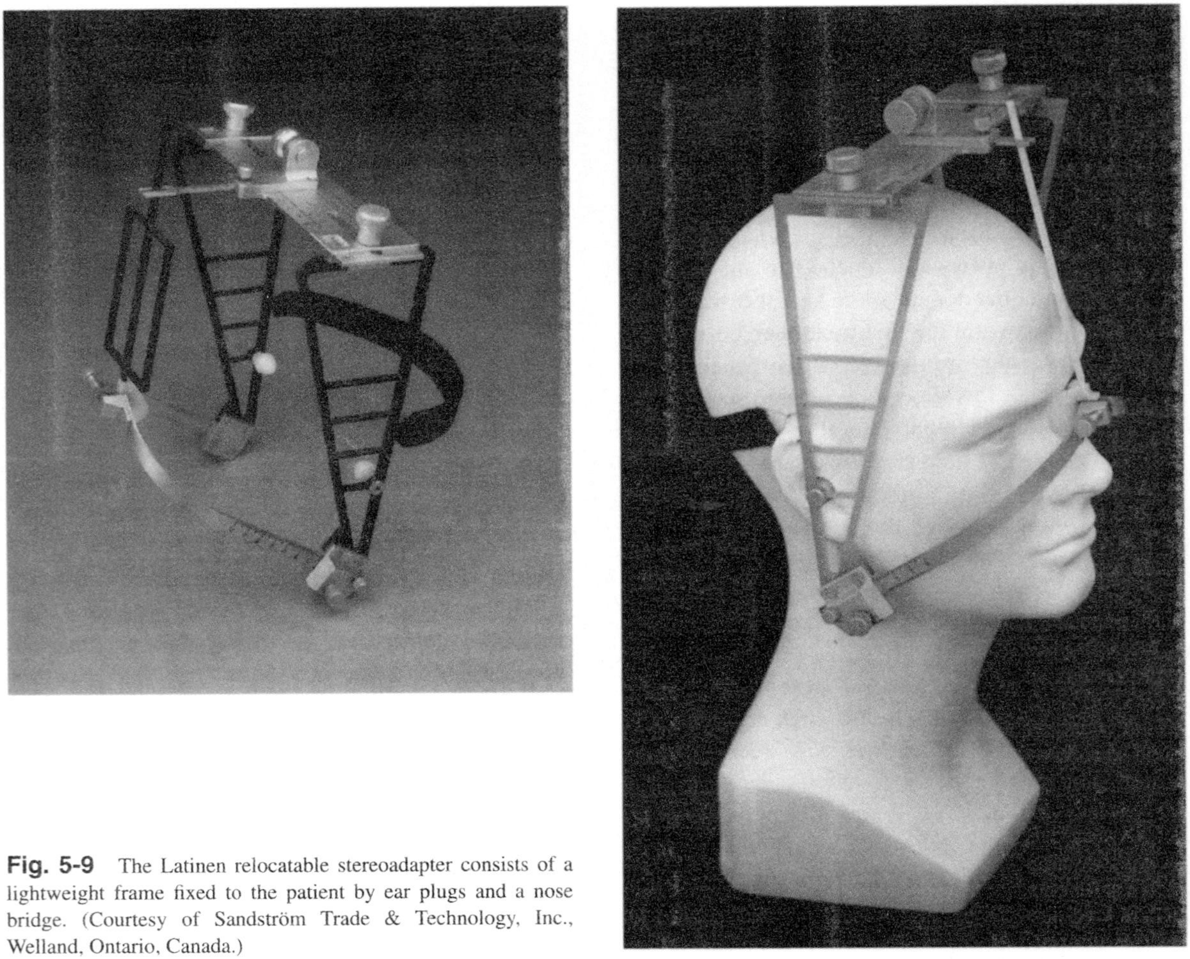

Fig. 5-9 The Latinen relocatable stereoadapter consists of a lightweight frame fixed to the patient by ear plugs and a nose bridge. (Courtesy of Sandström Trade & Technology, Inc., Welland, Ontario, Canada.)

onto two upright bars, which allow the center of the support to be positioned over the occipital protuberance. The bar assembly adapts easily to the particular head size. The oral appliance, made to conform to the upper dentition only, and the ring were designed to form a direct lock by means of internal sliders and locks. These modifications of the Gill-Thomas frame have been incorporated in the commercial version, recognized as the Gill-Thomas-Cosman (GTC) frame.*

*Radionics, Inc., Burlington, Massachusetts.

Most children under the age of 6 years require anesthesia, precluding the use of the oral appliance, which would prevent access to the airways. For these patients, yet another modification has been made consisting of ear canal supports, a premolded occipital support, and a glabellar support constructed from the malleable vinyl material. This modified GTC frame is referred to as the Boston Children's Hospital frame.

A depth-confirmation helmet is used with the GTC frame to confirm the relocatability of the frame for each treatment. The helmet consists of a hemispheric dome, resembling the device used for

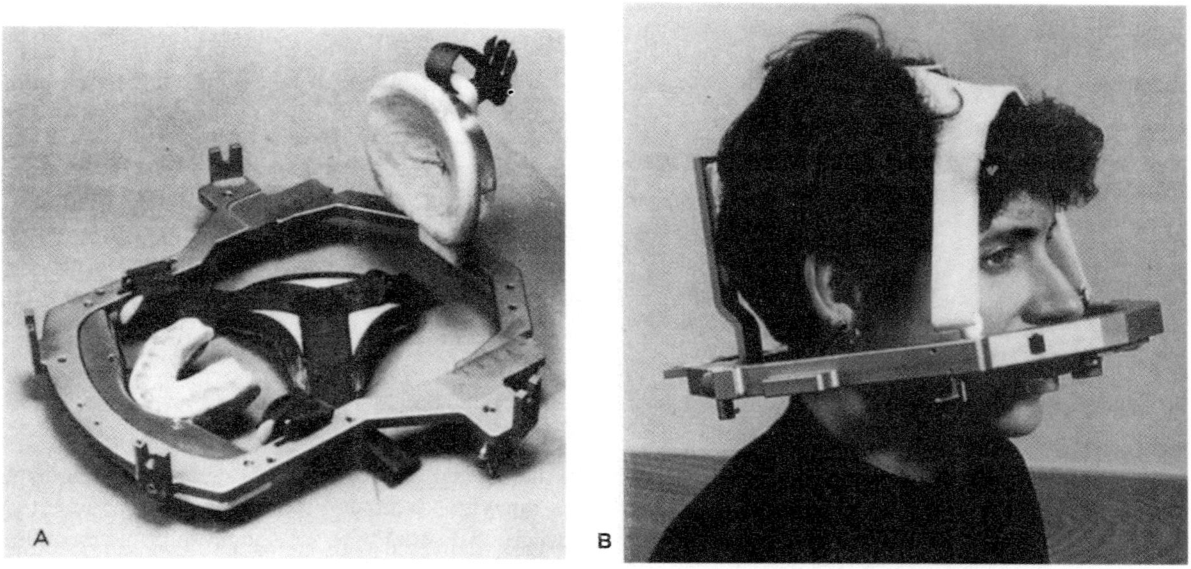

Fig. 5-10 *A*. The Gill-Thomas-Cosman (GTC) stereotactic frame consists of a dental impression and an occipital plate, formed to the posterior surface of the patient's head, and a strap that forces the impressions against the head. (Reprinted from Graham et al.,[35] with permission from Elsevier Science-NL, Amsterdam, Holland.) *B*. A GTC stereotactic frame affixed to a patient's head. (Courtesy of Radionics, Inc., Burlington, Massachusetts.)

Gamma Knife treatment planning, allowing measurement of the distance between the origin of the BRW coordinate system and the cranial surface. The measurements are obtained by insertion of a probe through a large number of holes in the helmet.

Both the modified GTC frame and the Boston Children's Hospital frame demonstrate a repeat repositioning of the frames with respect to the patient's anatomy with a standard deviation of 0.4 mm.[39,46] The GTC frame is not appropriate for single-fraction radiosurgery as a large setup error (>2 mm) for a single treatment cannot be excluded.[39]

In another study, the relocatability of the GTC frame was achieved within 1 mm when alignment lasers were used. When this is combined with a mean GTC frame locatability of 1 mm on the patient, a 2-mm allowance between the prescribed isodose surface and the defined target is recommended as a safety margin.[47]

4. A head fixation system* consisting of a full craniofacial cast custom-made of a self-hardening, low-density material† has also been described (Fig. 5-11). A small opening is left in the mask, under the nose, to facilitate easier breathing. Two L-shaped wooden support brackets (bows), duplicating the geometry of the stereotactic assembly, attach to fixed mounting posts on the casting table in the mold room. While the casting procedure is in progress, the casting strips are wrapped around the bows and then around the mask to affix the mask and the bows firmly together. After the mask hardens, it is cut open along the midcoronal plane, leaving approximately 10 cm uncut across the top of the head. This allows the mask to hinge open for patient

*The F. L. Fisher™ Mask System, Leibinger GmbH, Freiburg, Germany.

†Scotchcast™ Plus, 3M, St. Paul, Minnesota.

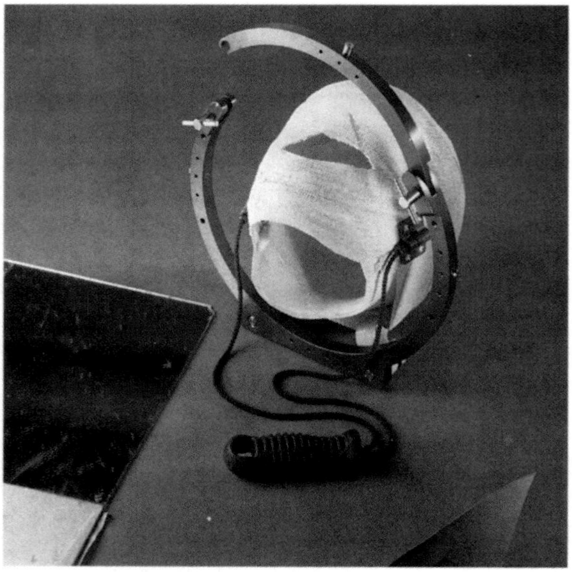

Fig. 5-11 A cranial-facial custom-made cast rigidly affixed to a stereotactic ring. The cast is hinged at the top of the head for patient access. (Courtesy of Howmedica Leibinger Inc., Dallas, Texas.)

access. Plastic hinge clasps are placed on each side of the head and the mask is locked by inserting pins into the hinges. The pins are connected to a string that the patient holds and can pull for quick release in case of an emergency. A modified stereotactic head ring, which is compatible with the SRS accessories, is used to register the marks with the stereotactic coordinate space. The L-shaped bows, which are an integral part of the mask, attach to fixed posts on the posterior aspect of the modified head ring. The anterior portion of the head ring is removable for patient access.

The accuracy of this device was measured in more than 100 setups by placing radiopaque spheres embedded in a custom mouthpiece. The standard deviation of the position of the treated isocenter in stereotactic coordinate space about its mean position was less than 1.4 mm in translation in any direction and less than 1° of rotation about any axis.

5. A similar device, also consisting of a thermoplastic facial mask and a stereotactic frame, that is used for single- or multifraction radiosurgical treatment has been described by Frankel et al.[48]

6. A mask system used for repeat fixation consists of posterior and anterior thermoplastic masks that, when locked together, form a full cranial encasement.* The mask is secured to a horseshoe-shaped noninvasive stereotactic frame which, in turn, is fixed to the end of the treatment couch. Thus, the device with the patient's head extends beyond the couch, allowing more freedom in arranging the beam orientation.

CRANIOSPINAL AXIS

Craniospinal irradiation (CSI) entails the treatment of the whole brain and the spinal axis. Treatment is usually delivered with the patient in prone position, opposed lateral brain fields, and one or two posterior spine fields matched in the spinal cord. Dose inhomogeneities almost always exist near the match lines between these fields. To reduce the magnitude of the dose inhomogeneities, the locations of the field junctions are usually shifted about 0.5 to 1 cm every 10 Gy.[49-51] Inadequate field design and inaccuracies of the setup of this complex field arrangement can result in overdosage in the spinal cord or underdosage in the target—both undesirable.[50,51] Thus, it is particularly important that patients be repositioned accurately and remain relatively motionless during each treatment.

An alternate technique, primarily used in infants and very small children, places the patient prone in a plaster shell with the head turned to the left and right on alternate treatments. A single field is used to treat the entire craniospinal axis, which is irradiated in a single field.[52] This treatment technique is not recommended unless compensators are utilized to provide a uniform dose.

In another technique, the patient is placed in the supine position with the head immobilized in a thermoplastic device similar to that described for head

*BrainLAB Mask System, BrainLAB, GmbH, Heimstetten, Germany.

and neck treatment. The brain and cervical spine are treated via opposed lateral fields and the spinal axis is irradiated by moving the patient (via in-out couch motion) past a stationary posterior treatment field.[53]

POSITION

Craniospinal irradiation most frequently requires that the patient be placed in the prone position, although small children may be treated in the supine position.[53] Treatment in the supine position, using posterior spinal fields, is limited in adult patients by the length of the window in the treatment couch. For most patients, the prone position is less comfortable than the supine; it is therefore less likely to be maintained during a treatment session. Many patients requiring CSI have neurologic deficits, compromising their mobility and their ability to remain motionless for prolonged periods of time. Children often move unintentionally, and if they are uncomfortable, the risk of movement is increased. A comfortable and effective positioning device that offers both adequate repositioning and stabilization may reduce the risk of motion.

IMMOBILIZATION DEVICES

Total-Body Plaster Shell. A total-body plaster shell, used for patients treated in the prone position, is constructed with the patient in the supine position and includes the anterior half of the body from the head to below the knees except for an opening for the mouth, nose, and eyes. The patient is covered by a protective layer of stockinette before the casting material is applied. Since the cast tends to shrink somewhat when it dries, it is recommended that two or three layers of protective stockinette be added around the head. A head cast that is too small may prevent the patient from repositioning his or her head properly in the cast. Prior to making the cast, the chin should be elevated slightly such that the posterior spinal field will not exit in the oral cavity. Too much chin elevation can cause skin folds in the posterior neck and also a more acute curve in the cervical spine. In some patients, a compromise between these effects may be necessary. An estimate of where the field junction between the lateral brain fields and the posterior spinal field will be placed and the approximate divergence of the posterior spinal field is necessary in order to select the optimal head position.

The casting material should be applied such that it covers the front and both sides of the patient's body and extends down to the surface of the couch. The extension of the cast to the couch top is necessary for subsequent leveling of the cast. It is particularly important that the cast be made strong at the junction between the head and torso, since the handling of the cumbersome cast during several weeks of treatment can cause a break between the two portions of the cast. The reproducibility of the head position relative to the torso would then be lost, resulting in difficulties with field matching in the cervical spine. It is also important to make the facial opening such that one can visualize the light field near the eyes during the setup of the lateral brain fields.

When the casting procedure is completed, the cast is carefully lifted off the patient and is then, with the patient removed, returned to the couch in the same position. Supports, or "feet," are then added anterior to the forehead, chest, and thighs (Fig. 5-12) such that when the cast is inverted and placed on its feet for prone treatment, the patient's dorsal surface is approximately horizontal. This is accomplished by first finding the "highest" point on the cast. Then, with the help of a long (~3 ft) piece of wood (or other rigid material) and a water level, the height needed to make the three supports horizontal is determined. By making the three supports (forehead, chest, thighs) such that they form a horizontal line, the patient's posterior surface will be approximately horizontal when the cast is inverted. A plaster cast can be quite heavy; therefore, these supports should be made from pieces of Styrofoam* of the type that is used in the casting of custom blocks. The supports are secured to the cast by strips of plaster. The cast requires approximately 1 h for fabrication (by three persons) and 24 to 48 h for drying at room temperature, but less if it is left outside on a sunny day.

*Dow Chemical, Midland, Michigan.

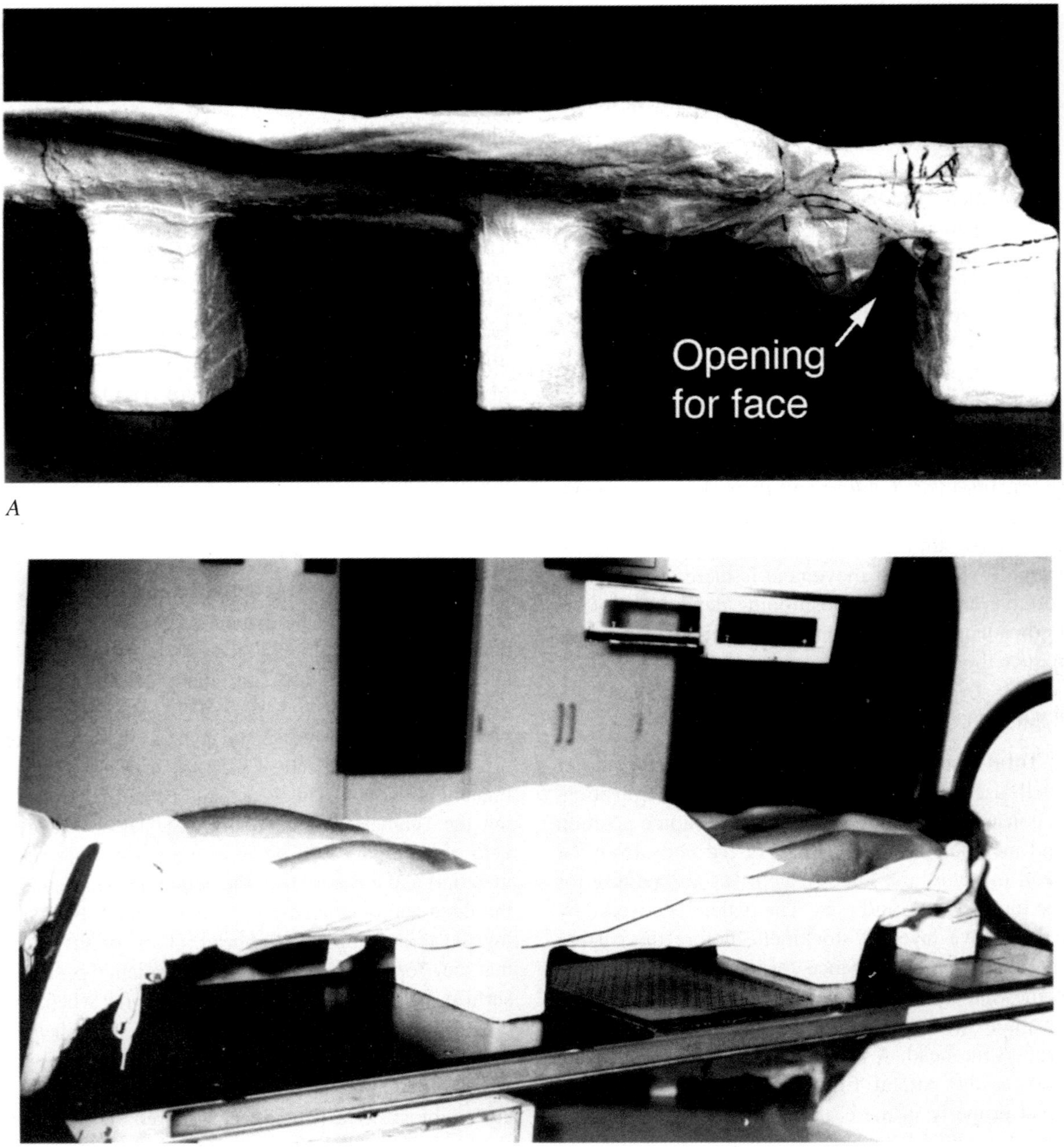

A

B

Fig. 5-12 *A*. Leveling supports added under the forehead, chest, and thighs of an almost full-body cast used for craniospinal irradiation. *B*. When the patient lies down prone in the inverted cast, the dorsal surface is approximately horizontal.

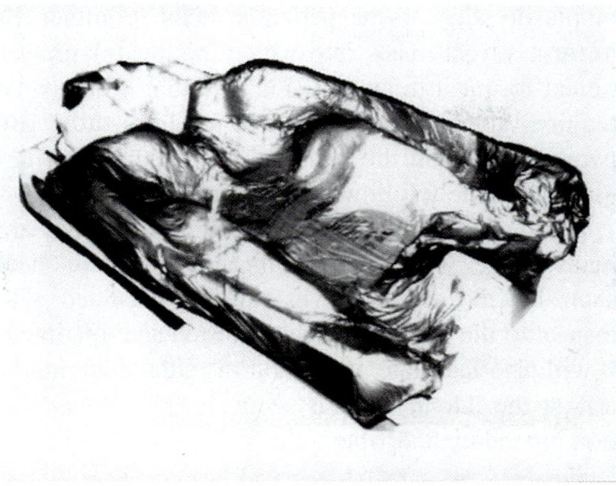

A

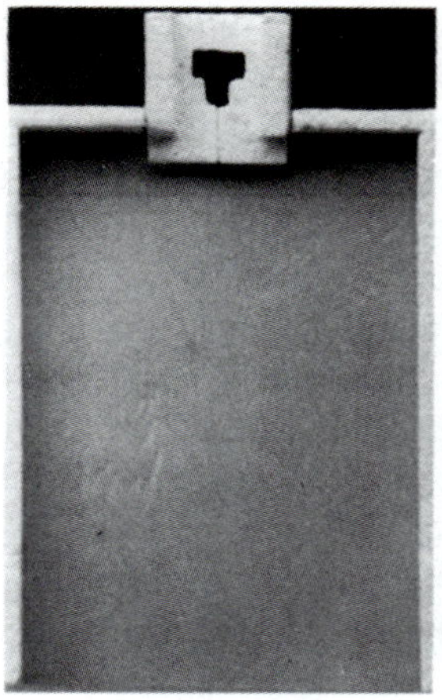

B

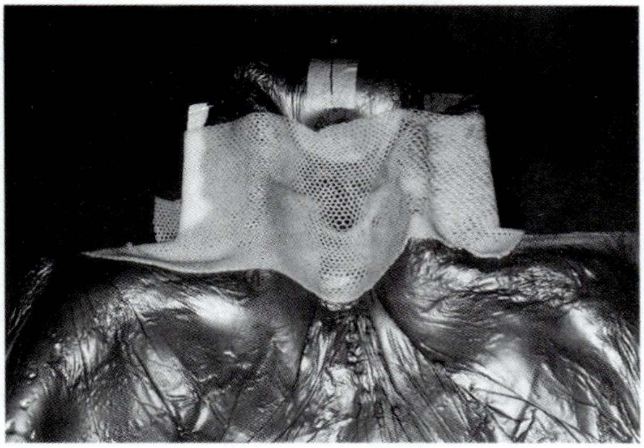

C

Fig. 5-13 *A*. An Alpha Cradle used for craniospinal irradiation. The sagittal setup line is marked on the mold above the head and between the knees. *B*. The mold is made from a shell resembling the shape of the patient's body and with an opening for the face. *C*. A softened thermoplastic sheet is draped across the face opening and is molded to the facial prominences.

Building total-body casts for small children presents special problems because these patients usually require general anesthesia. In them, the head may need to be positioned with the chin elevated to give the anesthesiologist better access to the airways. The facial opening may also need to be larger to facilitate an anesthesia mask. The "leveling" supports under the inverted cast may also need to be higher for an anesthetized child to allow more space for the anesthesiologist to work in.

For some patients, it can be quite difficult to get into and out of the cast. When the cast is placed on the lowered treatment couch, some patients may be able to climb into it from the side, while others may find it easier get into it from the foot-end of the couch. Due to the need for the patients to hold on to and brace themselves on the sides of the cast when getting into it, the cast needs to be very strong.

Total-Body Foam Mold. Patients requiring CSI are often treated on an emergent basis to relieve neurologic symptoms. For them, a device that allows the treatment to begin immediately and makes it easier for patients to get in and out of has also been described. Known as an Alpha Cradle,* it provides stabilization and aids in the repositioning of the head, torso, and thighs (Fig. 5-13*A*).

*Smithers Medical Products, Inc., North Canton, Ohio.

The Alpha Cradle consists of a Styrofoam shell that roughly matches the shape of the patient's head and torso and is covered by a polyvinyl sheet (Fig. 5-13*B*). The polyvinyl sheet covers the entire form and is secured by tape to the back of the Styrofoam shell except at the head portion. In this area, a hole is made in the sheet, leaving an opening for the patient's face. The sheet is then taped such that it forms a tube (channel) around the facial portion of the shell and with an opening on each side of the head. The openings should lead into the torso section of the shell under the polyvinyl sheet. Foaming agents are mixed and prepared as directed by the supplier and are poured into the shell under the polyvinyl sheet and into each opening of the channel surrounding the facial portion. It is important to pour about 30 mL into the channel and then manually guide the foam such that it is evenly distributed inside the channel.

The patient then lies down in the prone position on the polyvinyl sheet. Within a few minutes, the foam begins to expand and fill the space between the patient's body and the Styrofoam shell. The patient's head rests on the channel and the foam expands around the head, leaving an opening for the eyes, nose, and mouth. The diameter of the expanded channel should be about 1 in. If it is too large, the expanding foam may elevate the head too much, causing skin creases in the posterior portion of the neck. The polyvinyl sheet is pulled up between the patient's arms and torso, allowing the foam to expand and form a mold for the arms as well as for the torso. In some patients, it is necessary to elevate the torso so that the head and the torso lie on a horizontal line. This can be accomplished by placing a large piece of Styrofoam of appropriate thickness in the body part of the Styrofoam form prior to taping down the polyvinyl sheet.

Within a few minutes, when the foam has hardened, the patient's head is elevated from the facial support and a softened thermoplastic sheet is placed across the facial opening of the head support. The patient's head is then returned to the original position and, while one staff member ensures that the head is straight and with the chin elevated appropriately, another staff member gently contours the thermoplastic sheet to the patient's facial prominences to form a tight mask, into which the head is repositioned for each treatment (Fig. 5-13*C*). This device requires approximately 30 min for fabrication (by two persons) and the simulation procedure can begin immediately following fabrication.

During the simulation procedure, openings are made in the Styrofoam and the thermoplastic sheet such that the patient's eyes can be visualized with respect to the treatment field prior to each treatment. It will also facilitate placement of radiopaque markers on the lateral canthus, both during the simulation procedure and when port films are obtained.

Vacuum Bag Device. An immobilization system for craniospinal irradiation of pediatric patients in prone position consists of a bag with polystyrene beads and a prone head positioning device* (Fig. 5-14). The bag extends from the shoulders to the feet and is approximately 1 ft wider than the patient's torso. The patient lies prone on the bag and as the bag is molded to the patient's body, the air is removed, creating a firm mold. A thermoplastic mask draped over the posterior portion of the head fixes the head to the head immobilization device. This device facilitates immediate simulation and treatment.

Discussion. Due to the need for matching of several fields in the spinal cord during CSI, it is crucial that the patient's body within the irradiated area is fixed in a rigid fashion. It has also been shown that immobilization of areas away from the irradiated area improves setup reproducibility[54,55]; thus CSI immobilization devices should extend to below the knees. It is particularly important that the relationship between the head and the torso remain constant to assure reproducibility of the field matching in the cervical spine. It is important that the chin elevation remains constant to prevent inadvertent inclusion of the lens of the eyes in the lateral brain fields and also to prevent the posterior spinal field from inadvertently exiting in the oral cavity. The devices described above are designed to meet these objectives.

*MED-TEC, Inc., Orange City, Iowa.

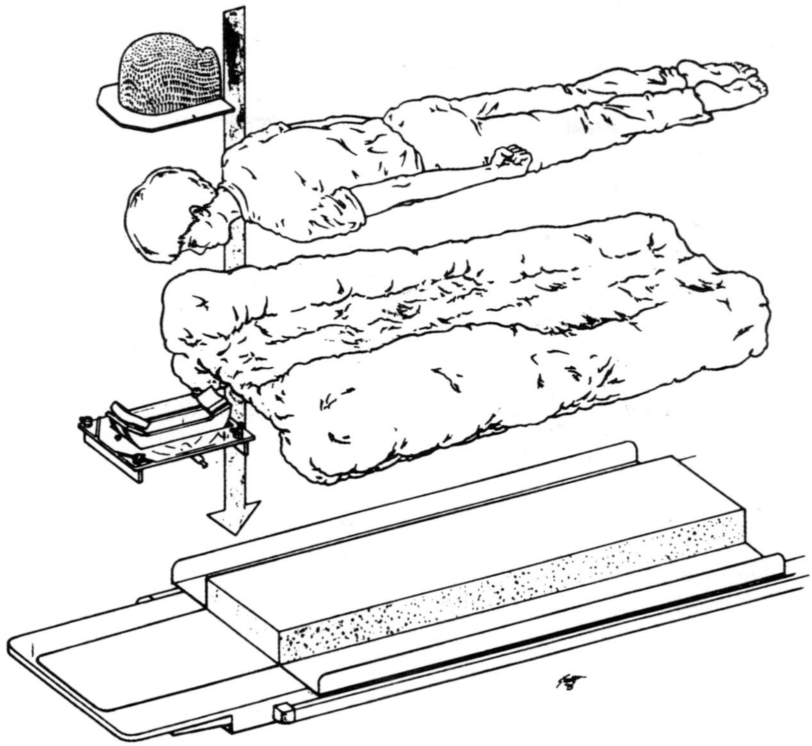

Fig. 5-14 Schematic of vacuum bag immobilization for craniospinal irradiation. (Courtesy of MED-TEC, Inc., Orange City, Iowa.)

The plaster cast requires more time for preparation (thus delaying initiation of the treatment by 1 to 2 days), is more fragile (particularly at the junction between the head and torso sections), more difficult for some patients to get in and out of, and is much heavier (even when dry) than the light foam cradle and vacuum bag. The warm foam in the cradle, on the other hand, causes some patients to feel very warm around the face when the foam inside the channel expands. Both the plaster cast and the foam mold devices become warm during the fabrication.

SPINAL IRRADIATION

Irradiation of part or all of the spinal column or spinal canal is frequently necessary, most commonly due to metastasis. This can be done with the patient in the supine or prone position. Many of these patients have received prior irradiation in the same region and the problem of matching fields arises. Commonly, the previous treatment was delivered with the patient in the supine position and with the arms down by the side of the torso. When the patient returns for spinal irradiation, it is common practice to deliver this treatment via a posterior field; in the lumbar region, an anterior field is sometimes also used. These treatments are commonly delivered with the patient in the prone position, making field matching with previous fields difficult.

Most patients are more comfortable in the supine position, and this position is also easier to reproduce and maintain. Some patients with spinal metastases may not be able to lie prone, and they often prefer to keep their arms raised above the head. Changing of the arm position as well as changing from the supine to the prone position causes shifts of internal organs, increasing the risks of overlaps in previously irradiated areas. Even in patients who have not had previous irradiation, the supine position is probably preferable; with modern technology, it is possible to treat posterior fields with the patient in the more reproducible supine position.

When only a posterior spinal field is to be matched with previous anterior and posterior fields, the optimal field matching is probably accomplished by placing the patient in the same position as during the previous treatment (usually supine). Under fluoroscopic guidance, the previous anterior field is recreated and marked on the patient's skin surface. The appropriate gap needed between the previous and the new field is then calculated (estimating the length of the new field) and is indicated on the anterior skin surface. The new field is then set to this mark, using the desired source-skin distance (SSD). The gantry is turned 180° to the posterior and, after adjusting the SSD, the posterior field is viewed under fluoroscopic guidance to assure no overlap with the previous field in the spinal cord. Small adjustments may be necessary due to possible changes in the length of the new field and so on. To aid in repositioning this new field in the treatment room, the posterior field can be marked on the anterior skin surface after rotating the simulator to the anterior position without changing the SSD, field size, etc. For each treatment, the field is then set to the marks on the anterior skin surface, after which the gantry is turned to the posterior position (SSD, etc., verified) and the field is treated.

EXTRACRANIAL STEREOTACTIC DEVICES

Stereotactic treatment techniques using head frames, described above, are an established clinical practice for irradiation of intracranial lesions. More recently, devices for stereotactic target localization and treatment of tumors in other parts of the body (abdomen, thorax, pelvis) have been developed.[56–58]

An extracranial stereotactic device* has been developed at the Karolinska Hospital in Stockholm (Fig. 5-15). This device, used for multifractional radiation therapy, consists of a rigid box (approximately 50 cm wide, 20 cm deep, and 100 cm long) that can be accommodated through the aperture of most CT scanners. A longitudinal ruler on each side and an arc ruler across the frame are used to reposition the patient and to accurately set up the treatment fields. A customized positioning mold for the patient's torso (supine or prone) is made inside the frame. Reproducible positioning can be achieved by using a marking system on the frame. This consists of a chest marker which is attached to the arc ruler and is used to align two skin marks over the patient's sternum. Skin marks on the lower legs over the tibia are also used to align the patient in the longitudinal direction. The coordinates used for patient positioning can be read on the arc ruler onto which the sternum marker is attached and on the longitudinal ruler on each side of the frame, along which the arc ruler can be moved. The frame has built-in reference indicators for CT or magnetic resonance imaging (MRI) determination of target coordinates. Using these external reference points, the coordinates of the target can be reproducibly localized during treatment setup.

A device, similar to the extracranial stereotactic device described above but accommodating the

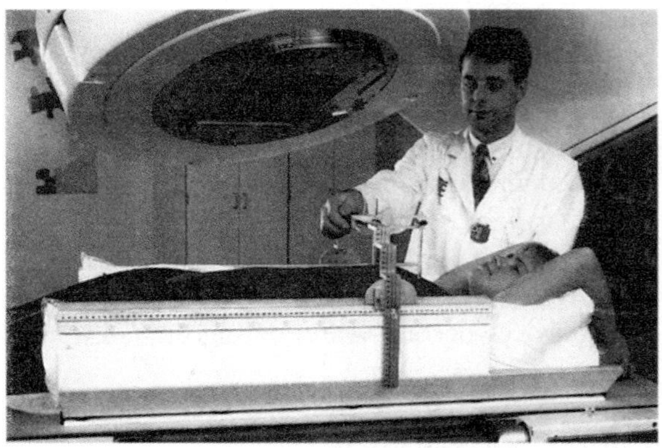

Fig. 5-15 An extracranial stereotactic device used for multifractional radiation therapy in the torso. This device has an external reference system facilitating precise targeting for each treatment. (Courtesy of Precision Therapy International, North Miami Beach, Florida.)

*The Stereotactic Body Frame™, Elekta Instrument AB, Stockholm, Sweden.

whole body, has also been developed at Karolinska Hospital in Stockholm.[59] The design of this frame is based on a unique concept where the alignment is made with the patient in an upright position (Fig. 5-16). The frame is placed vertically at the foot end of the treatment couch. The patient is placed in the frame in an upright position on a base plate and without shoes. After patient positioning and alignment, the frame is slowly tilted backward onto the treatment couch to a recumbent patient position. The frame is then advanced along the tabletop into treatment position via a very thin conveyor-type mat, eliminating the need for technologists having to move the patient into the beam. The center of rotation is approximately at the midbody of most adult patients (84 cm from the floor); thus, there is no sense of falling while the frame is being tilted. The stereotactic system described for the shorter frame can also be used with this whole-body frame. Both of these devices are compatible with CT, MRI, and positron emission tomography (PET) but require an aperture of ≥ 55 cm.

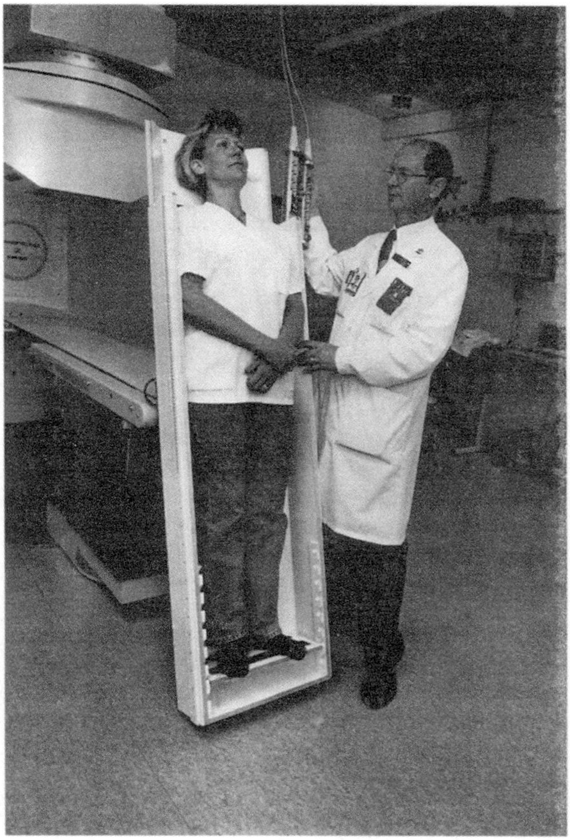

Fig. 5-16 A whole-body stereotactic frame where the patient is aligned in an upright position. The frame is placed at the foot end of the treatment couch; following patient positioning and alignment, it is slowly tilted to a horizontal position over the treatment couch. (Courtesy of Electa Oncology Systems, North Miami Beach, Florida, and of Ingemar Näslund, MD, and Ingmar Lax, PhD, Karolinska Hospital, Stockholm, Sweden.)

Horizontal positioning of these devices on the couch to compensate for sagging of the couch, etc., is achieved by adjusting the amount of air in small balloons under the frames. A Plexiglas plate, attached to the stereotactic frame, can be used to compress the diaphragm to reduce respiratory motion.

Although these extracranial stereotactic devices afford precise target localization, more generous margins may be needed when *extracranial* targets are irradiated due to organ motion (e.g., respiration, bowel motion, etc.).

Another extracranial stereotactic device has been developed at University of Arizona and has been used for single-fraction linear accelerator-based stereotactic radiosurgery of paraspinal neoplastic disease.[57] The device consists of a rigid box (approximately 50 cm wide, 18 cm deep, and 200 cm long), which can be accommodated within the aperture of most CT scanners. The frame also uses two semicircular metal arches that can be rigidly secured anywhere along the length of the device.

The patient is positioned prone inside the stereotactic frame. Clamps are attached to vertebral bodies above and below (cephalad and caudal) the target for both immobilization and localization. The frame is rigidly attached to the clamps during localization and treatment, analogous to the BRW cranial system. The treatment couch is then aligned so that the guide lasers are aligned on the target and the treatment is delivered. When the treatment is completed, the patient is returned to surgery for removal of the clamps.

REFERENCES

1. Das IJ, Cheng CW, Fein DA, et al: Dose estimation to critical organs from vertex field treatment of brain tumors. *Int J Radiat Oncol Biol Phys* 37:1023–1029, 1997.
2. Dong L, Shiu A, Tung S: Verification of radiosurgery target point alignment with an electronic portal imaging device (EPID). *Med Phys* 24:263–267, 1997.
3. Hartmann GH, Bauer-Kirpes B, Serago CF, Lorenz WJ: Precision and accuracy of stereotactic convergent beam irradiations from a linear accelerator. *Int J Radiat Oncol Biol Phys* 28:481–492, 1994.
4. Low DA, Li Z, Dryzmala RE: Minimization of target positioning error in accelerator-based radiosurgery. *Med Phys* 22:443–448, 1995.
5. Serago CF, Lewin AA, Houdek PV, et al: Stereotactic target point verification of an x-ray and CT localizer. *Int J Radiat Oncol Biol Phys* 20:517–523, 1991.
6. Serago CF, Lewin AA, Houdek PV, et al: Radiosurgery target point alignment errors detected with portal film verification. *Int J Radiat Oncol Biol Phys* 24:770–780, 1992.
7. Tsai JS, Buck BA, Svensson GK, et al: Quality assurance in stereotactic radiosurgery using a standard linear accelerator. *Int J Radiat Oncol Biol Phys* 21:737–738, 1991.
8. Yeung D, Palta J, Fontanesi J, Kun L: Systematic analysis of errors in target localization and treatment delivery in stereotactic radiosurgery (SRS). *Int J Radiat Oncol Biol Phys* 28:493–498, 1994.
9. Hamilton RJ, Kuchnir FT, Pelizzari CA, et al: Repositioning accuracy of a noninvasive head fixation system for stereotactic radiotherapy. *Med Phys* 23:1909–1917, 1996.
10. Lutz W, Winston KR, Maleki N: A system for stereotactic radiosurgery with a linear accelerator. *Int J Radiat Oncol Biol Phys* 14:373, 1988.
11. Phillips MH, Frankel KA, Lyman JT, et al: Comparison of different radiation types and irradiation geometries in stereotactic radiosurgery. *Int J Radiat Oncol Biol Phys* 18:211, 1990.
12. Saunders WM, Winston KR, Siddon RL, et al: Radiosurgery for arteriovenous malformations of the brain using a standard linear accelerator: Rationale and technique. *Int J Radiat Oncol Biol Phys* 15:441–447, 1988.
13. Maitz AH, Wu A, Lunsford LD, et al: Quality assurance for Gamma Knife stereotactic radiosurgery. *Int J Radiat Oncol Biol Phys* 32:1465–1471, 1995.
14. Becker G, Kortmann R, Kaulich TW, et al: Gamma Knife versus stereotactic linear accelerator: Utilization, clinical results and cost-benefit relations. *Radiologe* 36:345–353, 1996.
15. Maitz AH, Lunsford LD, Wu A, et al: Shielding requirements on-site loading and acceptance testing of the Leksell Gamma Knife. *Int J Radiat Oncol Biol Phys* 18:469–476, 1990.
16. Leksell L: A stereotactic apparatus for intracerebral surgery. *Acta Chir Scand* 99:229, 1949.
17. Leksell L: The stereotaxic method and radiosurgery of the brain. *Acta Chir Scand* 102:316, 1951.
18. Colombo F, Benedetti A, Pozza F, et al: Linear accelerator radiosurgery of cerebral arteriovenous malformations. *J Neurosurg* 24:833–840, 1989.
19. Engenhart R, Wowra B, Debus J, et al: The role of high-dose, single-fraction irradiation in small and large intracranial arteriovenous malformations. *Int J Radiat Oncol Biol Phys* 30:521–529, 1994.
20. Larson DA, Flickinger JC, Loeffler JS: The radiobiology of radiosurgery. *Int J Radiat Oncol Biol Phys* 25:557–561, 1993.
21. Loeffler JS, Alexander E, Siddon R, et al: Stereotactic radiosurgery for intracranial arteriovenous malformations using a standard linear accelerator. *Int J Radiat Oncol Biol Phys* 17:673–677, 1989.
22. Brown RA, Roberts TS, Osborn AG: A simplified CT-guided stereotaxic biopsy. *Am J Neurol Radiol* 2: 181–184, 1981.
23. Adler JR, Cox RS: Preliminary clinical experience with the Cyberknife: Image-guided stereotactic radiosurgery, in Alexander E, Kondziolka D, Loeffler JS (eds): *Radiosurgery.* Basel: Karger, 1996.
24. Murphy MJ, Cox RS: The accuracy of dose localization for an image-guided frameless radiosurgery system. *Med Phys* 23:2043–2049, 1996.
25. Murphy MJ: An automatic six-degree-of-freedom image registration algorithm for image-guided frameless stereotaxic radiosurgery. *Med Phys* 24:857–866, 1997.
26. Marks LB, Sherouse GW, Das S, et al: Conformal radiation therapy with fixed shaped coplanar or noncoplanar radiation beam bouquets: A possible alternative to radiosurgery. *Int J Radiat Oncol Biol Phys* 33:1209–1219, 1995.
27. Schwade JG, Houdek PV, Landy HJ, et al: Small-field stereotactic external-beam radiation therapy of intracranial lesions: Fractionated treatment with a fixed-halo immobilization device. *Radiology* 176:563–565, 1990.
28. Clark BG, Podgorsak EB, Souhami L, et al: A halo-ring technique for fractionated stereotactic radiotherapy. *Br J Radiol* 66:522–527, 1993.
29. Olivier A, Sadikot AF, Villemure JG, et al: Fractionated stereotactic radiotherapy for intracranial neoplasms. *Stereotact Funct Neurosurg* 59:193–198, 1992.
30. Souhami L, Olivier A, Podgorsak EB, et al: Fractionated stereotactic radiation therapy for intracranial tumors. *Cancer* 68:2101–2108, 1991.
31. Podgorsak EB, Souhami L, Caron JL, et al: A technique

for fractionated stereotactic radiotherapy in the treatment of intracranial tumors. *Int J Radiat Oncol Biol Phys* 27:1225–1230, 1993.

32. Gill SS, Thomas DGT, Warrington AP, Brada M: Relocatable frame for stereotactic external beam therapy. *Int J Radiat Oncol Biol Phys* 20:599–603, 1991.
33. Delannes M, Daly NJ, Bonnet J, et al: Fractionated radiotherapy of small inoperable lesions of the brain using a non-invasive stereotactic frame. *Int J Radiat Oncol Biol Phys* 21:749, 1991.
34. Gademann G, Schlegel W, Debus J, et al: Fractionated stereotactically guided radiotherapy of head and neck tumors: A report on clinical use of a new system in 195 cases. *Radiother Oncol* 29:205–213, 1993.
35. Graham JD, Warrington AP, Gill SS, Brada M: A non-invasive, relocatable stereotactic frame for fractionated radiotherapy and multiple imaging. *Radiother Oncol* 21:60–62, 1991.
36. Hariz MA, Fodstad H: Stereotactic localization of small subcortical brain tumors for open surgery. *Surg Neurol* 26:345–350, 1986.
37. Hariz MI, Henriksson R, Lofroth P, et al: A noninvasive method for fractionated stereotactic irradiation of brain tumors with a linear accelerator. *Radiother Oncol* 17:57–72, 1990.
38. Havelka C, Nelson LP, Shusterman S, Bellerive M: Custom oral appliance for noninvasive immobilization during stereotactic radiotherapy. *Pediatr Dent* 17:212–215, 1995.
39. Kooy HM, Dunbar SF, Tarbell NJ, et al: Adaptation and verification of the relocatable Gill-Thomas-Cosman frame in stereotactic radiotherapy. *Int J Radiat Oncol Biol Phys* 30:685–691, 1994.
40. Laing RW, Thompson V, Warrington AP, Brada M: Feasibility of patient immobilization for conventional cranial irradiation with a relocatable stereotactic frame. *Br J Radiol* 66:1020–1024, 1993.
41. Latinen LV, Liliequist B, Fagerland M, Eriksson AT: An adapter for computer tomography-guided stereotaxis. *Surg Neurol* 23:559–566, 1985.
42. Rosenthal SJ, Gall KP, Jackson M, Thornton AFJ: A precision cranial immobilization system for conformal stereotactic fractionated radiation therapy. *Int J Radiat Oncol Biol Phys* 33:1239–1245, 1995.
43. Schlegel W, Pastyr O, Bortfeld T, et al: Stereotactically guided fractionated radiotherapy: Technical aspects. *Radiother Oncol* 29:197–204, 1993.
44. Schlegel W, Pastyr O, Bortfeld T, et al: Computer systems and mechanical tools for stereotactically guided conformation therapy with linear accelerators. *Int J Radiat Oncol Biol Phys* 24:781–787, 1992.
45. Shrieve DC, Tarbell NJ, Alexander ER, et al: Stereotactic radiotherapy: A technique for dose optimization and escalation for intracranial tumors. *Acta Neurochir* suppl 62: 118–123, 1994.
46. Dunbar SF, Tarbell NJ, Kooy HM, et al: Stereotactic radiotherapy for pediatric and adult brain tumors: Preliminary report. *Int J Radiat Oncol Biol Phys* 30:531–539, 1994.
47. Warrington AP, Laing RW, Brada M: Quality assurance in fractionated stereotactic radiotherapy. *Radiother Oncol* 30:239–246, 1994.
48. Frankel KA, Levy RP, Fabrikant JI, Phillips MH: Heavy-charged-particle radiosurgery: Rationale and method, in Alexander E III, Loeffler JS, Lunsford LD (eds): *Stereotactic Radiosurgery*. New York: McGraw-Hill, 1993.
49. Bentel GC, Halperin EC: High dose areas are unintentionally created as a result of gap shifts when the prescribed doses in the two adjacent areas are different. *Med Dosim* 15:179, 1990.
50. Halperin EC: Impact of radiation technique upon the outcome of treatment for medulloblastoma. *Int J Radiat Oncol Biol Phys* 36:233–239, 1996.
51. Probst H, Griffiths S: Increasing the work speed of radiographers: The effect on the accuracy of a set-up of a complex shaped cranial field, part of a matched craniospinal junction. *Radiother Oncol* 38:241–245, 1996.
52. Glasgow GP, Marks JE: The dosimetry of a single "hockey stick" portal for treatment of tumors of the cranio-spinal axis. *Med Phys* 10:672, 1983.
53. Wara WM, Le QTX, Sneed PK, et al: Pattern of recurrence of medulloblastoma after low-dose craniospinal radiotherapy. *Int J Radiat Oncol Biol Phys* 30:551–556, 1994.
54. Bentel GC, Marks LB, Sherouse GW, et al: The effectiveness of immobilization during prostate irradiation. *Int J Radiat Oncol Biol Phys* 31:143–148, 1995.
55. Bentel GC, Marks LB, Krishnamurthy R, Prosnitz LR: Comparison of two repositioning devices used during radiation therapy for Hodgkin's disease. *Int J Radiat Oncol Biol Phys* 39:791–795, 1997.
56. Blomgren H, Lax I, Näslund I, Svanström R: Stereotactic high dose fraction radiation therapy of extracranial tumors using an accelerator: Clinical experience of the first thirty-one patients. *Acta Oncol* 34:861–870, 1995.
57. Hamilton AJ, Lulu BA, Fosmire H, et al: Preliminary clinical experience with linear accelerator-based spinal stereotactic radiosurgery. *Neurosurgery* 36:311–319, 1995.
58. Lax I, Blomgren H, Näslund I, Svanström R: Stereotactic radiotherapy of malignancies in the abdomen. *Acta Oncol* 33:677–683, 1994.
59. Näslund I, Lax I, Blomgren H, et al: New prostate repositioning paradigm—a whole body frame for conformal radiotherapy techniques, with vertical patient alignment and rotation to a horizontal position (abstr). *Int J Radiat Oncol Biol Phys* 39(suppl 2):328, 1997.

PROBLEMS

5-1 Patients treated for brain tumors are most commonly positioned
- (*a*) supine with the head flexed (forward)
- (*b*) prone with the head flexed
- (*c*) supine with the head in neutral position
- (*d*) supine with the chin extended

5-2 With the patient's head in the neutral position, the skull base lies at approximately
- (*a*) 20° off a vertical line
- (*b*) parallel with a vertical line
- (*c*) 20° off a horizontal line
- (*d*) parallel with a horizontal line

5-3 Organ motion in the brain
- (*a*) is of great concern because the margins are often small
- (*b*) is of little concern because the brain lies relatively fixed within the cranium
- (*c*) should be compensated for by increasing target margins
- (*d*) none of the above

5-4 Setup marks for brain fields
- (*a*) should always be made on the immobilization mask
- (*b*) are sometimes made on the scalp, where they are difficult to visualize and they tend to smear
- (*c*) should be made after the hair is shaved off
- (*d*) are very reliable because the patient's head is rigidly fixed

5-5 In single-fraction stereotactic radiosurgery
- (*a*) the target margins are generally large, since this is the only treatment and missing the target could be fatal
- (*b*) the target margins are generous, allowing room for setup errors and organ motion
- (*c*) the treatment fields are conformed to the shape of the target with a margin of 1 cm
- (*d*) the treatment is generally delivered without target margins

5-6 Target margins are generally
- (*a*) larger when the setup is less reproducible
- (*b*) smaller when a high-dose single-fraction treatment is delivered
- (*c*) based on ability to reproduce the treatment setup
- (*d*) all of the above

5-7 Craniospinal irradiation is usually delivered with the patient
- (*a*) supine with the chin extended
- (*b*) prone with the arms raised above the head
- (*c*) prone with the arms along the sides and the chin extended to avoid posterior beam exit in the mouth
- (*d*) all of the above

5-8 Comparing a plaster of paris craniospinal cast and a polyurethane mold, the cast
- (*a*) is heavier and breaks more easily

(*b*) takes longer to make and to dry
(*c*) delays initiation of therapy by a couple of days
(*d*) all of the above

5-9 A posterior spinal field used in treating metastatic disease adjacent to previously irradiated fields
(*a*) is less likely to cause overlap in the spine if it is treated with the patient in the same position as the previous fields (assuming that the gap is calculated and set correctly)
(*b*) is less likely to cause overlap in the spine if it is treated with the patient in prone position
(*c*) makes the patient's position irrelevant
(*d*) will overlap in the spine if it is treated with the patient in the same position as the previous fields

5-10 In treating brain tumors
(*a*) the patient's head position can be neutral and the beam direction achieved by compound couch, gantry, and collimator angles
(*b*) very large doses ($>$ 1000 cGy) can be delivered in a single fraction if the treatment field is very small ($<$ 5 cm in diameter)
(*c*) a stereotactic frame is sometimes screwed onto the head
(*d*) all of the above

CHAPTER

6

Thorax and Upper Abdomen

INTRODUCTION

Positioning and immobilization of patients receiving radiation therapy to the thorax and to the upper abdomen are similar and are therefore described together. Positioning and immobilization for patients with Hodgkin's disease and breast cancer are described in Chaps. 7 and 8, respectively. Tumors irradiated in the thorax include carcinoma of the esophagus, thymoma, germ cell tumors, lymphoma, metastatic disease, and, most commonly, lung cancer. Malignant tumors irradiated in the upper abdomen include carcinoma of the pancreas, gastric and hepatobiliary tumors, colon cancer, lymphoma, Wilms' tumor, and neuroblastoma. There are several tumors occurring in the pelvis (Chap. 9) that require irradiation of paraaortic lymph nodes or the whole abdomen, including seminoma and some gynecologic malignancies. Positioning and immobilization for patients undergoing irradiation for these tumors are discussed in Chap. 9.

Frequently, tumors in the thorax and the upper abdomen are initially irradiated via opposed anterior/posterior fields that may include critical normal structures (e.g., spinal cord, lungs, heart, esophagus, kidneys, liver, and bowel). When the radiation dose reaches the "tolerance" level of a particular organ, beams are adjusted (e.g., field size reduced or orientation changed) to exclude all (e.g., spinal cord) or most (e.g., lungs, liver, kidneys) of the organ. Alternatively, patients may be treated with multiple fields (e.g., anterior/posterior and obliques) throughout treatment. Reduced fields, usually referred to as *boost fields*, are often designed with small target margins and with beam edges close to critical normal tissues (Fig. 6-1). In all of these situations, patient repositioning and the patient's ability to maintain the position are crucial and may be improved by the use of an immobilization device.

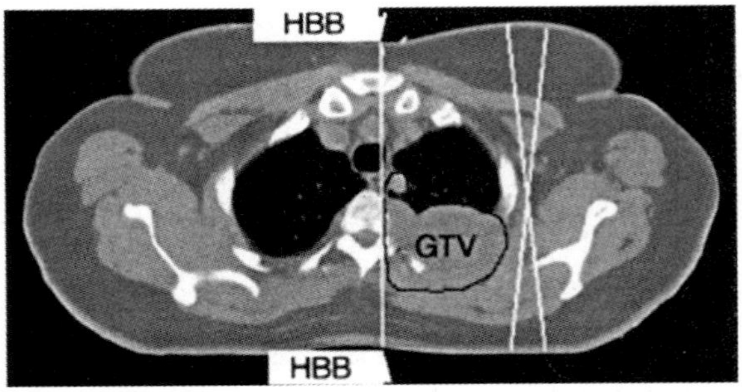

Fig. 6-1 Boost treatment fields are often designed with small target margins and with beam edges close to critical normal tissues, here illustrated by an extreme case. In these situations, patient repositioning and the patient's ability to maintain the position are crucial.

PATIENT POSITION

SUPINE VERSUS PRONE—ORGAN MOTION

In the majority of patients irradiated to the thorax or upper abdomen, the supine position is preferred, since it is usually more comfortable and reproducible than the prone position.[1,2] When prone, the head is usually turned and rests on the raised upper extremities. The prone position may be difficult to reproduce without a positioning aid (Fig. 6-2).

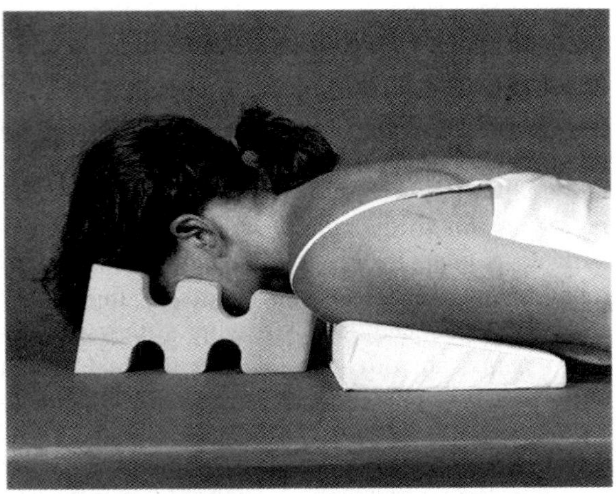

Fig. 6-2 A typical head support for the prone position with an opening for the nose and mouth facilitating respiration and a comfortable straight head position. (Courtesy of van Arsdale Innovative Products, Inc., Pensacola, Florida.)

Gravitational shifts of intrathoracic structures frequently occur when the patient's position is changed from supine to prone or vice versa. In a computed tomography (CT) study of position-induced organ motion, a ventral shift of hilar structures occurred in 36 of 38 patients when the position was changed from supine to prone, and the heart and great vessels shifted ventrally in all patients.[3] Within the upper abdomen, the prone position produced ventral and caudal shifts of both the liver and spleen in 34 of 38 patients. In all patients, a ventral and caudal shift of the kidney position was noted.[3] A ventral shift of the esophagus, increasing the distance between the spinal cord and the esophagus, may also occur in the prone position. The prone position may therefore be useful to facilitate delivery of radiation to an esophageal tumor while respecting spinal cord tolerance.[4,5] However, the gains from the small increase in distance may be compromised by the inferior repositioning capabilities and the patient's inability to maintain the position during the treatment. In the era of linear accelerators with small penumbras, customized beam shaping, and three-dimensional treatment planning (3DTP), the need for increased spinal cord distance is often not an issue.

Respiration-induced movement of intrathoracic and intraabdominal structures makes treatment of these areas challenging.[6,7] Field borders, e.g., margins, need to reflect organ motion.

It is important to recognize that both the target and normal tissues are mobile. Thus, as the target moves *out* of the field, normal tissues are moving *into* the field. Lung tumors, unlike tumors in the upper abdomen, are often visible on fluoroscopy and thus margins can be determined following observation of the magnitude and direction of the target motion during simulation. Making the field margins more generous to avoid underdosage in the target causes a larger volume of normal tissue to be irradiated; therefore, each situation should be evaluated individually.

ARM POSITION

Initial anterior/posterior fields are usually marked on the anterior chest, with the patient in the supine position and the arms along the sides of the torso. Boost fields, often utilized when spinal cord tolerance dose has been reached, are usually delivered via oblique or lateral fields with the patient's arms elevated above the head. This change in arm position typically causes the initial skin marks to shift 1 to 2 cm cephalad in the average patient. Internal organ shifts, such as changes in the curvature of the spine, may also occur as a result of changes in the arm position; however, this is more difficult to assess. In order to avoid discrepancies that might arise due to changes in arm position during treatment, the raised-arm position in an immobilization device can be implemented from the very beginning of radiation therapy.

HEAD POSITION

In patients requiring irradiation of the supraclavicular lymph nodes, or when the primary lesion lies in the lung apex, it may be necessary to extend the neck (typically by lowering the head support) to avoid inclusion of the chin. This is particularly important for a posterior field since its cephalad margin exits farther cranial than the entrance point of the anterior field (Fig. 6-3). Conversely, if the field extends into the upper neck, extension of the neck increases the volume of brain (posterior fossa) in the exit portion of the anterior field. Thus, each case must be considered separately.

In patients with severe kyphosis and patients with shortness of breath, it may be necessary to use a small tilt of the chest and a generous head support (Fig. 6-4). When the chest is elevated, it may be necessary to turn the couch 90° and rotate the gantry until the anterior/posterior fields are perpendicular to the chest.

PATIENT IMMOBILIZATION

Without a positioning device, alignment marks are limited to skin that might be mobile and thus marks are unreliable. In the chest and upper abdomen, skin marks also shift with the arm position. Thus, a customized positioning device on which alignment marks can be made and which improves repositioning of the chest/upper abdomen plus the upper extremities is desired.[8]

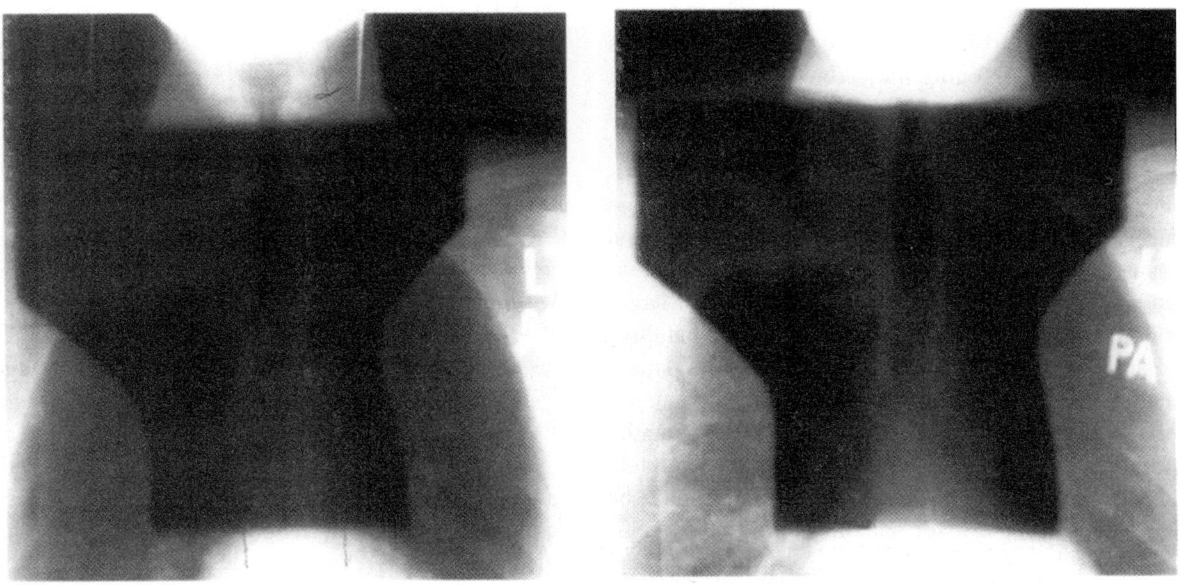

Fig. 6-3 The cephalad margin of a posterior lung field exits farther cranial, e.g., closer to the chin (*right*), than the entrance point of the anterior field (*left*).

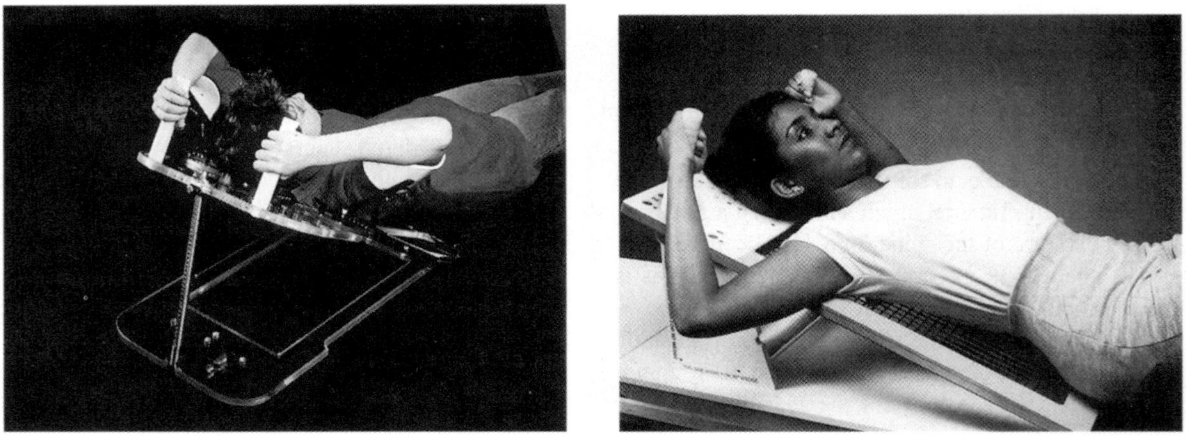

A *B*

Fig. 6-4 *A* and *B*. Two types of tilt boards used for patients requiring chest elevation. (Courtesy of MED-TEC, Inc., Orange City, Iowa.)

IMMOBILIZATION DEVICES

Immobilization devices for the thorax and upper abdomen have not been widely described and are not generally available commercially. This may be because many tumors in this area have traditionally been treated with generous margins, often due to respiratory motion and uncertainty of tumor extent; hence precise positioning has been considered less critical. This reasoning may, however, be flawed. It is important to recognize that the immobilization device is not intended to address the issues of organ motion and tumor extent. Failure to provide repositioning aids increases treatment uncertainties and necessitates larger field margins above and beyond what might be required due to organ motion and tumor extension. The clinical implications of a larger margin need to be considered in deciding what type, if any, of immobilization system to use. In a patient being treated palliatively for a central lung tumor, the treating physician often judges that the potential morbidity of a large field margin is minimal and that therefore an immobilization device may not be needed. Conversely, for patients being treated curatively in the modern era of improved imaging and three-dimensional treatment planning, margins are often tighter, making accurate patient repositioning important. Repositioning aids for patients undergoing radiation therapy to the thorax and upper abdomen are described below.

Simple Positioning Aids. A few simple devices that usually make patients more comfortable should be considered in almost all patients. For example, patients lying supine on a hard couch usually experience strain on the lower back. This can be eased by placing a pillow (foam rubber or regular bed pillow) under the patient's knees (Fig. 6-5*A*). Treatment couches are intentionally made narrow to prevent couch/gantry collisions and thus often cannot support the patient's arms. This can be addressed by placing a piece of Plexiglas under the chest that extends laterally beyond the couch to support the arms (Fig. 6-5*B*). The needed width of this support varies with patient size. Alternatively, a smaller support can be placed under each arm. However, this may be less reproducible than a single support (Fig. 6-5*A*).

Raised-Arm and Head Supports. The raised-arm position can be supported by a simple device consisting of a Plexiglas base plate with two hand grips (Fig. 6-6*A*). In some designs, there are also "wings" that support the arms as well as an indentation for a standard head support (Fig. 6-6*B*).

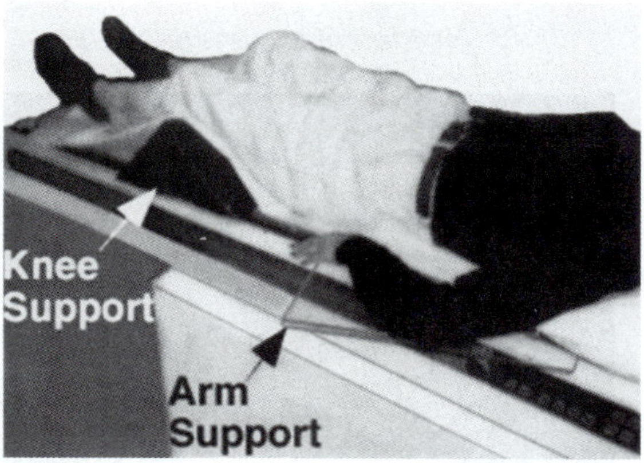

A

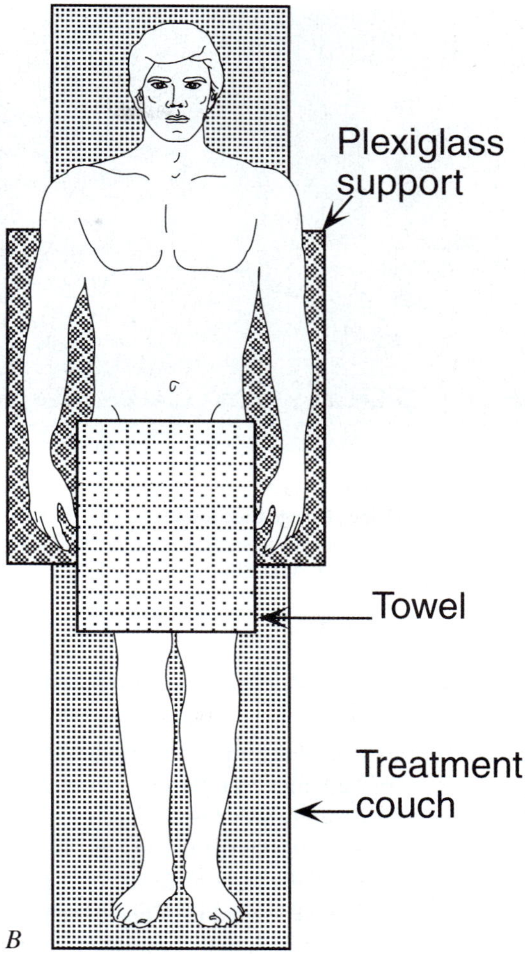

B

Fig. 6-5 *A*. Patients are generally more comfortable with a pillow placed under the bent knees when lying on a hard surface. When the couch is not sufficiently wide to support the arms, a piece of Plexiglas can be placed under each arm. The supports are secured by extending them under the chest. *B*. A more reproducible and symmetrical method of supporting the arms may be to use one large piece of Plexiglas under the patient's chest and arms.

Positioning Mold. When more accurate repositioning is desired, more extensive immobilization may be necessary. At Duke University Medical Center, all patients irradiated in the thorax and upper abdomen and whose treatment is planned using a 3DTP system, are immobilized in an Alpha Cradle™* extending from above the head to the knees (Fig. 6-7). A similar device is often used to aid in the repositioning of many other patients not having 3DTP where the target margins are small or it is crucial to avoid adjacent normal tissues (e.g., seminoma, pancreas, whole abdomen).

The immobilization device consists of foaming chemicals with several pieces of Styrofoam† that make the device sturdy and aid in containing the foam adjacent to the patient. The Styrofoam pieces are a base plate (approximately 60 in. long, 36 in. wide, and 1 in. thick), and three pieces (approximately 6 in. high and 1 in. thick) that are fastened to the base plate on each side and above the head of the patient such that they form a barrier for the chemicals (Fig. 6-8). The length of these pieces should approximate the dimensions of the base plate. A small piece of Styrofoam (approximately

*Smithers Medical Products, Inc., North Canton, Ohio.

†Dow Chemical, Midland, Michigan.

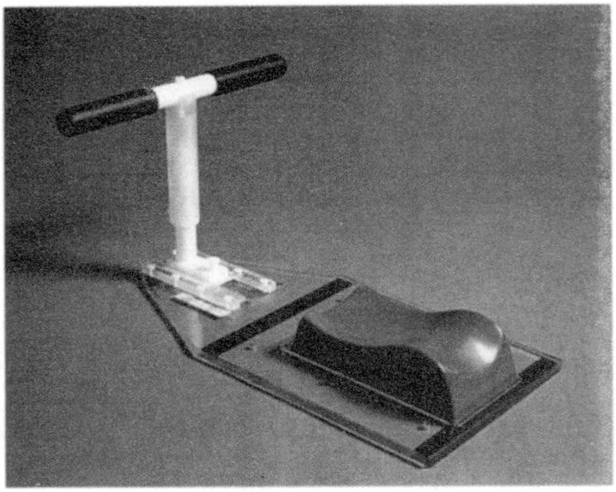

A

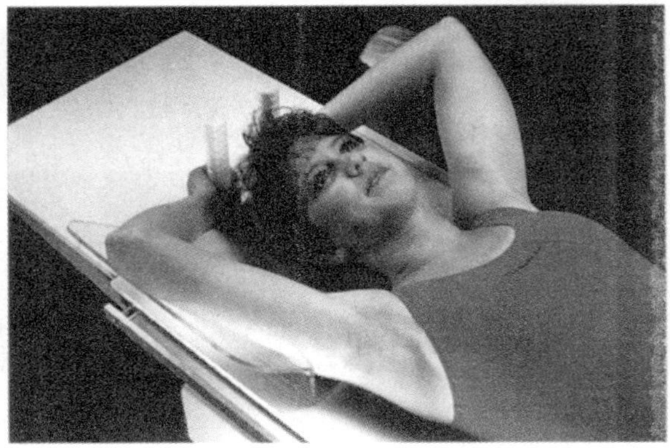

B

Fig. 6-6 *A*. A device to support the raised-arm position. This device also has an indentation in the base plate for precise repositioning of the head support. *B*. A similar device with "wings" supporting the arms. (Courtesy of MED-TEC, Inc., Orange City, Iowa.)

1 × 1 × 4 in.) is fastened to the base plate between the patient's knees to form an elevation on which alignment marks are later made. Optionally, small pieces can be placed under the knees to form an elevation for patient comfort.

The position of these Styrofoam pieces is determined and marked on the base plate with the patient in treatment position. The goal is to place the retaining walls as close to the patient as possible to help contain the chemicals close to the torso. With the patient removed, each Styrofoam piece is fastened, using adhesive tape, to the base plate. The excess width of the base plate is trimmed off to minimize the width of the finished mold. The trimmed-off Styrofoam, broken into smaller pieces, can be used to fill empty spaces on each side of the patient's head and under the raised arms. This will reduce the amount of chemicals needed to fill the spaces between the patient and the barriers. The entire Styrofoam shell is placed inside a polyvinyl bag approximately 2 ft wider and 2 ft longer than the shell. Approximately 600 to 900 mL of the foaming agents is mixed as directed by the manufacturer and poured evenly in the prepared shell inside the plastic bag. In general, the smaller amount of chemical is used for large patients, since they usually leave less space for the foam. Air is allowed to circulate inside the bag for a few seconds, following which excess air is squeezed out and the bag is securely sealed.

Immediately after sealing the bag, the mold is placed at the foot end of the couch. The patient, usually undressed above the waist and in a hospital gown, is positioned in the shell by first standing on a stepping stool at the end of the couch and then sitting down into the mold. The mold with the patient in it is then moved to the center of the couch and the patient assumes a supine position and elevates the arms above the head. The hospital gown is pulled up from under the patient such that the patient lies directly on the polyvinyl bag. It is important to make sure that the patient feels that he or she is lying flat and straight. A visual registration of the patient's straightness should also be made by the staff. (This can also be done with fluoroscopy if available). The polyvinyl bag is pulled up between the patient's knees to allow the foam to expand and form an elevation for making a sagittal alignment mark. The height of this elevation should be decided with the patient's agility in mind, since some patients may need to lift themselves over it on entering and leaving the mold.

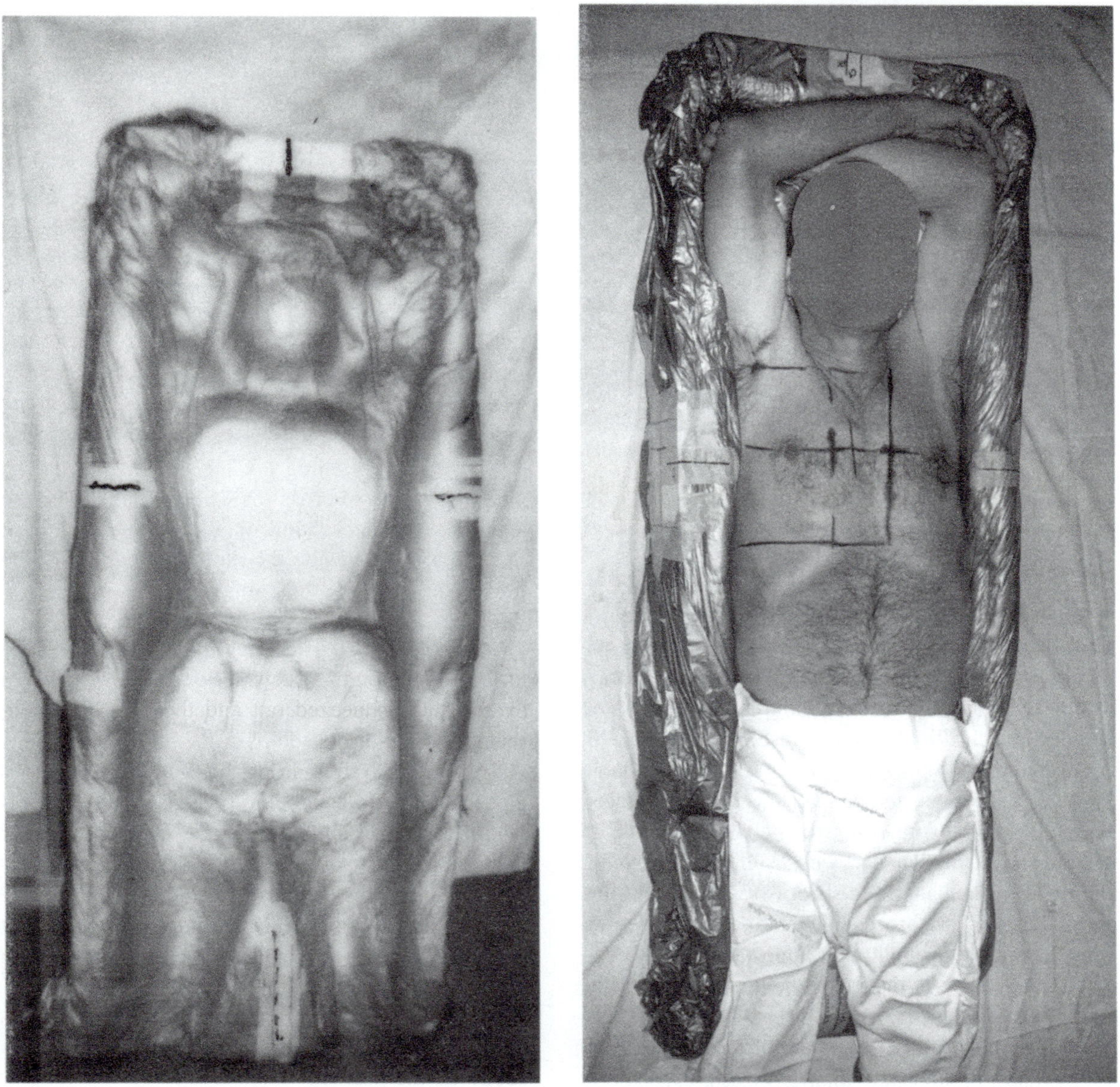

A *B*

Fig. 6-7 *A* and *B*. A positioning mold extending from above the head to the knees. Setup marks are made both on the patient and on the immobilization device. The sagittal alignment line is marked on the mold above the head and between the knees and the transverse line on each side of the patient's chest.

Since the foam is light and tends to expand in the direction of least resistance, it is often necessary to guide it up around the patient's head and arms such that it closely follows the patient's outline. Since the expanding foam tends to displace the side barriers away from the patient, an adhesive tape is stretched across the torso, pulling the two side pieces medially toward the torso. This forces the foam inside the polyvinyl bag to remain in contact with the patient as it expands and sets within approximately 7 to 10 min.

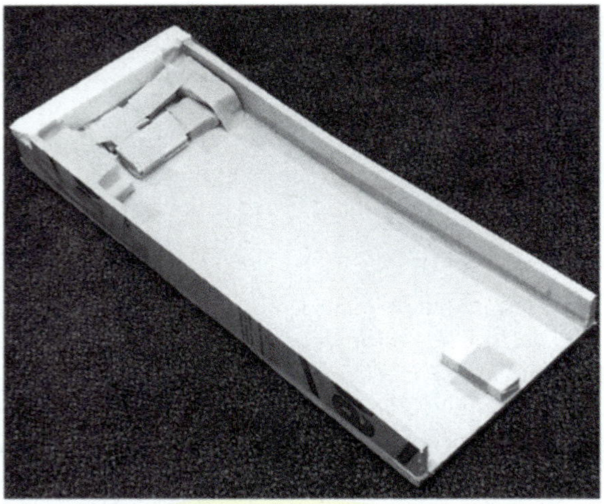

Fig. 6-8 Styrofoam pieces are fastened to the base plate on each side and above the head of the patient, forming a barrier for the expanding foam. Scrap pieces of Styrofoam are used to fill the spaces on each side of the head and under the raised arms.

Small amounts of foam may leak from the Styrofoam shell. Since the mold is often wider than the couch it is made on, the foam may form a "lip" around the couch. When the mold is later placed on a wider couch, this lip may cause an undesired tilt of the patient. To prevent formation of a lip, a large sheet of hardwood, wider than the mold, is placed under the base plate *prior* to making the mold to prevent any irregular surfaces from forming under the device. The hardwood sheet is removed after the foam has set. The process of making the device requires two persons and takes approximately 30 min. A similar device is made for patients treated in the prone position.

One advantage of using customized immobilization devices is the ability to make setup marks both on the rigid positioning device and on the skin, rather than on the mobile skin surface only. When discrepancies arise between these marks, the staff rely on the mold marks, since the skin is mobile. Setup marks on the mold are also useful in the event that skin marks become worn off or migrate during re-marking each day. Since misalignments are easier to detect in the periphery, sagittal alignment marks on the mold are separated by a long distance—e.g., above the head and between the knees. Since alignment systems may be less accurate farther from the isocenter, it is advisable to move the couch in and out (while at 0° rotation) such that each location to be marked is moved close to the isocenter; i.e., the couch is moved out from the gantry to mark above the head and in toward the gantry to mark between the knees. The transverse and coronal alignment lines are marked on each side of the mold. If the polyvinyl bag does not adhere to the foam where the marks are made, the bag needs to be peeled away and marks made directly on the foam, eliminating the risk of marks being displaced.

At Duke University Medical Center, this mold is most commonly made on the CT couch immediately prior to obtaining a CT scan for 3DTP. The patient is asked to cross his or her arms above the head (placing each hand on the opposite elbow); thus the arms fit inside the mold and can easily be moved through the scanning aperture of the CT unit.

Although the need for an immobilization device during irradiation of large anterior/posterior fields in patients with lung cancer may be considered unnecessary, its use during delivery of boost treatments, where smaller margins are utilized, is clearly beneficial (data summarized below).[8] Thus, if an immobilization device is planned for the boost portion of the treatment, it should be used throughout treatment such that its benefits can be realized during the entire treatment course. Furthermore, it ensures that the patient's position remains the same during both the initial and boost treatments.

EXTRACRANIAL STEREOTACTIC DEVICE

An extracranial stereotactic device, described in Chap. 5, has been used to treat intrathoracic and upper abdominal tumors.[9,10] The device consists of a rigid box, approximately 50 cm wide, 20 cm deep, and 100 cm long, with scales corresponding to CT [or magnetic resonance imaging (MRI)] indicators defining the stereotactic coordinate space. For targets affected by diaphragmatic motion, a Plexiglas plate is used to apply pressure on the upper abdomen. A mechanism to level the device on the treatment couch is used, thus counteracting possible sagging of the couch. Repositioning of the patient is achieved by a vacuum mold inside the box.

TREATMENT ACCURACY

We retrospectively reviewed the port films of 60 patients treated with or without the immobilization device described above.[8] The review included 726 port films from 60 patients representing 209 isocenter setups in the nonimmobilized and 229 in the immobilized group. Using the frequency of physician-requested isocenter shifts as a surrogate for setup reproducibility, the differences in the requested shifts in the two patient groups were compared using a two-tailed chi-square test (Table 6-1). Among routine port films (excluding the first set and port films obtained to verify a requested isocenter shift) representing 290 isocenter setups, the use of the mold reduced the number of requested isocenter shifts from 14.3 to 8.2%. This improvement was largest for the oblique treatments, where the frequency of isocenter shifts were reduced from 33 to 12% ($p = 0.038$).

In most other studies of treatment accuracy in the thorax, no immobilization device was used. Rabinowitz et al. studied treatment accuracy in several sites, including the thorax, and found the "worst-case" discrepancy value to be lowest in the head and neck (3.5 mm) and highest in the thorax (9.2 mm).[11] The average worst-case value for all sites studied was 7.7 mm. Rudat et al. reported a mean two-dimensional positioning error among 43 patients with tumors in the thorax and pelvis to be 5.5 (± 3.7) mm.[12] The authors also calculated the changes in tumor control probability (TCP) when the positioning errors were included and found a mean decrease in TCP of 2 and 5% for the gross tumor volume (GTV) and planning target volume (PTV), respectively, in a series of patients with esophageal carcinoma.

Reproducibility of the target, using the extracranial stereotactic devices described above, was studied in 72 CT examinations of the thorax and upper abdomen. Discrepancies include both organ motion and setup deviations. The mean deviation compared with the planning CT was 3.7 mm (95% ≤ 5 mm) and 5.7 mm (89% ≤ 8 mm) in the transverse and craniocaudal directions, respectively.

Utilizing 3DTP tools, dose-escalating trials in the treatment of lung cancer are under way in a few centers. In these studies, patient immobilization is important, since doses are high and normal tissue sparing is crucial.

Table 6-1 Comparison of the Frequency of Isocenter Shifts in Patients Treated with and without an Immobilization Device

	No Immobilization		Extended Mold		
Port Film Type	Number of Misalignments/ Number of Times Tested	Percent	Number of Misalignments/ Number of Times Tested	Percent	*p* value
AP/PA	9/95	9.5	4/89	4.5	0.219
Oblique	9/27	33.3	10/84	11.9	0.038
All routine	17/119[a]	14.3	14/171	8.2	0.139

[a]Shifts in more than one direction.

REFERENCES

1. Creutzberg CL, Visser AG, DePorre PMZR, et al: Accuracy of patient positioning in mantle field irradiation. *Radiother Oncol* 23:257, 1992.
2. Hulshof M, Vanuytsel L, van den Bogaert W, van der Schueren E: Localization errors in mantle-field irradiation for Hodgkin's disease. *Int J Radiat Oncol Biol Phys* 17: 679, 1989.
3. Ball WS, Wicks JD, Mettler FAJ: Prone-supine change in organ position: CT demonstration. *Am J Roentgenol* 135: 815–820, 1980.
4. Corn BW, Coia LR, Chu JCH: Significance of prone positioning in planning treatment for esophageal cancer. *Int J Radiat Oncol Biol Phys* 21:1303, 1991.
5. Vijayakumar S, Muller-Runkel R: Irradiation of the thoracic esophagus: Prone versus supine position. *Acta Radiol Oncol* 25:187, 1986.
6. Fontenla E, Pelizzari CA, Chen GT: Implications of 3-dimensional target shape and motion in aperture design. *Med Phys* 23:1431–1441, 1996.
7. Ten Haken RK, Balter JM, Marsh LH, et al: Potential benefits of eliminating planning target volume expansions for patient breathing in the treatment of liver tumors. *Int J Radiat Oncol Biol Phys* 38:613–617, 1997.
8. Bentel GC, Marks LB, Krishnamurthy R: Impact of cradle immobilization on setup reproducibility during external beam radiation therapy for lung cancer. *Int J Radiat Oncol Biol Phys* 38:527–531, 1997.
9. Blomgren H, Lax I, Näslund I, Svanström R: Stereotactic high dose fraction radiation therapy of extracranial tumors using an accelerator: Clinical experience of the first thirty-one patients. *Acta Oncol* 34:861–870, 1995.
10. Lax I, Blomgren H, Näslund I, Svanström R: Stereotactic radiotherapy of malignancies in the abdomen. *Acta Oncol* 33:677–683, 1994.
11. Rabinowitz I, Broomberg J, Goitein M, et al: Accuracy of radiation field alignment in clinical practice. *Int J Radiat Oncol Biol Phys* 11:1857, 1985.
12. Rudat V, Flentje M, Oetzel D, et al: Influence of the positioning error on 3D conformal dose distributions during fractionated radiotherapy. *Radiother Oncol* 33:56–63, 1994.

PROBLEMS

6-1 Respiration-induced organ motion in the upper abdomen
(*a*) is nothing to worry about because the diaphragm separates the chest from the abdomen
(*b*) should be considered when irradiating patients in the prone position only
(*c*) should be considered when shielding the kidneys
(*d*) does not exist

6-2 Lung tumors are almost invariably treated with the patient in
(*a*) supine position
(*b*) prone position
(*c*) prone position with the arms raised above the head
(*d*) decubitus position with the arms raised above the head

6-3 The arm position during thoracic irradiation
(*a*) should be consistent from treatment to treatment
(*b*) should be whatever the patient feels comfortable with
(*c*) is not important because it does not shift setup marks
(*d*) does not matter during simulation but should be consistent once treatment has started

6-4 Immobilization devices for thoracic irradiation are
(*a*) very common
(*b*) uncommon
(*c*) nonexistent
(*d*) never used

6-5 Using an immobilization device during thoracic irradiation
(*a*) facilitates using smaller target margins because it reduces organ motion

(*b*) facilitates using smaller target margins because it makes it easier to determine tumor extent
(*c*) does not affect the field margins
(*d*) facilitates using smaller target margins because it may improve patient repositioning

6-6 Using an extended positioning mold from above the head to the knees
(*a*) facilitates making sagittal alignment marks on the mold
(*b*) makes the patient comfortable and hence the respiratory motion is reduced
(*c*) should only be used in patients with very large tumors
(*d*) is unnecessary since these patients are incurable

6-7 Using an extended positioning mold from above the head to the knees
(*a*) reduced the frequency of requested isocenter shifts mostly on AP/PA fields
(*b*) reduced the frequency of requested isocenter shifts mostly among the oblique fields
(*c*) had no effect on the frequency of requested isocenter shifts
(*d*) increased the frequency of requested isocenter shifts among routine port films

CHAPTER

7

Hodgkin's Disease

INTRODUCTION

Hodgkin's disease is a curable disease that predominantly strikes individuals less than 35 years old. Great progress has been made in the management of Hodgkin's disease and the 10-year survival, combining all stages of the disease, is approximately 80%. The improved success rate in the management of patients with Hodgkin's disease can be attributed partly to improved radiation therapy techniques. The ability to customize the shape of the treatment fields, treat contiguous lymphatic sites in a single field, and treat large opposed fields without having to change the patient's position represent important improvements. However, serious attention must be given to precision in the delivery of the often complex radiation therapy treatment in these relatively young and curable patients who remain at risk for late adverse consequences for many years.

The extent of radiation therapy for Hodgkin's disease depends on the stage of the disease but usually involves treatment of all or some of the major lymph node sites and the splenic pedicle (or spleen if it is in situ). These treatment sites can be divided into three major regions: supradiaphragmatic, paraaortic, and pelvic. The supradiaphragmatic nodal sites (cervical, supraclavicular, infraclavicular, axillary, mediastinal, and hilar) are usually treated through large opposed anterior and posterior fields referred to as *mantle fields*. Paraaortic treatment fields include the abdominal paraaortic lymph nodes from the diaphragm to the pelvis and usually includes the splenic pedicle (or spleen). The pelvic field includes the pelvic and inguinal lymph nodes. The infradiaphragmatic sites are usually treated through opposed anterior and posterior fields.

The mantle field extends cephalad to include the submandibular lymph nodes, caudal to the level of the diaphragm, and lateral to include the axillary lymph nodes. The field is shaped by customized shielding blocks that protect the lung parenchyma, the humeral head, and the humeri bilaterally. Additional shielding blocks are added at appropriate dose levels to protect the left ventricle of the heart, the larynx, and the cervical spinal cord.

The infradiaphragmatic nodal sites usually include a large volume of bone marrow, which, if treated concurrently, may cause an hematopoietic depression. The infradiaphragmatic treatment sites are therefore sometimes treated sequentially; the paraaortic lymph nodes and the splenic pedicle are usually treated first and the pelvic and inguinal nodes following a recovery period. (The order may be reversed if the patient presents with pelvic nodal disease.) These fields are all custom-designed, using shielding blocks to protect as much as possible of bone marrow, liver, kidneys, bowel, and bladder.

Due to the proximity of many radiosensitive organs, the large size of the fields which, in the periphery, are very sensitive to small alignment errors (Fig. 7-1), and the need to match field borders between the adjacent areas, repositioning of these patients is extremely important. Rigid immobilization may improve repositioning and reduce risks of inadvertent mismatch of adjacent fields.

POSITION

The patient's position is usually supine, with the arms raised above the head and the chin extended (Fig. 7-2). The chin extension allows the submental, submandibular, and cervical lymph nodes to be treated while keeping the oral cavity out of the treatment field. The arms are elevated in an effort to move the axillary lymph nodes laterally and superiorly away from the lung parenchyma. This allows shielding of the lung tissue while simultaneously treating the axillary lymph nodes with adequate margins. In female patients, a larger volume of the breasts may be shielded by the lung blocks if the patient wears a brassiere during treatment.

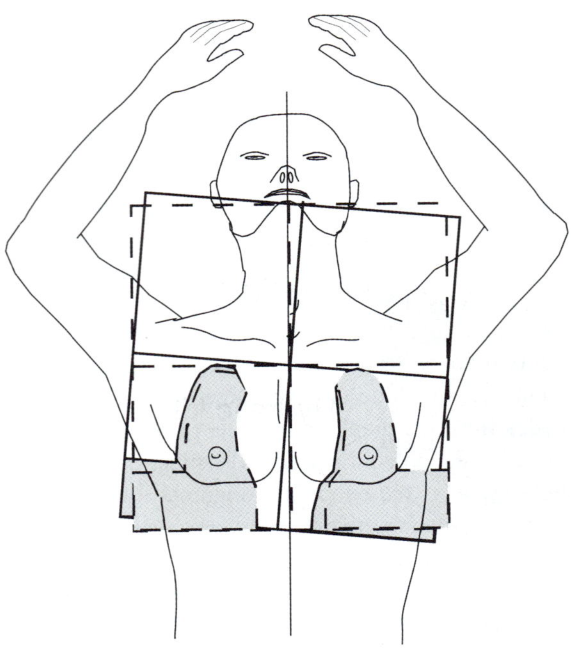

Fig. 7-1 Small rotational errors are easier to detect in large fields since the discrepancy becomes larger as the distance from the isocenter increases (in the periphery).

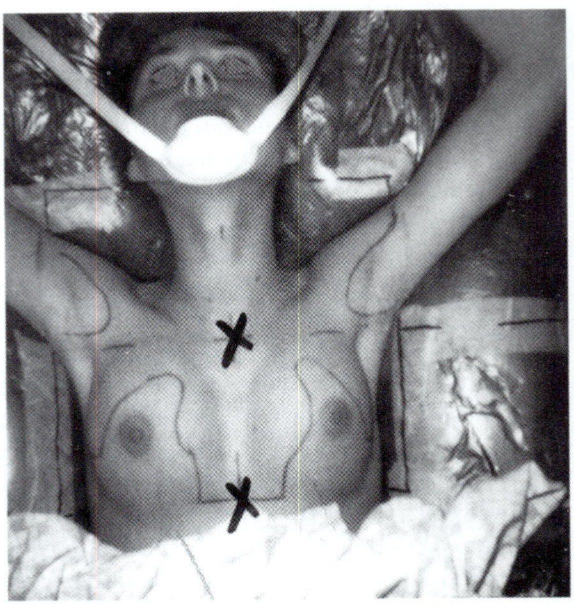

Fig. 7-2 Typical treatment position for mantle field irradiation; supine in positioning mold, arms raised, chin extended and supported by a chin strap.

Due to size limitations of the couch window in some treatment machines, patients may need to be placed in the prone position for the posterior mantle field. This is an undesirable situation, since changing the patient's position from supine to prone or vice versa causes shifts of internal organs and skin.[1] This may jeopardize the accuracy of matching adjacent fields, particularly since the curvature of the spine changes with the different positions. Furthermore, a larger field-placement error rate has been reported for posterior fields treated with the patient in the prone position.[2,3] Ideally, the supine position should be maintained during the treatment of all fields to eliminate these shifts. Organ motion and skin-mark shifts, although less obvious, also occur when the patient's arm position is changed from akimbo (hands on hips with elbows extended away from torso) to being elevated above the head.

ERECT POSITION

In rare situations, patients with Hodgkin's disease are treated in an upright position in an effort to reduce the width of the mediastinal target, allowing smaller fields to be used and thus sparing more of the lungs.[4] This position can be difficult to reproduce and maintain throughout treatment. Adequate supports must therefore be offered, both for the raised arms and for the elevated chin.

In treating their patients, Marcus et al. used a chair with adjustable hand and chin bars mounted on vertical rods (Fig. 7-3).[4] The position of the bars

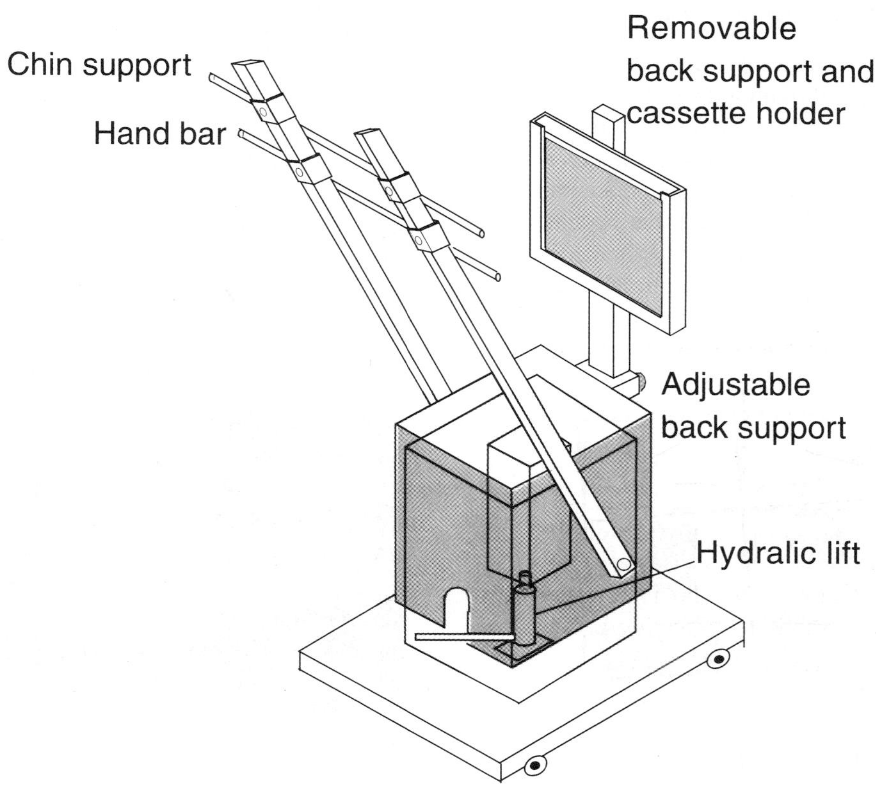

Fig. 7-3 A chair designed for treating patients in an upright position. The chair moves on casters and the height is adjusted by a hydraulic lift. The removable back support can be used as a cassette holder. The chair offers chin and arm supports. (Adapted from Marcus et al.[4])

can be reproduced daily by using scales on each side of the vertical rods. The patient is further supported by a back rest that can also hold a film cassette. The seat, back support, and adjustable hand and chin bars are mounted on a plywood box, 20 in. wide and 20 in. deep, with one side open. The open side fits over an insert mounted on a platform on wheels. The box can be moved vertically and the seat can be moved freely on the floor for each repositioning.

IMMOBILIZATION

It is fundamental to successful radiation therapy that the patient's position with respect to the radiation field be maintained during each treatment and from treatment to treatment. When the patient's position is unnatural (raised arms, extended chin, lying on a hard and flat surface), it may be uncomfortable and, as a result, the patient may move during the treatment. Without a positioning device, reproducing the patient's position for each treatment may be difficult, particularly since alignment marks can be made on only the mobile skin. Thus, a comfortable positioning device that stabilizes the patient's position and onto which alignment marks can be made is advocated. Surprisingly, descriptions in the literature of positioning and immobilization devices for patients undergoing radiation therapy for Hodgkin's disease are limited. Therefore, only the Duke University Medical Center experience is described.

POSITIONING MOLD

From the early 1970s until approximately 1983, patients irradiated for Hodgkin's disease at Duke University were positioned akimbo in an upper-torso Alpha Cradle™* supporting the head, chest, and arms and treated on a 4-MV linear accelerator. Since the size of the couch window on this machine was insufficient for the posterior field, patients were treated in the supine and prone positions for the anterior and posterior mantle fields, respectively. In the early 1980s, a policy of using the raised-arm position for all patients treated for Hodgkin's disease was introduced. The upper-torso mold appeared to give the arm position inadequate support; therefore, handles for the patients to hold onto were added to the device.[5] At approximately the same time, a new machine with a larger couch window was installed in the department, facilitating treatment of the anterior and posterior mantle and paraaortic fields in the supine position.

A retrospective review of port films, undertaken to assess the effectiveness of the addition of the handles, demonstrated a modest reduction in the frequency of physician-requested changes in mantle field position. A more significant finding during this port film review was an unacceptable frequency of positioning errors among port films of paraaortic and pelvic fields. This resulted in a decision to extend the immobilization device to also include the lower torso and thighs. Thus, the current immobilization device used for patients irradiated for Hodgkin's disease extends from above the head to the knees with built-in handles for arm position reproducibility (Fig. 7-4).

To assess the effectiveness of the extended mold (described below), the frequency of misalignments observed on port films of patients treated using this mold was compared with that of patients treated using the upper-torso mold with arm supports and handles but extending only to the waist. The retrospective review consisted of 782 port films representing 450 treatment setups—292 above and 158 below the diaphragm. The results are shown in Table 7-1. The frequency of misalignments among all setups was 20.3% (48/237) with the upper-torso mold and 9.9% (21/213) with the extended mold.[6]

Among the mantle fields, the frequency of misalignments was 13.4% (21/157) and 5.9% (8/135) using the upper-torso mold and the extended mold, respectively. The improvement seen in the setup of mantle fields was unexpected, since the only difference between the two molds was the extension to include the lower torso and thighs. It demonstrates that immobilizing the patient away from the treated area offers improved repositioning. This has also been shown in prostate treatment.[7] The frequency of misalignment in the infradiaphragmatic fields was 33.8% (27/80) and 16.7% (13/78) for the short and

*Smithers Medical Products, Inc., North Canton, Ohio.

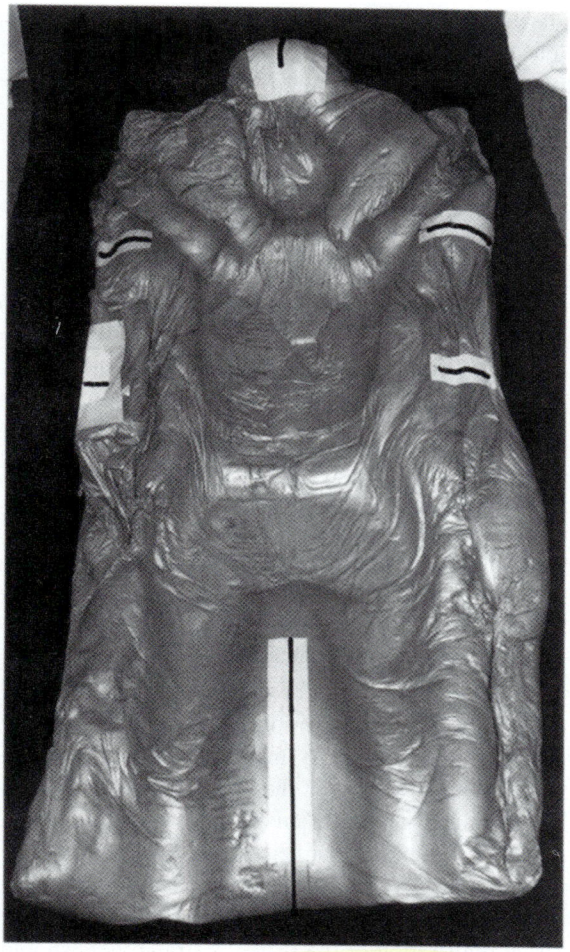

Fig. 7-4 Immobilization mold for patients undergoing irradiation for Hodgkin's disease. The extended mold includes handles for the patient's raised arms and facilitates extensive setup marking.

extended molds, respectively. A two-tailed chi-square test was used to compare the differences in requested shifts in the two patient groups.

FABRICATION OF THE POSITIONING MOLD

The immobilization device used for patients irradiated for Hodgkin's disease at Duke University Medical Center consists of a Styrofoam* shell that roughly matches the shape of the patient's body (Fig. 7-5), foaming chemicals, and a polyvinyl bag that is approximately 2 ft wider and 2 ft longer than the shell. The base plate of this shell is approximately 5 ft long, 2 ft wide, and 1 in. thick. A small rectangle of Styrofoam, approximately 2 in. wide, 4 in. long, and 1 in. high, is placed on the base plate between the patient's knees. This causes the foam to rise up between the knees and form an elevation on which the sagittal alignment line is later marked. Optionally, a small, triangular Styrofoam block can be placed under each knee to reduce the stress on the patient's lower back. In patients with whom the use of a scrotal shield is anticipated, the legs should be separated and a piece of Styrofoam of appropriate height placed between the legs to support the lead shield. Two cylinder-shaped pieces of Styrofoam, approximately 3 in. long and 1 in. in diameter, are placed in a separate small (3- to 4-gal) bag attached to the shell where the patient's raised arms and hands will be positioned. A retaining wall of

*Dow Chemical, Midland, Michigan.

Table 7-1 Comparison of the Frequency of Misalignments in Patients Treated with an Upper-Torso and an Extended Immobilization Mold

	Upper-Torso Mold		Extended Mold		
	Number of Misalignments/ Number of Times Tested	Percent	Number of Misalignments/ Number of Times Tested	Percent	*p* value
Mantle	21/157	13.4	8/135	5.9	0.054
Paraaortic	27/80	33.8	13/78	16.7	0.056
Both sites	48/237	20.3	21/213	9.9	0.009

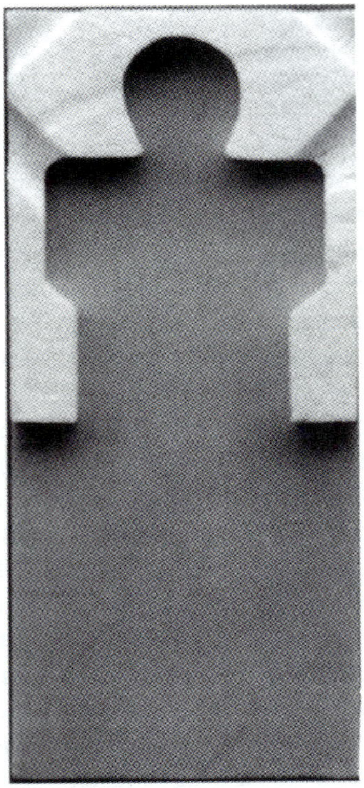

Fig. 7-5 The shell, forming the basis for the positioning mold, roughly matches the shape of the patient's body. Handles are added above the head, a small piece of Styrofoam is fastened between the knees, and side barriers are added to confine the foam. The foam is poured into the shell inside a large polyvinyl bag.

Styrofoam is added to each side of the base to contain the foam in close proximity to the patient's torso. The position of each piece of Styrofoam is determined with the patient in the shell but without the foam. This shell provides indentations for the elevated arms (45°) and offers a barrier for the foam as it expands inside the bag in the space between the Styrofoam and the patient.

With the patient removed, each piece of Styrofoam is fastened to the base with masking tape and the entire shell is placed inside the large protective polyvinyl bag. Before the patient is returned to the mold, one batch of foam (approximately 660 mL) is prepared as directed by the manufacturer. Approximately 100 mL is poured inside the arm-support bag holding the Styrofoam cylinders and the remainder is evenly distributed inside the shell. Several pinholes are made in the arm-support bag on the side toward the Styrofoam shell to allow some foam to leak and form an adhesive securing the small bag to the rest of the mold. Alternatively, a small amount of foam can be poured on top of the Styrofoam shell under the smaller bag.

After the air is allowed to circulate inside the bag for a few seconds, it is squeezed out, the bag is sealed, and the device is placed at the foot end of the couch. The patient, undressed except for underwear (unless a scrotal shield is used) and a hospital gown (open to the back), is returned to the shell by first standing on a stepping stool at the end of the couch and then sitting down in the shell. The shell with the patient in it is then moved to the center of the couch and the patient assumes a supine position, elevates the arms above the head, and extends the chin. A chin strap made of Velcro* can be used to help the patient maintain the chin extension. The two cylinders forming handles inside the bag and some of the foam are guided into the patient's hands. In male patients, the scrotal shield is positioned appropriately on the Styrofoam elevation so that the expanding foam forms an impression of the shield, thus facilitating repositioning. The hospital gown is pulled up from under the patient so that he or she lies directly on the polyvinyl bag. It is important to make sure that the patient feels that he or she is lying flat and straight. A visual registration of the patient's straightness should also be made by the staff. (This can also be done with fluoroscopy if available.) The plastic bag is pulled up between the patient's knees to allow the foam to expand and form an elevation for the sagittal alignment mark. The height of this elevation should be based on the patient's agility, as some patients may have difficulty lifting themselves over it when entering and leaving the mold for each treatment. Masking tape, fastened to the sides of the mold, is stretched anteriorly across the patient to force the foam medially toward the patient so as to form a tight-fitting mold. The foam stops expanding after approximately 7 to 10 min but requires an additional 10 min to become firm.

*Velcro USA, Manchester, New Hampshire.

A hardwood board, wider and longer than the mold, is placed on top of the couch *before* the fabrication is initiated to prevent leaking foam from forming a lip over the couch. Such a lip or other irregular surfaces under the mold could cause a tilt of the immobilization device, potentially giving rise to field misalignments.

To produce a tight-fitting mold, it is important that the patient wear minimal clothing during the mold fabrication. Since patients usually wear different clothing each day during the course of treatment, the mold may be too large on some days and too tight on other days. Both situations would compromise the ability to reposition the patient correctly. This mold is used during irradiation of both supra- and infradiaphragmatic sites.

SETUP MARKS

One important advantage of using a customized immobilization device is the ability to make setup marks on the rigid positioning device in addition to the mobile skin. Setup marks on the mold are also useful in the event that the skin marks should become worn off or migrate during re-marking each day. Since misalignments are easier to detect in the periphery (Fig. 7-1), sagittal alignment marks on the mold are separated by a long distance, e.g., above the head and between the knees. Since alignment systems may be less accurate farther from the isocenter, it is advisable to move the couch in and out (while at 0° rotation) such that each location to be marked is moved close to the isocenter; i.e., the couch is moved out from the gantry to mark above the head and in toward the gantry to mark between the knees. The transverse and coronal alignment lines are marked on each side of the mold. If the polyvinyl bag does not adhere to the foam where the marks are made, the bag needs to be peeled away and marks made directly on the foam, eliminating the risk of marks being displaced.

GONADAL PROTECTION

The dose to the gonads during radiation therapy is primarily caused by internal scatter but can also consist of primary and/or external scatter radiation. Elimination of the gonadal dose during pelvic and paraaortic irradiation is impossible; however, in patients where preservation of fertility is desired, efforts should be made to minimize the gonadal dose. In patients with Hodgkin's disease, the need for gonadal protection frequently arises, since most of these patients are young. Measures to reduce the gonadal dose depend on whether the dose is caused by internal or external scatter or primary beam and whether the patient is female or male.

In female patients, the ovaries are often moved medially or, less commonly, laterally to the pelvic brim (oophoropexy) during staging laparotomy to increase the distance between them and the pelvic lymph nodes. The new positions of the ovaries are marked with surgical clips to facilitate their shielding during pelvic radiation therapy.[8-11] This procedure is not always successful[9] and is sometimes performed unnecessarily since, at the time of the laparotomy, it is not clear whether the patient will need pelvic irradiation.[8]

Thomas et al. investigated reproductive and endocrine function in 22 female patients with Hodgkin's disease who had midline oophoropexies performed during staging laparotomy. Pregnancies occurred in 4 of 6 patients subsequently found not to require irradiation below the diaphragm. In the other 2 patients in this group, the menstrual history was unaffected and gonadotrophin concentrations remained normal. Among 4 patients receiving paraaortic lymph node irradiation (ovarian dose approximately 150 cGy), menstrual function and gonadotrophin levels were unaffected and 1 patient subsequently became pregnant. Of 12 patients who received paraaortic and pelvic irradiation with ovaries shielded by a lead block (ovarian dose ranged from 600 to 3500 cGy), 9 have persistent amenorrhea with elevated gonadotrophin levels, 1 became pregnant, and 1 resumed normal menstrual cycles and has normal gonadotrophin concentrations. The authors conclude that since oophoropexy does not appear to impair ovarian function, it should be performed even when it is uncertain whether pelvic irradiation will be necessary.[11]

In patients where the ovaries have been moved medially, the pelvic midline block, intended to shield the bladder and rectum, may also shield the ovaries without compromising coverage of pelvic and inguinal lymph nodes. If the ovaries were moved laterally, they would hopefully be outside the radiation field. Such ovarian displacement may prevent primary radiation and external scatter from reaching the ovaries; however, internal scatter is less affected by these measures. Internal scatter to the ovaries cannot be eliminated; however, some measures to reduce the dose may be considered, including use of a high-energy beam, maximizing the ovary-to-field edge distance, and the use of fields that are as small as possible.

In male patients, a small amount of dose to the testicles is unavoidable when pelvic and paraaortic fields are treated. However, if preservation of fertility is a concern, measures to reduce this dose should be implemented[12–15] and sperm banking offered. To reduce the testicular dose, a lead cup surrounding the scrotum is frequently used (Fig. 7-6). The primary purpose of this shield is to reduce the amount of internal scatter arriving at the testes during pelvic irradiation. The wall thickness of the clamshell shield (approximately one half-value layer) does not adequately attenuate the primary beam. Given the weight of the lead shield and the small space in which it needs to be placed, it can be difficult to position properly and may then be ineffective. The weight of the shield can be supported and the position adjusted when it is mounted on a platform with vertical (height adjustment) and a horizontal arm with a joint swivel (rotational adjustment). The shield surrounding the scrotum can also be built into an immobilization mold, as described above; thus the weight is supported by the mold and the repositioning is reliable. It is important that the internal dimensions of the lead shield be small to allow more room for thick walls. Shielding of the penis does not affect gonadal function and would only increase the size of the shield.

Additional methods to reduce the testicular dose have been described by Kubo and Shipley (Table 7-2).[15] They found the testicular dose to be 1.6% of the prescribed midplane dose when a 6-mm lead clamshell testicular shield was used during retroperitoneal irradiation with 10-MV photon beams. This dose was reduced to < 0.1% by using a testicular shield 1.2 cm thick designed with an opening for the scrotum and a hinged lid extending over this opening to minimize the risk of internal scatter reaching the testes, and two additional blocks upstream in the beam (Fig. 7-7). One block (block A) consists of caudal extension of the conventional field-shaping block beyond the field edge to cover the scrotum. Its purpose is to reduce the dose from primary beam leakage from the collimator. The second block (block B), 10 cm thick, was placed on a platform (1.5-cm acrylic) about 7 cm above the patient and just outside the caudal margin of the radiation field and covering the scrotum. Its purpose is to eliminate secondary scatter off the collimator.

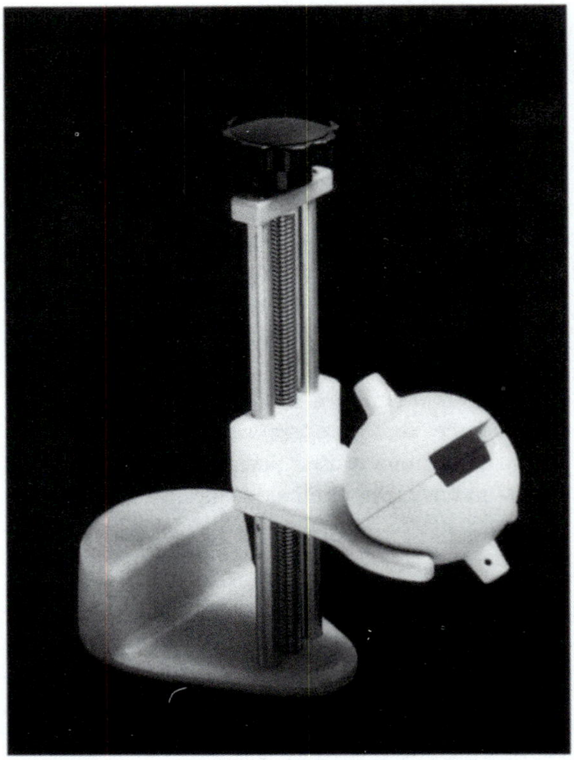

Fig. 7-6 A testicular shield mounted on a stand that facilitates height and angle adjustments. A counterweight at the base of the stand stabilizes the position of the shield. (Courtesy of MED-TEC, Inc., Orange City, Iowa.)

Table 7-2 Scrotal Dose Measured in Phantom

Type of Shield Used	External Dose, %	Internal Scatter, %	Total Dose, %[a]
Collimator only	3.5	1.0	4.5
Block A (Fig. 7-7)	1.4	0.9	2.3
Blocks A + B (Fig. 7-7)	0.05	0.8	0.85
Blocks A + B + clamshell	0.05	0.5	0.55

[a]Percent of prescribed midplane dose.
Source: Modified from Kubo and Shipley.[15]

Precautions should be taken to prevent inadvertent irradiation of the gonads. For example, when an anterior pelvic field designed to exclude the scrotum is opposed by a posterior field, the diverging caudal margin of the posterior field may include the testicles (Fig. 7-7). Similarly, when the ovaries are excluded from the anterior field, they may inadvertently be included in the posterior beam. Another situation where inadvertent gonadal irradiation may occur is during port filming. Routinely, port films are obtained by using a double-exposure technique, where the second exposure is made with beam-shaping blocks removed and the collimator opening increased so that bony anatomy in the vicinity can be visualized. This procedure may cause the primary beam to include the gonads (female and male), thus defeating the purpose of shielding. Even if the gonadal shield is in place during port filming, the scrotal shield is not, as noted above, able to attenuate the primary beam. In patients where preservation of fertility is important, routine port filming procedures may therefore need to be modified—for example, by using a single exposure of the treatment field only or by placing a block or independent jaw over the testicles.

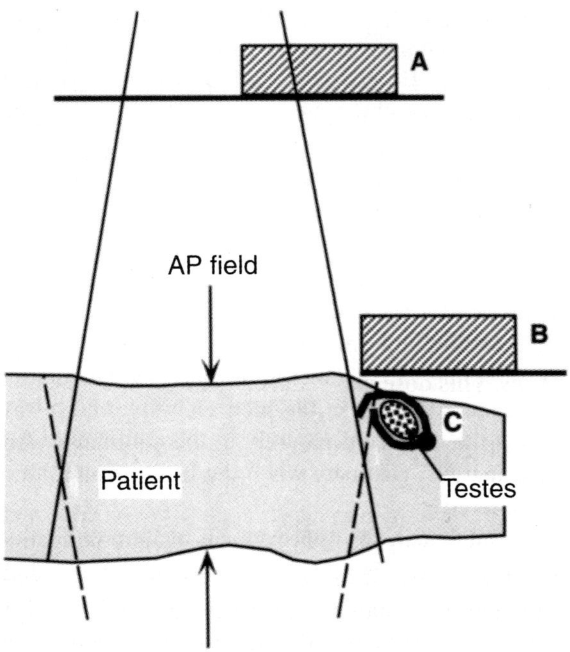

Fig. 7-7 Three testicular shielding devices: an extension of the field-shaping block caudally over the scrotum (A), a 10-cm-thick lead block mounted about 7 cm above the patient (B), and a scrotal shield with a hinged lid extending over the opening for the scrotum, providing nearly complete shielding from internal scatter (C). The posterior field, diverging caudally, may need to be adjusted to prevent direct irradiation of the testes.

TREATMENT ACCURACY

Several authors have reported data regarding the accuracy of treatment delivery and marginal failures in Hodgkin's disease. Marginal failures in mantle field irradiation may have causes other than misplacement of treatment fields and/or shielding blocks, such as uncertainties regarding tumor extent, respiratory motion, and beam characteristics (penumbra, beam flatness). These factors should be considered when treatment margins are decided.

Taylor et al. have reported on the frequency of mantle field misalignment and found that 15% of 1186 port films from 28 patients were in error by more than 5 mm.[16] No target areas were inadvertently shielded in these misaligned fields and only 1% of the ports were considered unacceptable. The anterior field was treated with the patient supine and immobilized using a bite-block and face-mask system, while the posterior field was treated with the patient prone and positioned in a polyurethane body mold.

In a retrospective review of port films representing 902 setups on 99 patients with Hodgkin's disease and other lymphomas, Marks et al. reported that 36% of the treatment fields were erroneously placed.[17] In 10 of 99 patients, disease was not controlled locally. Two of these failures were at the margins of the fields and were shown by portal films to be correlated with positioning errors, leading to reduced dose at the sites of recurrence. One might conclude that errors in treatment delivery, including positioning errors, may be a significant cause of marginal recurrences.

Hulshof et al. studied patient positioning and custom shielding-block errors in 216 mantle setups of 102 nonimmobilized patients treated supine and prone. On the first port film at the start of the treatment, 50% of the setups were in error by >5 mm and 13% by >10 mm.[2] The clinical relevance of these geometric errors was evaluated using a clinical scoring system considering the target margins. Based on the clinical scoring system, corrections were made to the patient's position (79%) or the shielding blocks (21%) when the setup was considered inadequate. Creutzberg et al. compared 94 megavoltage portal films with 26 simulation films and found that alignment errors in excess of 10 mm occurred in 7.2% of cases.[3] Both Hulshof and Creutzberg reported a larger field-placement error rate observed on posterior fields treated with the patient in the prone position. It therefore appears that maintaining the patient's position supine for all fields improves setup reproducibility. In addition, as alluded to earlier, it also reduces dose uncertainties across the junction of adjacent fields.

Kinzie et al.,[18] in a Patterns of Care study, reviewed port films of 181 patients with Hodgkin's disease treated in four major American university medical centers to assess the relapse rates and adequacy of portals. The adequacy criteria were as follows: an inadequate field that was corrected on subsequent treatments was considered adequate. Inadequate fields were those where a shielding block consistently touched the edge of known disease or overlapped it, blocks consistently covered uninvolved supraclavicular or axillary nodes that were intended for treatment, and abdominal node groups intended for treatment were clearly not in the fields. The investigators found that treatment portal films did not adequately encompass the disease in 66 patients. When this occurred, there was a 50% overall relapse rate with 32% recurrences either in-field or marginal. Postulating that chemotherapy might obscure inadequate technology, the relapse rate among patients treated with radiation therapy alone was determined. When 26 patients receiving chemotherapy were excluded, the overall relapse rate was 54% among patients with inadequate margins: 33% of those were in-field or marginal. When the port films were judged to be adequate, the overall relapse rate was 14%, with only 7% being in-field or marginal recurrences.

The findings in these studies indicate the need for periodic in-house evaluation of technical aspects of radiation therapy. Questions to be asked during such evaluations should include the following: Can patient positioning and immobilization be improved? Is shielding block fabrication and implementation adequate? Are blocks fastened securely onto a tray, and is the tray fixed securely to the collimator? Are field margins adequate when the beam penumbra is considered?

In our search for improvement of immobilization in patients with Hodgkin's disease, such an evaluation led to an impressive improvement when an Alpha Cradle was extended from the waist to the knees. This change in patient immobilization may lead to improved survival among these often young and curable patients with Hodgkin's disease.[6] It also convinced us of the need to use extended immobilization devices in other sites as well (prostate, breast, and thorax).

REFERENCES

1. Ball WS, Wicks JD, Mettler FAJ: Prone-supine change in organ position: CT demonstration. *Am J Roentgenol* 135: 815–820, 1980.
2. Hulshof M, Vanuytsel L, van den Bogaert W, van der Schueren E: Localization error in mantle-field irradiation for Hodgkin's disease. *Int J Radiat Oncol Biol Phys* 17: 679, 1989.
3. Creutzberg CL, Visser AG, DePorre PMZR, et al: Accuracy of patient positioning in mantle field irradiation. *Radiother Oncol* 23:257, 1992.
4. Marcus KC, Svensson G, Rhodes LP, Mauch PM: Mantle irradiation in the upright position: A technique to reduce the volume of lung irradiated in patients with bulky mediastinal Hodgkin's disease. *Int J Radiat Oncol Biol Phys* 23:443, 1992.
5. Bentel GC: Positioning and immobilization of patients undergoing radiation therapy for Hodgkin's disease. *Med Dosim* 16:111, 1991.
6. Bentel GC, Marks LB, Krishnamurthy R, Prosnitz LR: Comparison of two repositioning devices used during radiation therapy for Hodgkin's disease. *Int J Radiat Oncol Biol Phys* 39:791–795, 1997.
7. Bentel GC, Marks LB, Sherouse GW, et al: The effectiveness of immobilization during prostate irradiation. *Int J Radiat Oncol Biol Phys* 31:143–148, 1995.
8. Gabriel DA, Bernard SA, Lambert J, Croom RD: Oophoropexy and the management of Hodgkin's disease: A reevaluation of the risks and benefits. *Arch Surg* 121: 1083–1085, 1986.
9. Hunter MC, Glees JP, Gazet JC: Oophoropexy and ovarian function in the treatment of Hodgkin's disease. *Clin Radiol* 31:21–26, 1980.
10. Ray GR, Trueblood HW, Enright LP, et al: Oophoropexy: A means of preserving ovarian function following pelvic megavoltage radiotherapy for Hodgkin's disease. *Radiology* 96:175–180, 1970.
11. Thomas PR, Winstanly D, Peckham MJ, et al: Reproductive and endocrine function in patients with Hodgkin's disease: Effects of oophoropexy and irradiation. *Br J Cancer* 33:226–231, 1976.
12. Bentel GC: *Radiation Therapy Planning,* 2nd ed. New York: McGraw-Hill, 1996.
13. Fraass BA, Kinsella TJ, Harrington FS, Glatstein E: Peripheral dose to the testes: The design and clinical use of a practical and effective gonadal shield. *Int J Radiat Oncol Biol Phys* 11:609, 1985.
14. Harter DJ, Hussey DH, Delclos L, et al: Device to position and shield the testicle during irradiation. *Int J Radiat Oncol Biol Phys* 1:361, 1976.
15. Kubo HD, Shipley WU: Reduction of the scatter dose to the testicle outside the radiation treatment field. *Int J Radiat Oncol Biol Phys* 8:1741, 1982.
16. Taylor BW, Mendenhall NP, Million RR: Reproducibility of mantle irradiation with daily imaging. *Int J Radiat Oncol Biol Phys* 19:149, 1990.
17. Marks JE, Haus AG, Sutton HG, Griem ML: Localization error in the radiotherapy of Hodgkin's disease and malignant lymphoma with extended mantle fields. *Cancer* 34: 83, 1974.
18. Kinzie JJ, Hanks GE, MacLean CJ, Kramer S: Patterns of Care study: Hodgkin's disease relapse rates and adequacy of portals. *Cancer* 52:2223, 1983.

PROBLEMS

7-1 Hodgkin's disease is most common in
(*a*) females over 50 years of age
(*b*) males over 50 years of age
(*c*) males and females under the age of 35 years
(*d*) age and gender is not a factor

7-2 Mantle and paraaortic fields are usually treated with the patient in
(*a*) supine position with the arms along the sides and the chin raised
(*b*) supine position for the anterior and prone for the posterior fields
(*c*) supine position with the arms raised above the head and the chin elevated
(*d*) supine position with hands on hips, elbows extended, and legs spread

7-3 Mantle fields are sometimes treated with the patient sitting in a chair to
(*a*) reduce the width of the mediastinum
(*b*) improve field matching between mantle and paraaortic fields
(*c*) improve setup reproducibility
(*d*) make it easier for the patient to breathe

7-4 Immobilizing patients with Hodgkin's disease in an extended rather than an upper-torso mold
(*a*) increases setup uncertainties of both mantle and paraaortic fields
(*b*) improves reproducibility of mantle but not paraaortic field setups
(*c*) has no impact on setup reproducibility
(*d*) improves reproducibility of mantle and paraaortic field setups

7-5 Immobilizing patients with Hodgkin's disease in an extended mold
(*a*) facilitates making reliable setup marks on the mold
(*b*) causes setup lines on the mold to shift
(*c*) makes setup marks obsolete
(*d*) prevents marking of setup lines

7-6 Radiation dose to the testicles from pelvic lymph node irradiation consists of
(*a*) primary radiation only
(*b*) external scatter only
(*c*) primarily of internal scatter
(*d*) primarily of primary radiation

7-7 Gonadal protection in patients with Hodgkin's disease is
(*a*) unnecessary since all patients are over 50 years of age
(*b*) a desirable goal since most patients are young
(*c*) impossible to accomplish due to the patient's position
(*d*) can be achieved only in male patients

7-8 Measures to reduce radiation to the ovaries consist of
(*a*) moving the ovaries away from the radiation field
(*b*) placing a lead apron over the ovaries during irradiation
(*c*) delivering all treatments with the patient in the prone position
(*d*) all of the above

7-9 Field placement errors may be due to
(*a*) patient positioning
(*b*) skin marks shifting
(*c*) discrepancies between simulator and treatment tabletops
(*d*) all of the above

7-10 Periodic in-house testing of setup reproducibility is
(*a*) an excellent method to determine how well the technologists can reposition the patients
(*b*) not a good idea, because it is too much work and does not yield enough information
(*c*) a good idea, since it would demonstrate weaknesses in patient immobilization and hopefully lead to improvements
(*d*) too costly and therefore not worthwhile

CHAPTER

8

Breast

INTRODUCTION

In recent years, the trend of breast cancer management has been toward breast conservation, with the surgical intervention being limited to "lumpectomy" (tumor removal), usually followed by radiation therapy. Recent data have reaffirmed the role of radiation therapy following mastectomy as well. Thus, an increasing number of patients are receiving radiation therapy for breast cancer. Delivery of radiation therapy in such patients is complex, and it can be challenging, with respect to both dose delivery and patient positioning. This is especially true in patients with large breasts.

Radiation therapy for the patient with an intact breast usually involves treating the breast and the underlying chest wall and, following mastectomy, only the chest wall with or without the regional lymph nodes (internal mammary, supraclavicular, and axillary). The field arrangement commonly consists of opposed tangential fields including the breast/chest wall and sometimes also the internal mammary nodes. When the internal mammary nodes cannot be included within the tangential fields, a separate anterior field, adjacent to the medial tangential field, can be used. Supraclavicular nodes, with or without the axillary lymph nodes, are treated via an anterior oblique field adjacent to the cephalad margin of the tangential fields and angled (anterior/medial) to avoid the spinal cord. A posterior axillary field is occasionally used to boost the dose in the axilla. Matching of multiple fields with different orientations is complex and requires careful treatment planning and implementation.

POSITION

PATIENT POSITION

The usual patient position during breast/chest wall irradiation is supine with the arm on the involved side (ipsilateral) raised to facilitate tangential fields across the chest without irradiating the arm. The face is usually turned toward the contralateral side with the head extended to maximize the distance between the face and the radiation beam (Fig. 8-1). This distance can be increased by reducing the size of the head support (pillow) or removing it.

The raised-arm position may give rise to unsatisfactory repositioning, since the patient tends to rotate her torso as she raises her arm. For this and other reasons, it may be advantageous to elevate both arms with the head straight in order to follow the convention used in most other sites, where the patient is placed in a symmetrical and basically straight position (Fig. 8-2).[1] Many patients are more comfortable and relaxed with both arms elevated because they can then clasp their hands together. Another potential advantage of a symmetrical position is the ability to match adjacent fields should the patient return for future treatments in the upper torso (e.g., mediastinal or spinal lesions). Repositioning the patient, maybe years later, in the asymmetrical position used during breast irradiation and using tattoos for field matching may create uncertainties.

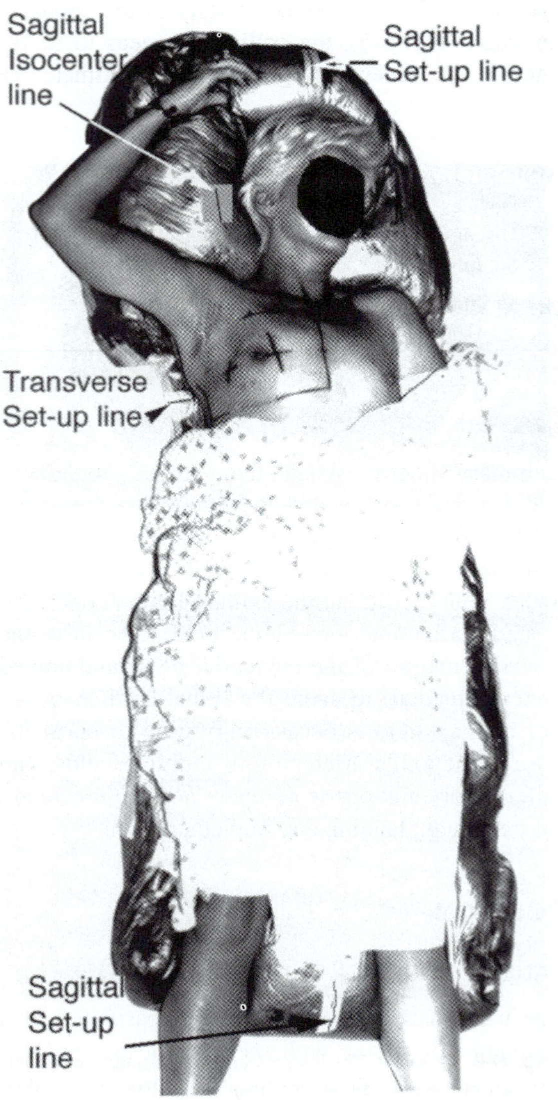

Fig. 8-1 A patient in a typical position for breast irradiation—supine, with the arm on the involved side raised and the face turned toward the opposite side.

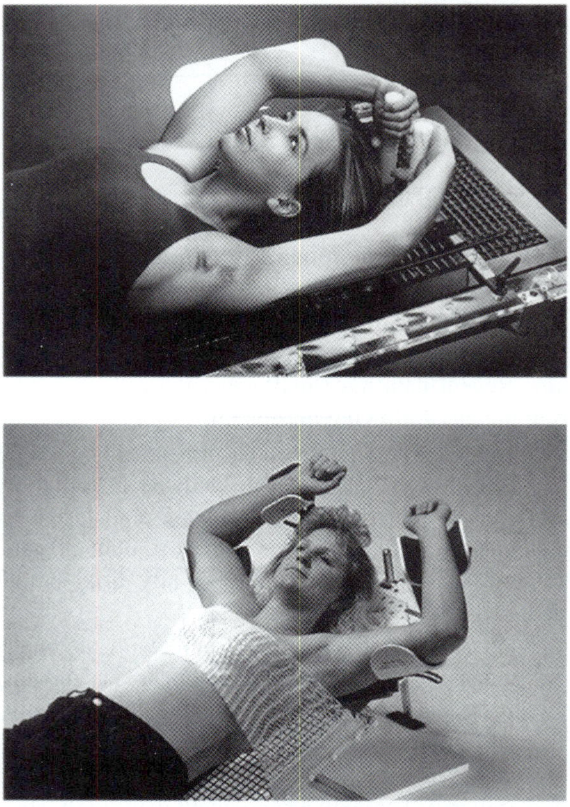

Fig. 8-2 Placing the patient in a symmetrical position with both arms raised and the head straight may reduce field-matching problems should the patient return for future treatments. (Courtesy of MED-TEC, Inc., Orange City, Iowa.)

The angle at which an arm is elevated depends on several factors: the patient's ability to elevate the arm without discomfort, the extent to which the arm can be elevated without causing skin folds in the supraclavicular area, and, when computed tomography (CT)-based treatment planning is used, the ability to move the patient through the CT aperture. The aperture of many CT units has an hourglass shape (as seen in cross section from above), with the scanning section at the narrowest portion. Thus, it is often possible to scan the chest while the patient's raised arms are within the wider part of the hourglass (e.g., patients raise their arms after being moved through the narrowest part of the aperture) (Fig. 8-3*A*). When only one arm is raised, most patients can be moved into the scanner with the arm elevated by being positioned off center on the couch (Fig. 8-3*B*). When tangential fields only are used, concerns with respect to skin folds in the supraclavicular region are eliminated; thus the arm elevation may be increased to facilitate motion through the CT aperture.

The tangential fields are usually designed to include approximately 1 to 3 cm of the lung silhouette, depending on the target (breast/chest wall with or without internal mammary lymph nodes) and the shape of the lung contour in the transverse plane (Fig. 8-4). Since the lung contour in the beam's-eye view (BEV) curves posteriorly in the cephalad direction (Fig. 8-5), the collimator needs to be rotated if the "deep" margin is to approximate the

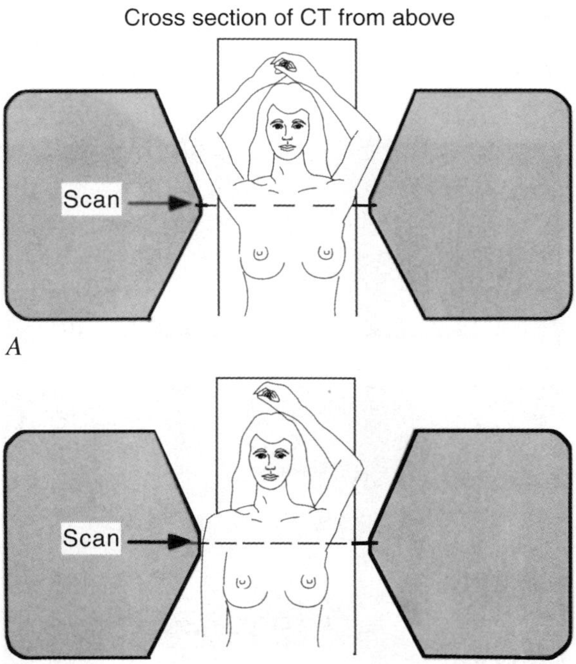

A

B

Fig. 8-3 *A*. Some CT units facilitate obtaining a chest scan of a patient with both arms raised above the head. The patient's arms are raised after being moved through the narrowest part of the aperture. *B*. When only one arm is raised, the patient can be moved off center on the couch and the arm can remain raised while moving through the aperture.

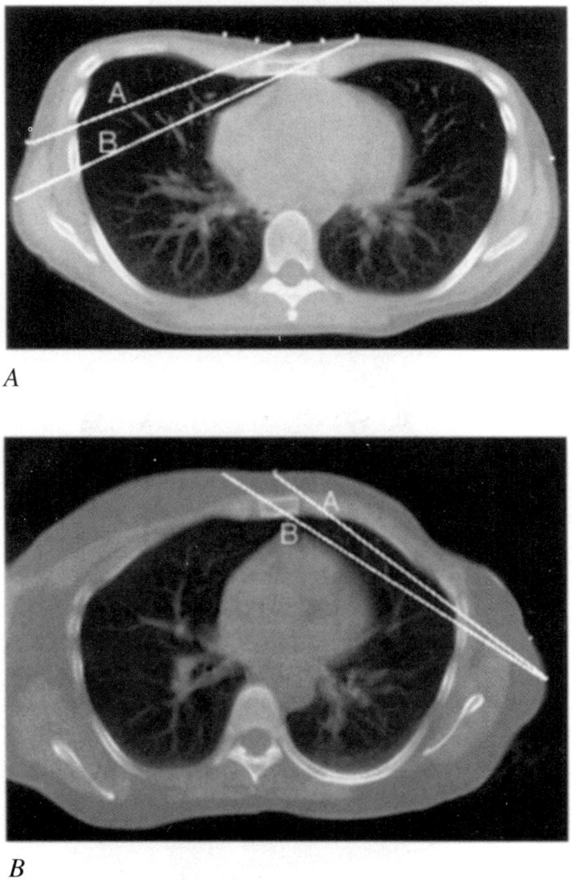

A

B

Fig. 8-4 *A* and *B*. The lung thickness within tangential fields depends on whether the internal mammary lymph nodes (IMN) are included. (Line *A* without the IMN, and line *B* with the IMN.) The lung thickness also depends on the shape of the lung contour in the transverse plane, as demonstrated by these two patients.

lung contour (Fig. 8-6). The collimator angle causes the cephalad field margin to transect the patient at an angle, preventing field matching with the straight half-beam blocked vertical (nondivergent) caudal margin of the supraclavicular field (Fig. 8-6). When this method is used, the tangential field needs to overlap the supraclavicular field and the overlapping portions of the tangential fields are blocked to match the caudal margin of the supraclavicular field (Fig. 8-7). In some treatment techniques, the upper torso is instead elevated to make the chest wall approximately horizontal, eliminating the need for a collimator angle (Fig. 8-8). A disadvantage of tilting the patient's chest when a supraclavicular field is used is the increased lung tissue volume within this field (Fig. 8-9). In another technique, the patient lies flat on the couch and the "deep" field margin is

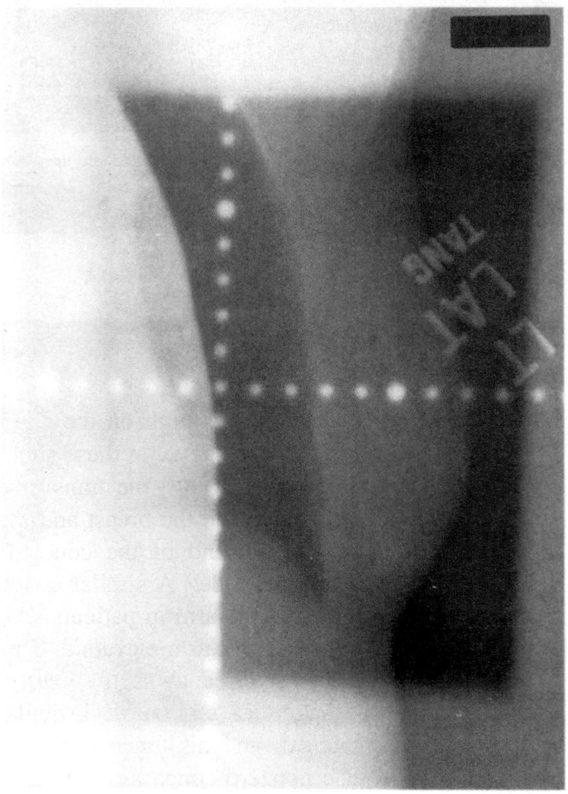

Fig. 8-5 The lung contour in the cephalad portions of tangential fields usually curves posteriorly when seen in the beam's-eye view. In this patient, a shielding block is customized to the shape of the lung contour to prevent unnecessary lung irradiation.

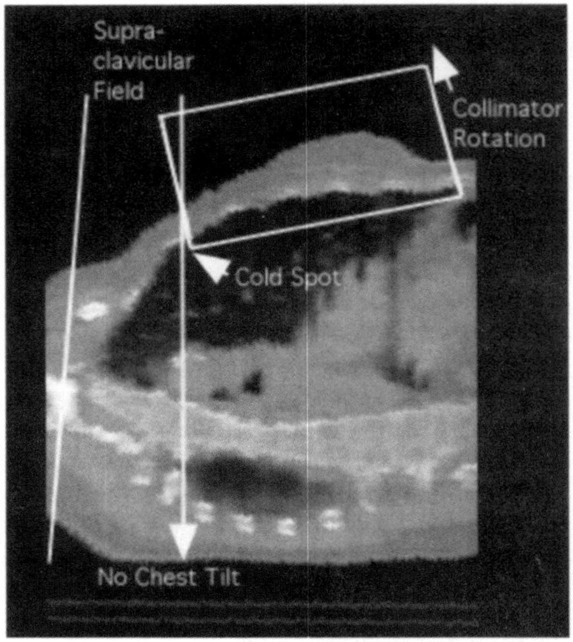

Fig. 8-6 Collimator rotation, sometimes used to make the "deep" tangential field margin approximate the lung contour, causes difficulties with matching the caudal supraclavicular field margin.

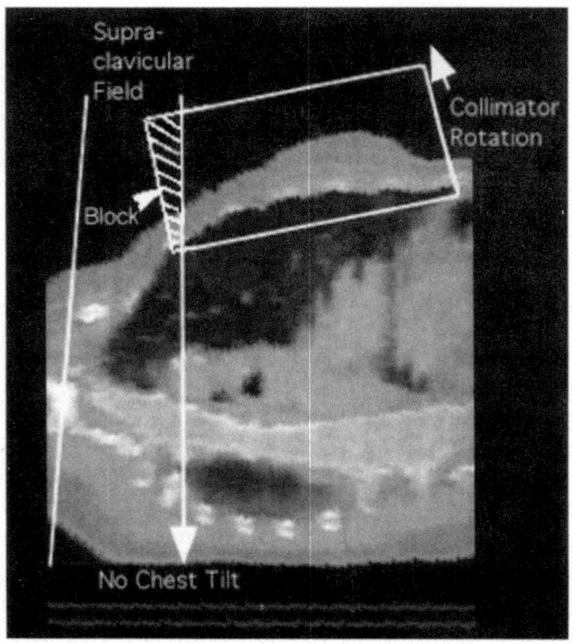

Fig. 8-7 To match the supraclavicular/tangential field margins, the tangential fields extend into the supraclavicular field and the overlap region is blocked.

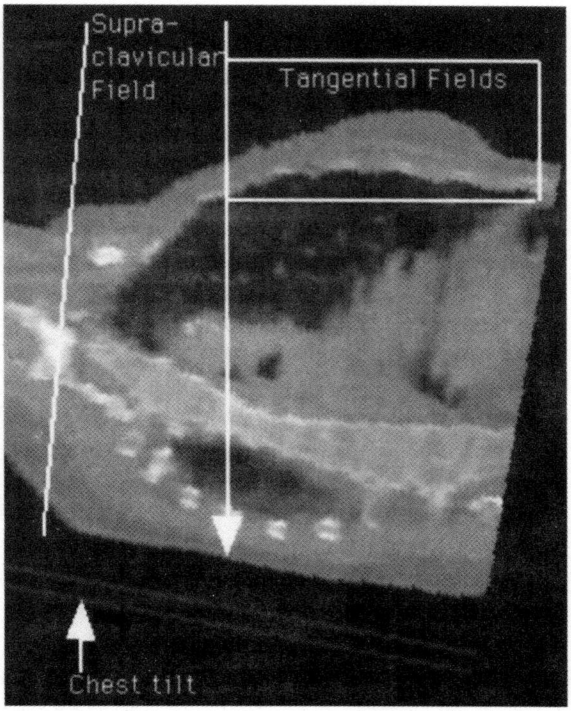

Fig. 8-8 Tilting the patient's chest until the chest wall/lung contour lies on a horizontal line may eliminate collimator rotation and blocking.

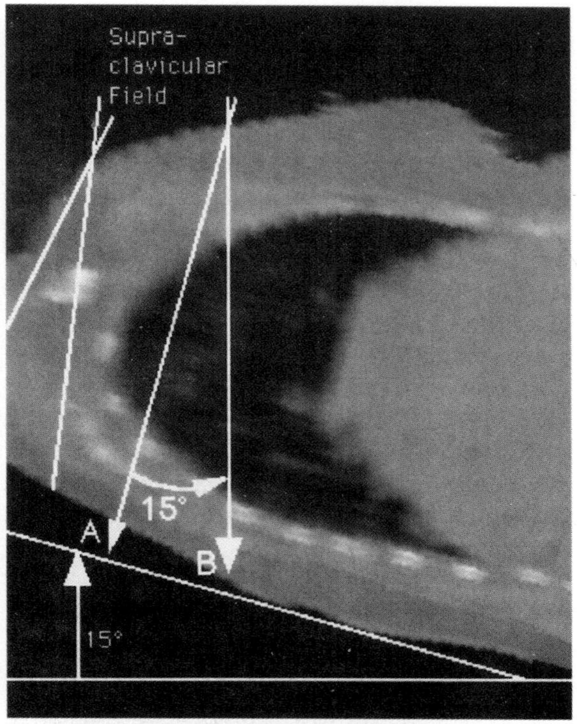

Fig. 8-9 Tilting the patient's chest causes a larger lung volume to lie within the supraclavicular field. The lung volume between the caudal margin of the supraclavicular field when the patient's chest is horizontal (line *A*) and with a 15° tilt (line *B*) is added when the chest is tilted.

shaped to the lung contour by a customized lung-shielding block (Fig. 8-5).

The treatment couch is turned in opposite directions for the tangential fields (foot end away from the collimator) to make the cephalad margins coplanar and thus prevent divergence into the supraclavicular field. This geometric arrangement would be "perfect" only if the tangential fields were at right angles to the supraclavicular field. Since they are not (tangential fields are generally angled 45 to 55° off vertical), a perfect match can be achieved only with a small (2 to 3°) collimator angle.[2] Given the uncertainties associated with this field matching (moving skin marks, thickness of skin marks and laser alignment lines, respiration), this collimator angle is sometimes ignored.

Following an axillary dissection, exclusion of the axilla from the tangential fields is usually desired. In patients where the breast lies high on the chest wall, this may be difficult to achieve. In these situations, the couch can be turned until the transverse alignment line transects between the breast and the axilla (Fig. 8-10). (The foot end of the couch is turned toward the ipsilateral side.) A similar couch angle can be used to avoid the arm in patients who are unable to achieve sufficient arm elevation. This nonzero couch angle is referred to as the *neutral* couch angle. The tangential and supraclavicular fields are then matched on this unconventional "transverse" line. The nonzero couch angle is used in the same way as the conventional zero-degree setting; e.g., the couch is turned in the opposite direction with respect to the neutral angle to prevent beam divergence into the supraclavicular field.

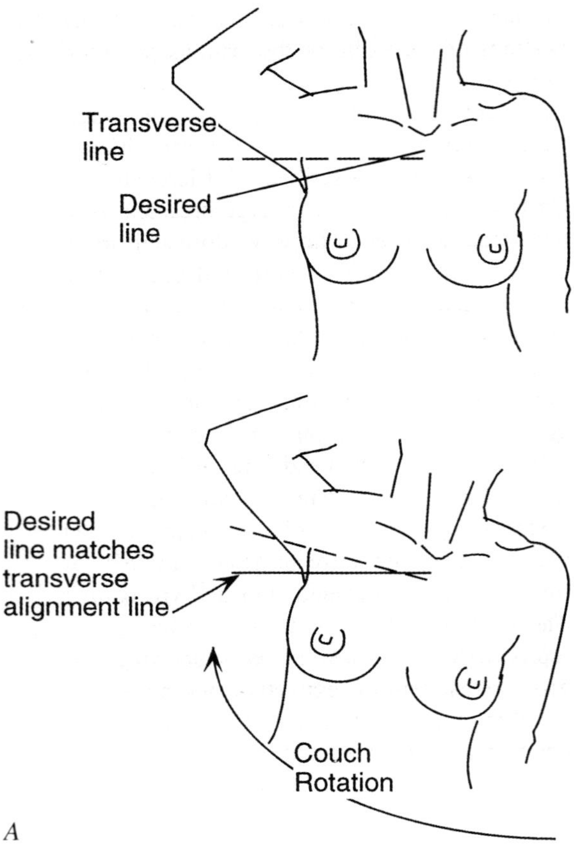

A

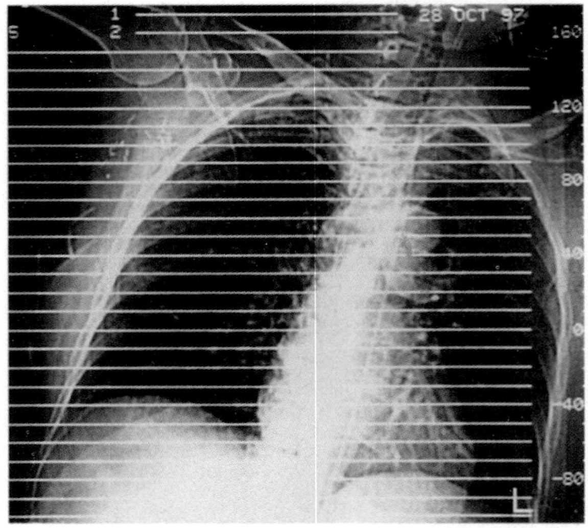

B

Fig. 8-10 *A* and *B*. Traditionally, the cephalad margin of the tangential fields traverses the chest perpendicular to the patient's midline. In some patients where the breast lies high on the chest or the patient is unable to raise the arm sufficiently for tangential fields to clear the arm and axilla, the couch can be turned until the breast is included while the arm/axilla are excluded (*desired line*). The desired cephalad tangential field margin is now aligned with the transverse line.

In some patients, breast tissues may extend over the supraclavicular fossa; thus, inclusion of the entire breast within tangential fields may be impossible even when the nonzero couch angle is used. However, the most cephalad portion of the breast would usually be included with a supraclavicular field. When a supraclavicular field is not contemplated and irradiation of this portion of the breast is clinically indicated, it can be treated via an *en face* electron field.

An alternative to the neutral couch angle is to purposely place the patient (preferably in a positioning device) at an angle on the couch, as is necessary on the CT table, where couch angles are not possible. Turning the patient a few degrees on the couch rather than turning the couch is more difficult to reproduce unless reliable sagittal alignment marks can be made on the positioning device and/or the patient's skin.

In rare situations, it may be necessary to treat patients with breast cancer in the erect position, especially when the patient is morbidly obese with large, pendulous breasts (Fig. 8-11). For the patient shown in Fig. 8-11, a sitting position was found to be the most satisfactory, though not ideal. A Styrofoam* "tray," attached by a strap around the chest, was used to separate the breast from the abdominal surface and to elevate the breast. The enormous difficulties encountered with this patient's pendulous breast can be appreciated by observing the contralateral breast.

*Dow Chemical, Midland, Michigan.

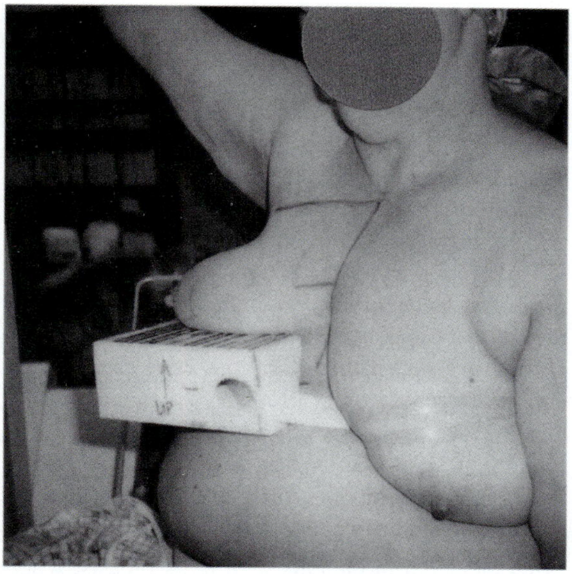

Fig. 8-11 Large-breasted and/or obese patients may benefit from being treated in an upright position. This patient was treated while sitting on the treatment couch—not an ideal position, but for this patient the optimal solution. To separate the breast from the abdominal surface, the breast was supported by a Styrofoam "tray" attached by a strap around the chest.

Prone and decubitus treatment positions have been described for patients with large, pendulous breasts. These positions are described below.

BREAST POSITION

Patients irradiated with an intact breast often require consideration of the breast position on the involved side; in some patients, it may also be necessary to displace the uninvolved breast away from the radiation fields. This is especially true for patients with large, pendulous, or flaccid breasts, who often present difficulties due to the presence of skin folds and/or an unusual breast position. It is important to recognize that a *large patient* is not always synonymous with a *large breast,* and vice versa. Large or flaccid breasts frequently lie too far lateral on the chest for tangential fields to include them without also including a large volume of lung tissue.[3] In other patients, the breast may be too high (cephalad) to treat with tangential fields without also including portions of the axilla or the arm, as previously addressed.

To solve some of these problems, alternative patient positions and methods of repositioning the breast have been described.[3–6] Merchant and McCormick describe treating large-breasted patients in the prone position to improve dose uniformity. Patients are placed prone on a platform on the treatment couch with the breast and a portion of the chest wall protruding through an aperture in the platform (Fig. 8-12).[5] Cross et al. describe breast treatment in the decubitus position with the breast against the couch top and the arm on the involved side raised above the head (Fig. 8-13).[4] The torso is rolled slightly on the couch to shift the contralateral breast away from the radiation beam. The patient's position is supported by an Alpha Cradle™* and the treated breast is molded into a Styrofoam cutout. The authors surmise that this position offers good reproducibility; however, no supporting data are given. Treatment of regional lymph nodes and field matching with the patient in the decubitus or prone position have not been addressed.

Another technique, used at Duke University since 1991, places the patient in the supine position with a

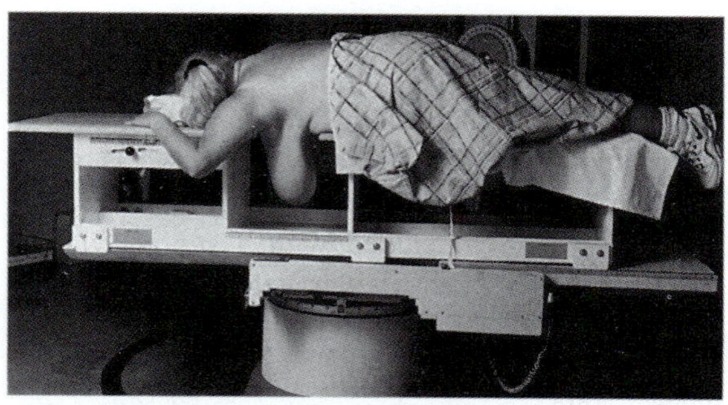

Fig. 8-12 Patient treated in the prone position on a platform facilitating unobstructed gravitational shift of the breast. The breast and a portion of the chest wall protrudes through an opening in the platform. (Courtesy of Nuclear Associates, Carle Place, New York.)

*Smithers Medical Products, Inc., North Canton, Ohio.

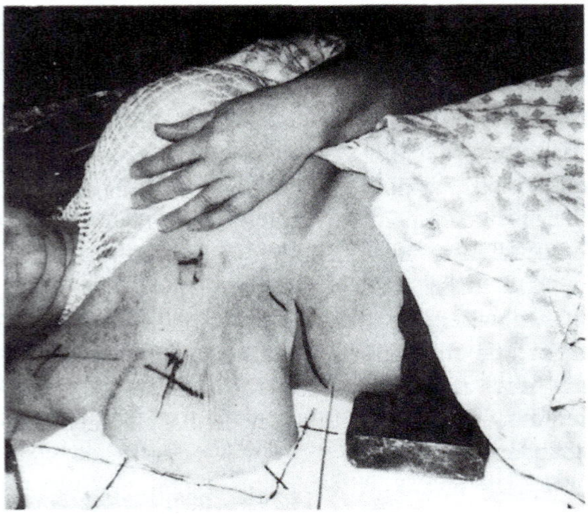

Fig. 8-13 Patient treated in decubitus position with the breast, molded to a Styrofoam cutout, on the couch top. The torso is rolled slightly to shift the contralateral breast away from the tangential fields. (From Cross et al.,[4] reprinted with permission of Elsevier Science, Inc., New York.)

breast-positioning ring (Fig. 8-14) that is used to move the breast to a more central position on the chest.[3] This ring also reduces skin folds commonly seen in large-breasted women as well as the volume of lung/heart in the tangential fields. This method is described in more detail below. Use of a thermoplastic mask to place the breast in the desired position and to displace the uninvolved breast away from the radiation fields has also been described (Fig. 8-15).[6,7] With this approach, care should be taken to assure that the thermoplastic mask does not flatten the breast, thereby making it wider and possibly aggravating the problem.

The need to lower the breast on the chest wall occurs most frequently in patients with large breasts. Elevation of the upper torso, taking advantage of gravity, may lower the breast to a more caudal position on the chest wall. However, a lowered pendulous breast may touch the abdominal surface, thus creating a skin fold. When a radiation beam traverses a skin fold, its skin-sparing effects are reduced. Thus, skin reaction (moist desquamation) is often observed in patients with large breasts, where skin folds are common. Utilization of the breast-positioning ring and/or placing Styrofoam pieces (or the "popcorn" used in packing) in skin folds to separate the surfaces may reduce the skin reaction. In patients where the cephalad portion of the breast cannot be included in tangential fields and irradiation of the entire breast is clinically indicated, the excluded portion may be irradiated via a planned supraclavicular/axillary field or an *en face* electron field.

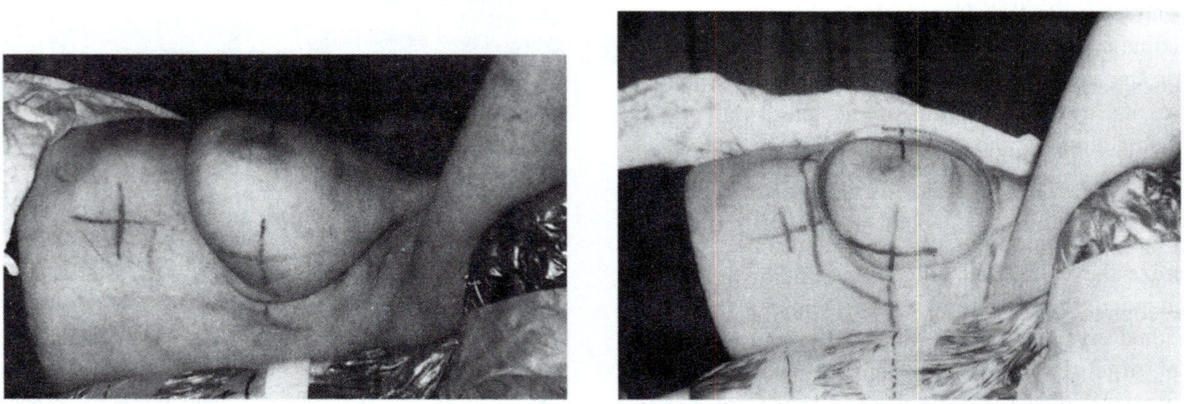

Fig. 8-14 A breast that lies too far lateral (*left*) can be moved to a more central position on the chest wall by placing a polyvinyl ring, supported by a strap, around the base of the breast (*right*). The breast position is adjusted by tightening or loosening the strap.

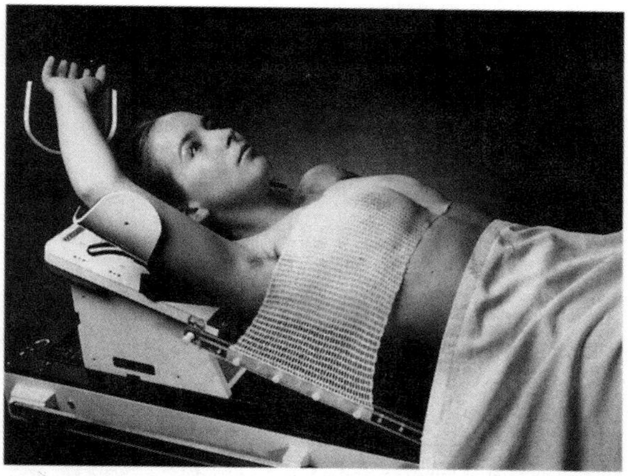

Fig. 8-15 A thermoplastic mask can be used to reposition the breast in desired position and to move the contralateral breast farther from the radiation beam. (Courtesy of MED-TEC, Inc., Orange City, Iowa.)

IMMOBILIZATION

The orientation of multiple matched fields from different directions onto an irregularly shaped surface such as the breast/neck region is complex and requires care and repositioning aids. Small repositioning discrepancies can result in overlap at the junction between fields or exclusion of target tissues. A small misalignment of the patient with the sagittal alignment line can cause the internal mammary field to be misaligned with the sternum; hence, the abutting tangential and supraclavicular fields also become misaligned. When the patient's body is rotated on the sagittal axis and the fields are set to the skin marks, the deep margin of the tangential fields is changed; thus the thickness of lung shadow observed on port films varies. When the internal mammary lymph nodes are included in the tangential fields, the margin is often small in order to minimize the volume of lung tissue and/or the need to avoid the contralateral breast. Thus, a small rotational error (patient or gantry) can cause exclusion of target tissue or inadvertent inclusion of the contralateral breast.[8] The ability to reposition patients treated for breast cancer is therefore extremely important.

POSITIONING AND IMMOBILIZATION DEVICES

Arm Board. An arm-positioning board, consisting of an L-shaped aluminum or Plexiglas support with an adjustable hand grip, can be used to support the patient's elevated arm (Fig. 8-16). The horizontal, flat portion of the board is placed under the chest and upper arm on the involved side and the perpendicular portion with the hand grip extends upward along the lower arm. This board, when placed under the chest, tends to rotate the torso, is frequently the cause of gantry collisions, and usually does not fit through a CT aperture. For these reasons, the use of this device has largely been abandoned.

Breast Boards. A popular positioning device used for patients undergoing breast irradiation is referred to as a *breast board* (Fig. 8-17). The variations in the design of breast boards are too numerous to be outlined in this text; thus, only the basic principles will be described. A breast board usually consists of an acrylic base plate under the chest and head. Attached to this base plate is a head support,

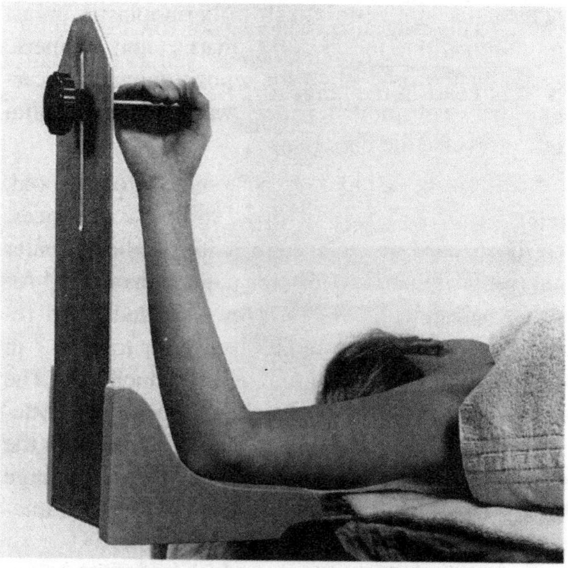

Fig. 8-16 An L-shaped arm board with a hand grip to support the extended arm and hand. (Courtesy of Smithers Medical Products, Inc., North Canton, Ohio, and Van Arsdale Innovative Products, Inc., Pensacola, Florida.)

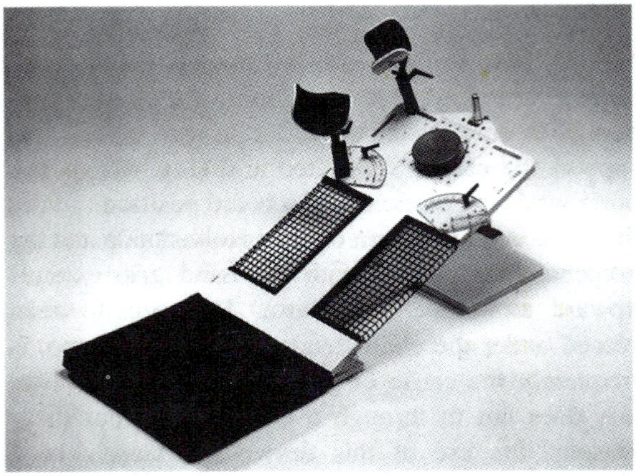

Fig. 8-17 A breast board featuring adjustable arm and head supports, removable replacement panels for tangential fields, and facilitating a chest tilt. (Courtesy of MED-TEC, Inc., Orange City, Iowa.)

with or without a hand grip for the elevated arm or arms. The arm supports can be adjusted in terms of location, rotation, and height to each particular patient's need. Most breast boards also offer the capability of elevating the upper torso. Other variables include the ability to attach a thermoplastic breast immobilization mask, grid marks and numeric scales on the base plate for repositioning, and carbon-fiber replacement panels where the tangential fields traverse the base plate.

Positioning Mold. A customized foam mold, extending from above the head to below the knees, has been used at Duke University Medical Center since approximately 1991 for patients irradiated for breast cancer (Fig. 8-18). This extended mold replaced an upper-torso mold, used prior to 1991,[9] in the hope that it would improve reproducibility. The tight-fitting mold is an excellent repositioning device that allows alignment marks to be made on the it—an important consideration in treating a large breast, where skin marks can move several centimeters and therefore are relatively unreliable.

The extended positioning device consists of a Styrofoam shell that roughly matches the shape of the patient (Fig. 8-19), foaming agents, and a polyvinyl bag. The base plate of the shell is approximately 5 ft long, 2 ft wide, and about 1 in. thick. Before the mold is actually made, the patient, undressed above the waist and in a hospital gown open at the back, lies down on the base plate in treatment position to assess the needed arm elevation, chest elevation, and head rotation. Several pieces of Styrofoam are fastened to the base plate to support the patient's position and form barriers to prevent the expanding foam from escaping. These pieces of

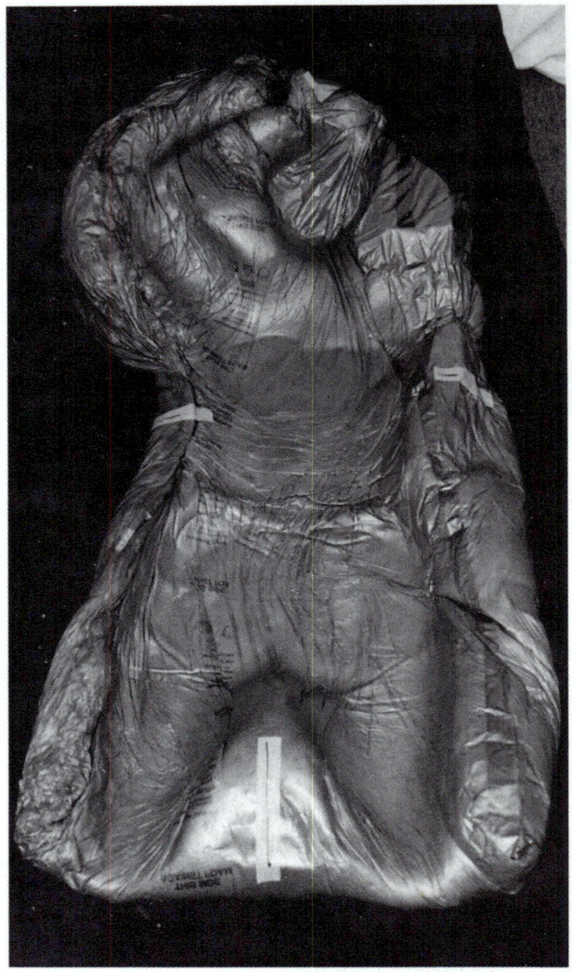

Fig. 8-18 A customized positioning mold, used for patients undergoing breast irradiation, extends from above the head and raised arm to the knees. A handle aids in reproducing the arm elevation and relaxing the patient. The sagittal alignment line is marked above the head and between the knees.

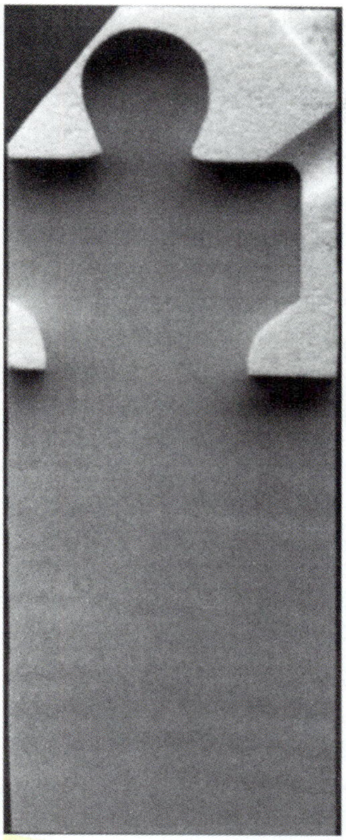

Fig. 8-19 The shell used for building the extended mold for breast patients. (Courtesy of Smithers Medical Products, Inc, North Canton, Ohio.)

Styrofoam become an integral part of the finished positioning device (i.e., they cannot be removed). The position of each piece of Styrofoam is determined with the patient in the shell but without the foam.

A retaining wall of Styrofoam is added to each side of the base plate to contain the foam in close proximity to the patient's torso. A small rectangle of Styrofoam (approximately 2 × 4 × 1 in.) is fastened to the base plate between the patient's knees. This aids in forming an elevation between the knees on which the sagittal alignment line is later marked. Optionally, a small triangular Styrofoam piece can be placed under each knee to reduce the stress on the patient's lower back. In patients requiring a chest tilt, an angled piece of Styrofoam is placed inside the shell to provide the desired tilt. A cylindrical piece of Styrofoam, approximately 3 in. long and 1 in. in diameter, is placed in a separate small (3- to 4-gal) bag attached to the shell where the patient's raised arm and hand will be positioned. This piece of Styrofoam forms a handle for the patient to hold onto during each treatment and aids in reproducing the arm elevation from treatment to treatment. This bag needs to be fixed to the shell to prevent shifts that would lead to altered arm position. The fixation can be achieved by taping the bag to the shell, pouring a small amount of foam between the shell and the bag, or making a few pinholes in the bag to allow a small amount of the foam to leak out onto the shell to expand and set, forming an adhesion. The purpose of the smaller bag is to contain the foaming chemicals near the handle.[9]

With the patient removed, each piece of Styrofoam is fastened to the base plate, using masking tape. A section of the base plate is removed on the ipsilateral side to allow visualization of the lateral tangential field on the skin and to prevent the radiation beam from traversing the mold. In other sites, radiation beams often traverse the mold with minimal adverse effects. However, in breast irradiation, skin sparing is already compromised by the tangential beam path; thus measures should be taken to prevent further reduction of skin sparing in these patients.

The Styrofoam shell is placed inside the large polyvinyl bag and approximately 600 mL of foaming chemicals, after being mixed and prepared as directed, is poured into the shell inside the protective bag. Approximately 50 mL of the foam is poured into the smaller bag with the Styrofoam handle. The foam should be generously distributed near the elevated arm to form an effective arm support. The foam is then evenly distributed on each side of the patient's torso and between the knees. To prevent the foam from rising more than a couple of inches where the tangential fields are anticipated, the polyvinyl bag is taped down in this area. With only a small barrier in this region, the lateral tangential field can usually be visualized and does not intercept the foam.

After the air is allowed to circulate inside the bag for a few seconds, it is squeezed out, the bag is sealed, and the device is placed at the foot end of the couch. The patient is returned to the shell by first standing on a stepping stool at the end of the couch and then sitting down into the shell. The shell, with the patient in it, is then moved to the center of the couch and the patient assumes the treatment position. The foam expands inside the bag and fills the space between the shell and the patient's body. The cylinder, forming the handle inside the smaller bag, and some of the foam are guided into the patient's hand. The hospital gown is pulled up from under the patient such that the patient lies directly on the polyvinyl bag. It is important to make sure that the patient feels that she is lying flat and straight. A visual registration of the patient's straightness should also be made by the staff. (This can also be done by fluoroscopy if available.) The polyvinyl bag is pulled up between the knees to allow the foam to expand and form an elevation for the sagittal alignment mark. The height of this elevation should be based on the patient's agility, as some patients may need to lift themselves over it when entering and leaving the mold for each treatment.

To make an effective mold, it is important that the polyvinyl bag be about 2 ft longer and 2 ft wider than the shell to allow space for the foam to expand without being restricted by the bag. Masking tape, fastened to each side of the shell and stretched anteriorly across the patient, forces the foam medially toward the patient, forming a tight-fitting mold. To produce a tight-fitting mold, it is important that the patient wear minimal clothing during the fabrication. Patients' clothing usually varies during the treatment course, causing the mold to be too tight one day and too loose on another day; either situation compromises repositioning ability. The foam stops expanding after approximately 7 to 10 min but requires an additional 10 min to become firm.

A flat hardwood board, wider and longer than the mold, is placed on top of the couch *before* the fabrication is initiated to prevent leaking foam from forming a lip over the couch. Such a lip or other irregular surface under the mold can cause the immobilization device to tilt, potentially giving rise to field misalignments.

Breast-Immobilization Devices. A polyvinyl ring, wrapped around the base of the breast and fastened to a Velcro* strap around the chest, is used to reposition the breast on the chest wall (Fig. 8-20). The desired breast position is accomplished by adjusting the Velcro strap.[3] In some patients, a Styrofoam barrier is fastened to the breast ring to prevent the breast from assuming a mushroom-like shape (Fig. 8-20). Such pieces of Styrofoam can also be used to adjust the breast position in the cephalad/caudal direction (Fig. 8-21) and to displace the contralateral breast farther from the radiation beams. Another method of repositioning the breast on the chest is the use of thermoplastic material (Fig. 8-2)[6] or a plastic mask.[7] Treating through a breast positioning device may reduce the skin sparing, possibly resulting in a higher incidence of moist desquamation.[7]

DISCUSSION

Except for the extended mold, immobilization devices are discussed only briefly due to the large variety of designs. Although breast boards help to reposition the patient in a given position, they offer minimal support during the treatment. Supporting the body in the treatment position may contribute to the patient's ability to relax and maintain the position. The customized mold both offers an *aid to repositioning* and *supports the patient during the treatment.* Furthermore, it offers the patient a personalized positioning device. Setup marks can be made on the immobilization device, unlike the breast board—a potentially superior alignment method, since skin marks tend to move with respect to underlying anatomy, particularly on the breast. The size of the extended mold may appear excessive. However, it has been shown that immobilizing/stabilizing the patient's body away from the treated area improves repositioning in prostate cancer and Hodgkin's disease,[10,11] and this approach is logical for breast cancer as well.

*Velcro USA, Manchester, New Hampshire.

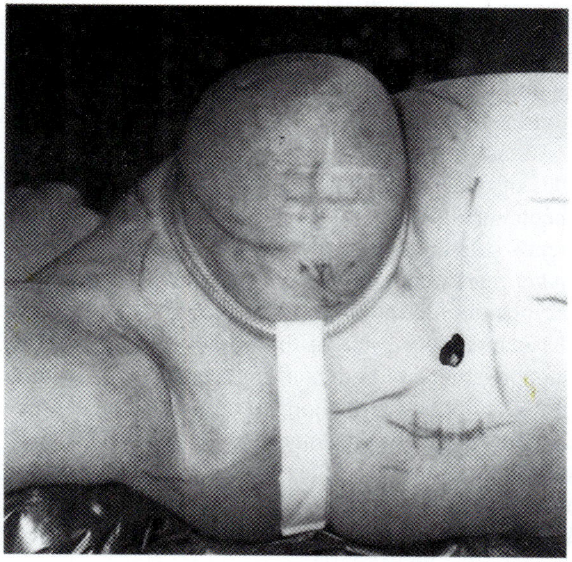

A

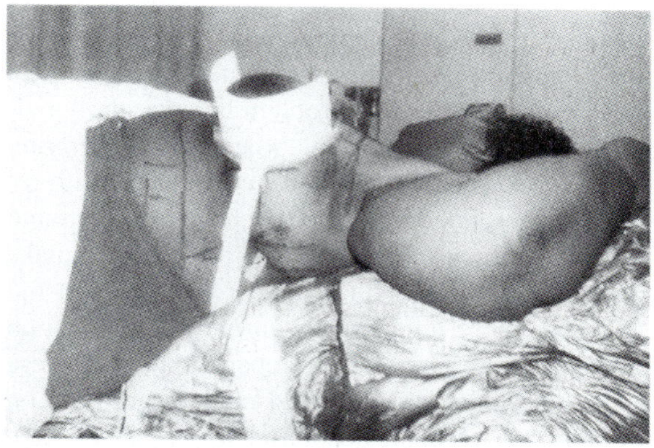

B

Fig. 8-20 *A*. Breast-positioning ring supported by a strap around the patient's chest. *B*. A support to prevent the breast from assuming a "mushroom-like" shape can be made from a piece of Styrofoam fastened to the positioning ring.

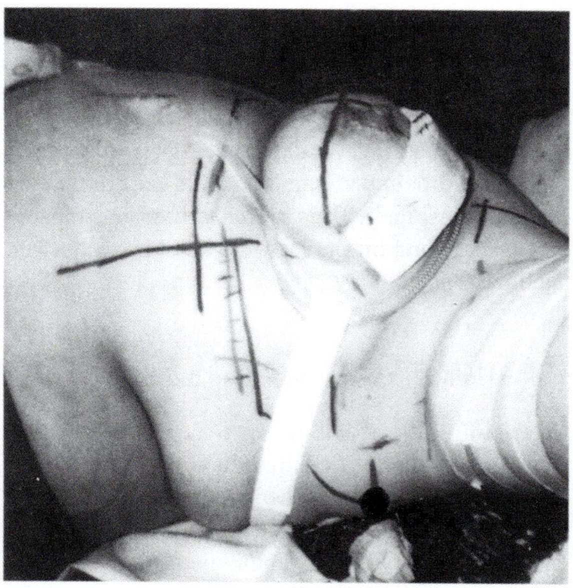

Fig. 8-21 The breast may be shifted caudally by taping a piece of Styrofoam to the breast-positioning ring and such that caudal traction is exerted.

Some caution should be used with regard to the loss of skin sparing when the beam traverses devices, since skin sparing may be already compromised by the tangential beam path. The lightweight material in the mold does not appear to have an adverse effect on the skin; however, the possibility of the beam traversing the foam should be minimized. The customized device is lightweight and strong, and it does not break when accidentally dropped.

The use of the breast-positioning ring does not appear to have an adverse acute or late effect on the irradiated breast tissues, although this is difficult to assess. In a review of 56 patients irradiated and using the positioning ring, 60.7% had moist desquamation, most commonly in the inframammary fold. Of 45 patients who were followed for a year or more, all reported good or excellent cosmetic results.[12] Surface dose under two polyvinyl breast-positioning rings with the same inner diameter (1/4 in.) but with different outer dimensions (7/16 and 6/16 in.) was measured using 6-MV photons. The surface dose was 85 and 80% of the D_{max} dose for the larger and smaller rings, respectively, compared with 35% for an open field.

SETUP MARKS

In most areas of the human body, skin moves over underlying tissues; thus, setup marks on the skin may be unreliable. This problem is particularly evident in the breast region, where skin overlying breast tissues can move several centimeters with respect to the underlying chest wall. In the treatment of an intact breast, it is therefore important to make setup marks on the skin distant from the breast tissues and, more importantly, on the immobilization device. When there is a discrepancy between these marks, the marks on the mold rather than those on the skin are used. In postmastectomy patients, the chest-wall skin is usually firm and setup marks on the chest wall are relatively reliable.

Prior to each treatment, it is essential that the patient be aligned on the couch in precisely the same position as during simulation. This is true for any treatment but is stressed in breast treatment, where compound angles are often used. Alignment marks, used only for the purpose of aligning the patient (positioning mold) on the couch, are therefore made after positioning the patient on the simulator couch and prior to simulation. The sagittal alignment line is marked on the positioning mold above the head and between the knees and on the chest. The transverse alignment line is marked on the right and left sides of the mold and on the patient's skin (Fig. 8-1). To ensure freedom from patient rotation along the sagittal axis, a coronal (horizontal) alignment mark is made on each side on the mold and on the patient's chest. Since a portion of the mold is removed for the tangential fields, the marks on the ipsilateral side are marked on the mold cephalad, caudal, and posterior to the opening (Fig. 8-22). On the contralateral side, the patient's arm is briefly moved to facilitate marking. These marks, used to align the patient correctly on the couch prior to simulation and treatment, *do not* represent the isocenter. Instead, these marks are made at a location where the skin appears relatively immobile. This aspect of the treatment is essential for treatment accuracy, as a misalignment of the patient on the couch has the same effect as a couch, gantry, or collimator rotation.

Breast treatment usually requires compound angles of couch, gantry and collimator, causing alignment lines and treatment fields to intercept the patient's skin in many locations. This usually results in many marks being made both on the patient and on the positioning mold. To reduce the risks of confusing marks, only some of these lines may be marked and different colored marking pens may be used. For example, for the tangential fields, where the couch is turned to prevent divergence into the supraclavicular field, the lines indicating the isocenter when the couch is in the neutral position only may be marked. Since the isocenters of tangential fields are usually off the midline, extending and marking the sagittal setup line on the mold caudally may require briefly moving the patient's leg out of the mold. Cranially, this line can be marked on the mold above the shoulder and on the skin surface caudal to the breast, where skin often is less mobile. Since alignment systems often are less accurate away from the isocenter, marks made at a distance—e.g., above the head and between the knees—should be made with the point to be marked close to the machine isocenter. This is accomplished by moving the couch in toward the gantry for marking caudally and out for marking cephalad. Although alignment marks are often made on the breast, these lines are usually also indicated on the mold and on the less mobile skin away from the breast.

TREATMENT ACCURACY

Determining reproducibility of treatment fields used for breast irradiation is extremely difficult. Inconsistencies between the planned treatment (simulation radiograph) and the actual treatment (port film), often reported for the tangential fields only, can be caused by rotation of the patient's torso as well as by translational errors and respiratory motion.[13] Determination of setup reproducibility is often based

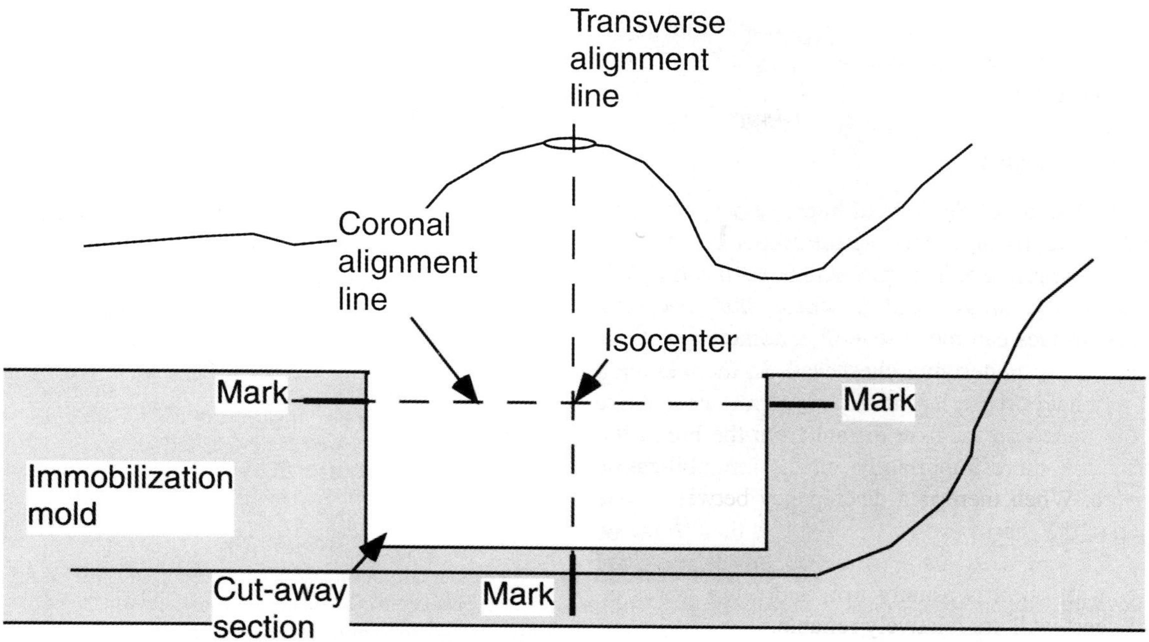

Fig. 8-22 Since a portion of the mold is removed for the tangential fields, three alignment marks can be made on the mold distant to the isocenter (cephalad, caudal, and posterior).

on measurements related only to the ventral/dorsal position of the tangential fields with respect to the lung and external breast tissue. However, it is important to recognize that a cephalad/caudal shift of the tangential fields may also cause a change in the ventral/dorsal distances (Fig. 8-19). Measurements are usually obtained on a plane through the central axis of the beams and, in some reports, also near the cephalad and caudal margins. These measurements, obtained at a fixed point with respect to the fields rather than to the patient, usually describe the position of the "deep" field margin with respect to the lung and external surface shadows. However, a field shift in the cephalad/caudal direction only may cause these distances to appear different because the field now lies over a different portion of the curving lung shadow and a different region of the irregularly shaped breast tissue (Fig. 8-23).

Numerous authors have shown that uncertainties exist in the position of patients undergoing tangential breast irradiation.[7,14–21] Creutzberg et al. found that the ventral border of the breast in the ventral/dorsal direction yielded variations of 3.2 and 4.6 mm, respectively, with and without a breast-positioning mask. Westbrook et al. found similar measurements to be within ±5 mm in 88% of all cases. In a report by Carter et al., the height of the lung shadow, measured on the central axis plane, was within 3 mm of that prescribed (simulator radiograph) in 42% of 172 port films studied and in error by more than 10 mm in 6% among patients treated in the extended mold described above.[14]

In a study by Das et al., where the patients underwent a second simulation procedure (mock treatment), the frequency of variations in the setup parameters between the second simulation and treatment was significantly reduced from the changes that occurred between the first and second simulation in 95% of the patients.[15] Das et al. also studied the effect of setup errors on the dose distributions; isocenter shifts up to ±1.0 cm changed the dose by ±2%, while gantry variations up to ±4° produced a

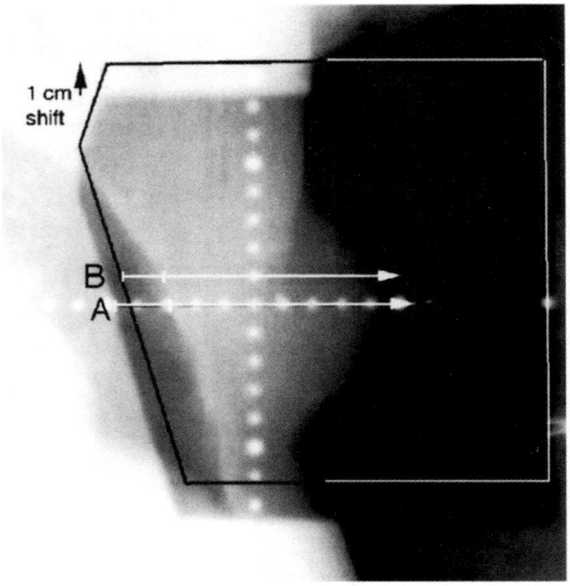

Fig. 8-23 Setup reproducibility of tangential fields is usually determined by measuring the ventral/dorsal distances from the deep field margin to the lung contour and the external breast tissues. These distances may change when the field position is in error in the cephalad/caudal direction only (*hatched lines*), leading to the erroneous conclusion that the field misalignment was in the ventral/dorsal direction.

change less than ±5% of the dose within the target. This variation of gantry angle resulted in additional tissue irradiation outside the desired field of about 10 cm^3 in a large patient. A gantry angle variation of ±6° produced a change in the volume of tissue that receives the prescribed dose by at least ±10%.[15]

Uncertainties in repositioning of patients undergoing breast irradiation cannot be eliminated, although the use of improved patient immobilization methods may be prudent.

REFERENCES

1. Gagliardi G, Lax I, Rutqvist LE: Radiation therapy of stage I breast cancer: Analysis of treatment technique accuracy using three-dimensional treatment planning tools. *Radiother Oncol* 24:94–101, 1992.
2. Siddon RL, Buck BA, Harris JR, Svensson GK: Three-field technique for breast irradiation using tangential field corner blocks. *Int J Radiat Oncol Biol Phys* 9:583–588, 1983.
3. Bentel GC, Marks LB: A simple device to position large/flaccid breasts during tangential breast irradiation. *Int J Radiat Oncol Biol Phys* 29:879, 1994.
4. Cross MA, Elson HR, Aron BS: Breast conservation radiation therapy technique for women with large breasts. *Int J Radiat Oncol Biol Phys* 17:199–203, 1989.
5. Merchant TE, McCormick B: Prone position breast irradiation. *Int J Radiat Oncol Biol Phys* 30:197–202, 1994.
6. Zierhut D, Flentje M, Frank C, et al: Conservative treatment of breast cancer: Modified irradiation technique for women with large breasts. *Radiother Oncol* 31:256–261, 1994.
7. Creutzberg AL, Althof VG, Huizenga H, Visser AG: Quality assurance using portal imaging: The accuracy of patient positioning in irradiation of breast cancer. *Int J Radiat Oncol Biol Phys* 25:529–539, 1993.
8. Warlick WB, O'Rear JH, Earley L, et al: Dose to the contralateral breast: A comparison of two techniques using the enhanced dynamic wedge versus a standard wedge. *Med Dosim* 22:185–191, 1997.
9 Bentel GC: Positioning and immobilization device for patients receiving radiation therapy for carcinoma of the breast. *Med Dosim* 15:3, 1990.
10. Bentel GC, Marks LB, Sherouse GW, et al: The effectiveness of immobilization during prostate irradiation. *Int J Radiat Oncol Biol Phys* 31:143–148, 1995.
11. Bentel GC, Marks LB, Krishnamurthy R, Prosnitz LR: Comparison of two repositioning devices used during radiation therapy for Hodgkin's disease. *Int J Radiat Oncol Biol Phys* 39:791–795, 1997.
12. Bentel GC, Marks LB, Whiddon CS, Prosnitz LR: Acute and late morbidity of radiation therapy in women with large pendulous breasts treated with a breast positioning ring. (abstr). *Int J Radiat Oncol Biol Phys* 39(suppl 2): 267, 1997.
13. Bonetta A, Zingoni A, Lambertini D, et al: Radiotherapy of the breast: Changes in the volume of the lung covered in the treatment fields and resulting changes in dose distribution. *Radiol Med* 92:634–637, 1996.
14. Carter DL, Marks LB, Bentel GC: Impact of setup variability on incidental lung irradiation during tangential breast irradiation. *Int J Radiat Oncol Biol Phys* 38: 109–115, 1997.
15. Das IJ, Cheng CW, Fosmire H, et al: Tolerances in setup and dosimetric errors in the radiation treatment of breast cancer. *Int J Radiat Oncol Biol Phys* 26:883–890, 1993.
16. Fein DA, McGee KP, Schultheiss TE, et al: Intra- and interfractional reproducibility of tangential breast fields: A prospective on-line portal imaging study. *Int J Radiat Oncol Biol Phys* 30(suppl 1):230, 1994.
17. McGee KP, Fein DA, Hanlon AL, et al: The value of setup portal films as an estimate of a patient's position throughout fractionated tangential breast irradiation: An on-line study. *Int J Radiat Oncol Biol Phys* 37:223–228, 1997.

18. Pouliot J, Lirette A: Verification and correction of setup deviations in tangential breast irradiation using EPID: Gain versus workload. *Med Phys* 23:1393–1398, 1996.
19. Valdagni R, Italia C: Early breast cancer irradiation after conservative surgery: Quality control by portal localization films. *Radiother Oncol* 22:311, 1991.
20. van Tienhoven G, Lanson JH, Crabeels D, et al: Accuracy in tangential breast treatment set-up: A portal imaging study. *Radiother Oncol* 22:317–322, 1991.
21. Westbrook C, Gildersleve J, Yarnold J: Quality assurance in daily treatment procedure: Patient movement during tangential field treatment. *Radiother Oncol* 22:299, 1991.

PROBLEMS

8-1 The usual position for breast treatment is
(*a*) supine with the contralateral arm raised and head turned toward the affected side
(*b*) supine with the ipsilateral arm raised and the head turned away from the affected side
(*c*) supine with both arms raised and the head straight
(*d*) supine with the ipsilateral arm raised and the head turned toward the affected side

8-2 The angle of arm elevation depends on
(*a*) the patient's ability to elevate the arm and the angle of the medial tangential field
(*b*) the angle of the medial tangential field and the ability to move through the CT aperture
(*c*) the patient's ability to raise the arm and the amount of skin folds in the supraclavicular area
(*d*) all of the above
(*e*) none of the above

8-3 The "deep" margin of tangential fields approximates the lung contour in the beam's-eye view when
(*a*) the patient lies flat on the couch and the collimator is turned a few degrees
(*b*) the patient's chest is elevated at an angle and the collimator is not turned
(*c*) the patient lies on a flat couch or is elevated and a customized lung-shielding block is used
(*d*) all of the above
(*e*) none of the above

8-4 The neutral couch angle is the angle necessary for
(*a*) the supraclavicular field to include the most cephalad portion of the breast tissue
(*b*) the transverse alignment line to transect between the breast and the axilla
(*c*) achieving a "perfect" geometric match between tangential and supraclavicular fields
(*d*) achieving a "perfect" geometric match between tangential and axillary fields

8-5 Patients undergoing irradiation for breast cancer can be treated
(*a*) in supine or lithotomy position
(*b*) in supine position only
(*c*) in prone position only
(*d*) in supine, prone, or decubitus position

8-6 During breast irradiation, the breast position
(*a*) is always acceptable
(*b*) can be adjusted by using a thermoplastic mask or a breast-positioning ring
(*c*) is always lowered (caudal) by elevating the patient's chest
(*d*) is always acceptable if the patient is treated in an erect position

8-7 Skin folds can be reduced or eliminated by
(*a*) placing a piece of Styrofoam or "popcorns" used in packing in the folds
(*b*) having the patient turn slightly to the side
(*c*) having the patient raise the arm up higher
(*d*) moving the other breast farther away from the beam

8-8 Positioning molds for breast cancer treatment
(*a*) are unnecessary because setup marks on the breast are very reliable
(*b*) are beneficial because setup marks can be made on the device
(*c*) are unnecessary because these patients are easy to reposition
(*d*) are beneficial because they help patients to relax and the positions are reproducible
(*e*) (*a*) and (*b*) are true
(*f*) (*a*), (*c*), and (*d*) are true
(*g*) (*b*) and (*d*) are true
(*h*) (*a*) and (*c*) are true

8-9 In making a positioning mold
(*a*) the foam never touches the patient's skin
(*b*) the polyvinyl bag should be much larger than the shell
(*c*) the foam needs to be guided into the hand and on each side of the raised arm
(*d*) all of the above
(*e*) none of the above

8-10 When patients are simulated for breast treatment
(*a*) only lines indicating the alignment on the couch, isocenters, and treatment fields (tangential fields in neutral position only) should be marked
(*b*) using different colored marking pens is a good idea
(*c*) setup lines should be extended and marked distant to the breast
(*d*) all of the above
(*e*) none of the above

8-11 In determining setup accuracy of tangential fields
(*a*) only ventral/dorsal shifts are important
(*b*) only cephalad/caudal shifts are important
(*c*) a cephalad/caudal shift can appear as a ventral/dorsal shift
(*d*) ventral/dorsal shifts are usually larger than cephalad/caudal shifts

8-12 Field misplacements can occur because
(*a*) skin marks have shifted
(*b*) the patient's torso is "rolled" around the sagittal axis
(*c*) the patient is not aligned correctly on the couch
(*d*) all of the above
(*e*) none of the above

8-13 Errors in field placement
(*a*) have no impact on dose distribution
(*b*) have no impact on the amount of dose
(*c*) are of no concern because discrepancies in dose distribution are compensated for in the next treatment
(*d*) all of the above
(*e*) none of the above

8-14 Patients with breast cancer are

(*a*) easy to treat because they are always treated with tangential fields only and they always have small breasts or have had a mastectomy

(*b*) difficult to treat because field matching is complex and the breast size and position vary

(*c*) difficult to treat because they are always treated with tangential, supraclavicular, axillary, and internal mammary fields and they always have lots of skin folds

(*d*) easy to treat because they can always raise the arm sufficiently and maintain the position without support.

CHAPTER

9

Pelvis and Abdomen

INTRODUCTION

The most commonly irradiated diseases in the lower abdomen and pelvis are gynecologic, prostate, and colorectal carcinoma. Other tumors irradiated in this region include bladder cancer, lymphoma, sarcoma, and bone metastases.

Normal tissue sparing, a common concern in radiation therapy, is critical in the pelvis, where cancerocidal doses often are higher than the tolerance of neighboring normal organs. For example, in the treatment of uterine cervix carcinoma, doses in excess of 80 Gy are often required, far exceeding the tolerance of the neighboring rectal mucosa. A large fraction of this dose is therefore delivered via intracavitary brachytherapy, limiting the dose to the rectum. In the treatment of prostate carcinoma, where the doses usually exceed rectal tolerance, it is nearly impossible to irradiate the target without also including the anterior rectal wall. In this setting it is critical to minimize the *volume* of rectal mucosa within the high-dose region.

Immobilization is always important for setup reproducibility. In many pelvic treatments, as for gynecologic and rectal cancers, special immobilization devices are often not used. This may be because these fields are often large; however, this reasoning may be flawed. The target margins are often the same size as those in small fields, thus requiring the same treatment accuracy. Some prostate treatment techniques utilize very small margins, making immobilization crucial. In these techniques, treatment fields designed with three-dimensional treatment planning (3DTP) tools are shaped to conform to the target in the beam's-eye view (BEV) to minimize rectal volume (Fig. 9-1). More elaborate treatment techniques include intensity-modulated radiation therapy (IMRT), which attempts to conform the high-dose region to the geometry of the target in three dimensions while excluding all of the rectal mucosa from the high-dose region. With IMRT, the dose "intensity" within each field is intentionally varied depending on what tissues lie within the beam.[1,2] In areas within a treatment field where the target (prostate) and a dose-limiting organ (rectum) are superimposed in the beam's-eye view, a lower dose is delivered. The lower dose delivered to this portion of the prostate is compensated for by increasing the dose to this region from another beam direction whose trajectory does not include the rectum. In this fashion, using multiple beams, the dose to the rectum is reduced and uniform high doses are delivered to the prostate. Variations in dose intensity are achieved either by inserting a beam attenuator of varying thickness (compensator) within the field or by using dynamic or static multileaf collimation, where the dose is varied by moving the leaves in and out of the field. Intensity-modulated radiation therapy is clearly sensitive to setup accuracy and requires effective immobilization methods.

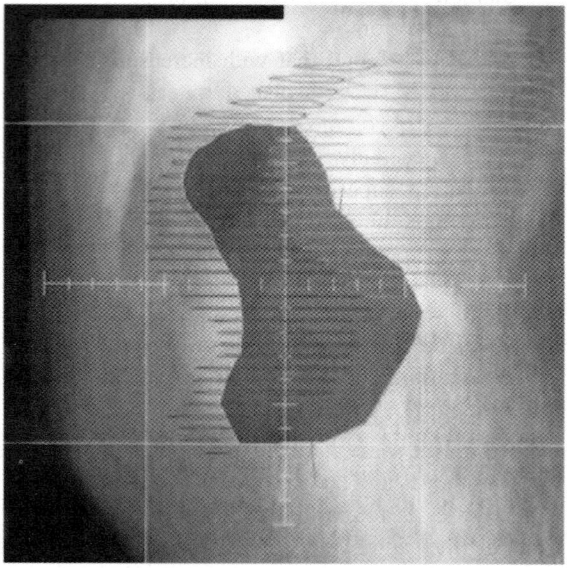

Fig. 9-1 Digitally reconstructed radiograph of a conformal lateral prostate treatment field.

The use of conformal target-dose distributions has raised concerns regarding the ability to accurately and reproducibly deliver the intended dose to the target and the clinical implications of failure to do so.[3] Because of variations in registration of the radiation field with respect to the target, the dose received by the target and adjacent normal organs may not be as planned. Such variations may be due to a number of sources, including errors in patient positioning or field placement as well as organ motion relative to bony structures and/or skin marks used to register the field position. Failure to appreciate the extent of disease is another source of treatment uncertainty. Because treatment plans are almost invariably based upon only one computed tomography (CT) scan session done prior to treatment, motion of the target within the body can lead to systematic errors throughout the course of treatment, resulting in underdosage to the target and an overdose to the adjacent normal tissues. Therefore it is critical to fully understand the extent of target and normal organ motion when delivering high doses of radiation using small margins.

ORGAN MOTION AND DISPLACEMENT

Organ *motion* in the pelvis and lower abdomen appears intimately related to the fullness of the bladder and rectum. Such physiologic motion, where the target (e.g., prostate) may move out and normal tissues (e.g., rectum) into the radiation field during the treatment, are *undesired* and difficult to *prevent.* Desired organ *displacements,* on the other hand, can be difficult to *induce.* Such intentional displacements are sometimes attempted by changes in patient position to avoid irradiation of normal tissues (e.g., small bowel).

PROSTATE

The precise position of the prostate, bladder, and rectum is difficult to ascertain since these organs are not discernible on plain radiographs. The inner dimensions of the bladder and rectum can be visualized when filled with contrast material. The position of the prostate is presumptive without a three-dimensional imaging study such as CT. Prostate movement is often described with respect to the bladder and rectum; however, these organs may expand and contract and are thus also mobile. Bony anatomy may therefore be the most reliable reference by which prostate motion should be assessed.

In some patients, the distance between the prostate and rectum appears to be larger in the prone versus supine position.[4] Likewise, the fullness of the bladder and rectum appears to cause shifts in the prostate position. Since it is difficult to control the fullness from treatment to treatment and small tumor margins are often used in prostate irradiation, precise conformal treatment is very difficult. It is important to develop an understanding of the sources and magnitude of positional changes of the prostate and seminal vesicles so that adequate margins can be used.

Pelvic organ motion during irradiation of prostate cancer has been extensively studied (Table 9-1).[5-15] Melian et al. obtained CT scans on four different treatment days in 13 patients irradiated in the prone position for prostate cancer to assess motion of the planning target volume (PTV) related to variations of bladder and rectal fullness.[11] The average displacement (over all patients and scans) from the planning scan "center of mass" was 0.03, 0.07, and 0.04 cm in the mediolateral, anterior/posterior, and cephalad/caudal directions, respectively. The effect of the motion on the target dose was measured and found to cause a median of 6% of the PTV to receive less than 95% of the planned dose for any given treatment day.

Table 9-1 Magnitude and Direction of Prostate Motion Specified as One Standard Deviation (cm)

	Directions		
Author	Mediolateral	Anterior/ Posterior	Cephalad/ Caudal
Melian[11a]	0.12	0.40	0.31
Roeske[16]	0.07	0.39	0.32
van Herk[15]	0.09	0.27	0.17
Balter[7]	0.08	0.22	0.18
Althof[5]	0.08	0.15	0.17

[a]Prone position.

In a similar study by van Herk et al., the authors reported the standard deviation displacement of the prostate/seminal vesicles center to be 0.09, 0.27, and 0.17 cm in the mediolateral, anterior/posterior, and cephalad/caudal directions, respectively.[15] In this study, the patients were scanned and treated in the supine position. In another study by Beard et al., two sequential supine CT studies were obtained in 30 patients to quantify prostate and seminal vesicle positional changes between treatment planning and delivery.[9] Positional changes were generally small (<0.5 cm) but maximum displacements of 1.5 to 2.2 cm occurred. Bladder volume did not appear to correlate with target motion; however, rectal volume and diameter correlated with both prostate and seminal vesicle motion.

Melian et al. found that with increased rectal volume, the PTV was displaced anteriorly; with increased bladder volume, the PTV was displaced posteriorly and caudally.[11] The largest variability in the PTV occurred superior (cranial) to the base of the bladder (i.e., at the seminal vesicles). It appears possible that the superior portion of the prostate and seminal vesicles is more mobile than the remainder of the gland and more likely to move with changes in rectal and bladder filling. The investigators also observed variation in the distance between the anterior and posterior borders of the prostate, among different scan sequences of the same patient, implying that the prostate not only moves as a body but also changes shape.

Melian et al. found that the changes in PTV position in the anterior/posterior direction appeared to be equally strongly correlated with changes in both the rectal and bladder volumes.[11] Planning target-volume shifts in the cephalad/caudal direction appeared to correlate more with changes in the bladder volume than in the rectal volume. The authors postulate that in their patients treated in the prone position, the influence of the bladder on prostate position may be greater than it is in patients treated in the supine position. This may be because of more limited space for bladder expansion anteriorly, forcing the bladder to expand posteriorly and caudally.

Roeske et al. obtained weekly CT scans of 10 prostate cancer patients to document the location of the prostate, seminal vesicles, bladder, and rectum during a course of treatment.[16] Shifts of the prostate "center of mass" were minimal (<1 mm) in the mediolateral direction, while in the anterior/posterior and cephalad/caudal directions the movements ranged from 0 to ±1 cm. The movement of the seminal vesicles showed a similar trend.

Other authors have measured prostate shifts by implanting radiopaque markers in the prostate that were visible on port films.[5,7,17,18] Balter et al., in a study of 15 patients, measured prostate shifts on port films over the treatment course.[7] It yielded one standard deviation in the prostate position of 0.08, 0.22, and 0.18 cm in the mediolateral, anterior/posterior, and cephalad/caudal directions, respectively.[7] In a similar study, prostate shifts with respect to bony anatomy were assessed using seeds of iodine 125 from a permanent implant in nine patients. One standard deviation of the normal distribution function was 0.08, 0.15, and 0.17 cm in the mediolateral, anterior/posterior, and cephalad/caudal directions, respectively.[5] Anterior/posterior motion of the prostate and seminal vesicles correlated strongly with the rectal diameter over the length of these organs. Caudal enlargement of the bladder caused a posterior/caudal displacement of the prostate.

As shown by these studies, the prostate is not a static organ but rather has some limited motion in the pelvis secondary to changes in the bladder and rectal volumes. Typical prostate displacements are <5 mm. However, occasionally larger shifts may occur. The findings in the studies described above may provide a guide for placement of treatment borders and assist in determining actual dose to the target and normal structures in the vicinity.

LIVER, SPLEEN, KIDNEYS, HEPATOBILIARY TREE, AND COLON

Organ motion in the abdomen (e.g., liver, kidneys, hepatobiliary tree, colon) is related to respiratory movements, peristaltic activity,[19-26] and positional changes.[6] The focus on abdominal organ motion has been on the kidneys, due to their relative radiosensitivity. The magnitude of cephalad/caudal kidney motion, under normal and forced respiratory conditions, can be up to 35 and 86 mm, respectively.[23] Schwartz et al., using fast magnetic resonance imaging (MRI), studied kidney motion during deep inspiration and expiration in a series of 14 patients. The maximal vertical motion of the superior pole from its end-expiratory to its end-inspiratory position was 39 mm (43 mm for the inferior pole).[25] Positional changes from supine to prone caused ventral/caudal shifts of both the liver and spleen in 34 of 38 and of the kidneys in 38 of 38 patients.[6] The transverse and sigmoid colon are freely mobile except for the proximal and distal segments, while the ascending and descending colon and the hepatic and splenic flexures are relatively immobile.[22]

SMALL BOWEL

It is frequently desired to displace small bowel away from the treatment fields during pelvic irradiation due to this organ's limited tolerance. Several methods, described later in this chapter, can reduce the small bowel volume within pelvic radiation therapy fields: prone position with a false tabletop ("belly board") or abdominal wall compression and bladder distention.[27-34] Surgical displacement methods have also been used.[35-38]

Small bowel mobility may vary among patients, depending on several factors. Adhesions related to prior pelvic surgery may cause loops of small bowel to be fixed to other pelvic structures.[22] A greater incidence of relatively immobile small bowel and a larger amount of small bowel in the pelvis has been observed especially in female, thin, and elderly patients.[29] No demonstrable alteration in small bowel mobility following 40 to 46 Gy to the whole pelvis has been demonstrated.[39]

POSITION

SUPINE, PRONE, DECUBITUS, OR LITHOTOMY

The patient position used during pelvic radiation therapy depends largely on field sizes, beam directions, and the prescribed dose. In pelvic and lower abdomen irradiation, the supine and prone positions are most commonly used. However, a decubitus position is sometimes used in an effort to displace small bowel away from a lateralized abdominal field. The lithotomy position may be used when perineal fields are treated. The ability to position an elderly, ill, or postsurgical patient may be limited due to pain or lack of agility.

It is important to place the patient in a comfortable and reproducible position that allows optimal treatment to be delivered. The supine position is usually more comfortable and reproducible than prone and generally is preferred. When prone, some patients are more comfortable holding their arms above their heads. The degree of arm elevation and the side to which the head is turned are important for setup reproducibility, as variations may cause changes in the relationship between skin marks and underlying anatomy.

Gynecologic Disease. In external beam irradiation for the majority of gynecologic diseases, the whole pelvis is treated to moderate doses (45 to 50 Gy) using a four-field technique. These treatments are usually delivered with the patient in the supine position. For patients where whole-pelvis irradiation to doses exceeding small bowel tolerance are simulated, oral barium sulfate* (about 1 pint) is usually given prior to the simulation to make the small bowel visible on the radiographs. Details of small bowel localization procedures have been described by Gunderson et al.[22] Loops of small bowel that lie within the anterior/posterior fields can usually be avoided with the lateral fields by using customized shielding blocks. By excluding the small bowel from the lateral fields, its dose is reduced by approximately 50%. In patients where small bowel shielding in the lateral fields is not possible, a prone position may be tried, utilizing gravitational position shifts of the small bowel out of the treatment fields.

Obese patients and/or those with large abdominal skin folds are difficult to treat due to the loss of skin sparing in the folds; variability of the patient's thickness, causing dose uncertainties; and unreliable skin marks. In the supine patient, straps and tapes may be used to reduce the skin folds, or the patient can be asked to pull the tissues superiorly away from the field. These methods are often unsatisfactory because they may cause the patient's thickness and the delivered dose to vary from treatment to treatment or even during a treatment if the patient's hold should slip. Another major difficulty is the uncertainty of field placement, since skin marks may shift by several centimeters.[24] A prone position may therefore be preferred in these patients. Skin folds may be reduced by having the patient pull skin folds superiorly while getting into the prone position. This, hopefully, will shift the folds superiorly and away from pelvic treatment fields. In the prone position, the abdomen is usually flattened against the hard treatment couch, making the patient's thickness more consistent and perhaps reduced.[40] The reliability of skin marks may also be improved, since the posterior skin surface is often more flat and less mobile.[40]

Rectal Carcinoma. In patients irradiated for rectal carcinoma, a three- or four-field technique is usually used. The prone position is often used to facilitate the lateral fields that extend far posterior and, in some patients, flash over the buttocks. When such fields are treated in the supine position, portions of the couch top also lie within the lateral fields, generating secondary scatter that reduces skin sparing. Loss of skin sparing in the gluteal fold is also a concern. In the supine position, the buttocks are often pressed together. Skin sparing observed in the buildup region of radiation beams is lost when the beam exits one buttock and immediately enters the other (Fig. 9-2).[22] In the prone position, the gluteal fold is often reduced and, if needed, can be further reduced by taping the buttocks apart.

*E-Z Paque barium sulfate for suspension, E-Z-EM, Inc., Westbury, New York.

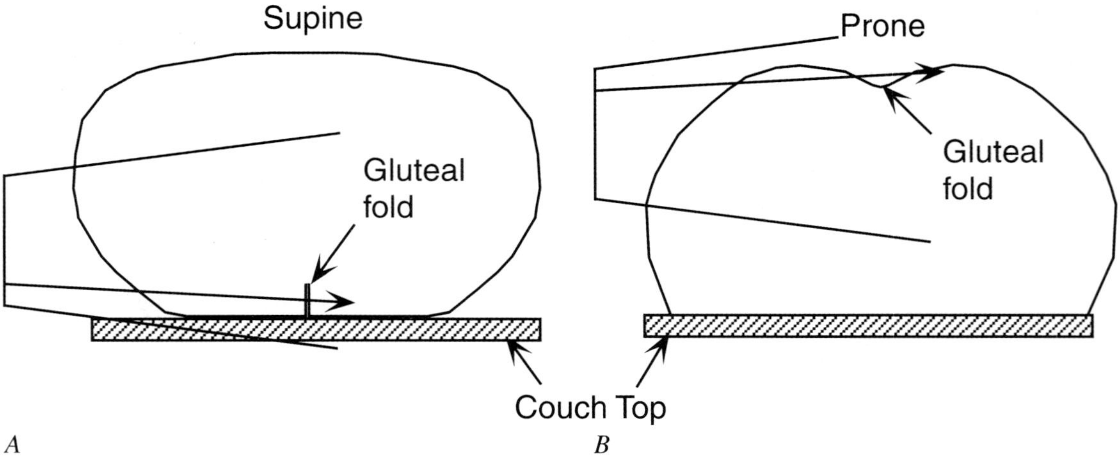

Fig. 9-2. *A.* In a supine patient, the buttocks are often pressed together. When a lateral pelvic field traverses the gluteal fold, skin sparing may be lost. Scatter of the couch may also contribute to increased skin dose in this region. *B.* In the prone position, the gluteal fold is often reduced and scatter off the treatment couch is eliminated.

Small-bowel sparing is often not a problem in patients treated preoperatively for rectal cancer since lateral fields, being relatively far posterior, usually can be shaped such that small bowel is excluded. In the postoperative setting, however, the volume of small bowel in the pelvis may be increased.[22]

Prostate Carcinoma. Both the supine and prone positions have been advocated for prostate irradiation.[11,14,41,42] In an unpublished survey of prostate treatment position in the United States, Canada, and Australia, 89% reported using supine, 9% prone, and 2% either supine or prone positions during prostate irradiation.[43] In general, the supine position is more comfortable and reproducible, but it may cause a larger rectal volume to lie within the lateral prostate fields.

In a prospective study to assess the effect of supine versus prone position on the dose to normal tissues in 26 patients with prostate carcinoma, using conformal treatment techniques, the prone position was found to be the more optimal in the majority of patients.[14] Based on dose-volume histograms (DVH), the prone position was associated with lower rectal doses in nearly 50% of the patients as compared with the supine position. In the prone position, the average dose to the rectal wall and the volume of rectal wall receiving 95% of the prescription dose was 64 and 24%, respectively, compared with 72 and 29%, respectively, for the supine position. The average rectal wall dose was lower in the prone versus the supine position in 14 of 26 patients as compared with 1 patient who demonstrated an advantage for the supine position. Similarly, when the volume of rectal wall receiving 95% of the prescribed dose was used as an endpoint, 15 patients had an advantage of the prone position compared with 1 who demonstrated an advantage for the supine position. An advantage was scored if the absolute dose in a particular normal tissue structure was decreased by $\geq$5%. The effect of treatment position on the rectal wall dose was most pronounced in the region of the seminal vesicles. The treatment position had no significant impact on the dose to the bladder wall.

It is not clear whether the advantage of the prone position is due to an anterior shift of the prostate or an anterior displacement of the rectum in the supine position. It appears that in the supine patient, the buttock muscles are forced anteriorly and thus displace the rectum anteriorly. In an ongoing study to address this issue at Duke University Medical Center, pelvic CT scans were obtained of 9 patients in both supine and prone positions. For each position, an additional scan was made with an opening (belly board) under the buttocks (supine) and abdomen (prone), respectively, to assess the impact of pressure from the tabletop. Preliminary results indicate that in the supine position, the presence of the tabletop displaces the inferior rectum anteriorly as compared with the CT with the opening. The bladder, rectum, and prostate appeared to move together when the position was changed from supine to prone.

Abdominal Irradiation. During whole-abdomen irradiation, the supine position is generally used, since it is usually more comfortable and practical than the prone. The patient's arms may need to be extended out away from the torso or raised above the head to minimize the risks of direct and scattered radiation to the arms. When a portion of the abdomen is irradiated, reduction of the small-bowel volume within the fields may be a desirable goal. A decubitus position, taking advantage of gravitational shifts, may be a feasible option in some patients.

Perineal Irradiation. A treatment field oriented directly toward the perineum may be used for low pelvic or perineal tumors (e.g., of the prostate, anus, vulva, buttock), often using electron beams. For this treatment, a lithotomy position, where the leg position is supported by stirrups, may be used (Fig. 9-3). Depending on the patient's agility, the treatment equipment available, and the precise location of the target, a decubitus position with the hips and knees bent may be an alternative. This position, often assumed during sleep, resembles a sitting position; however, in this situation the patient is lying down on his or her side (Fig. 9-4). The knee-chest position may also be used with perineal fields to treat anal lesions (Fig. 9-5).

Testicular Irradiation. In some patients efforts are made to *minimize* the testicular dose, while in

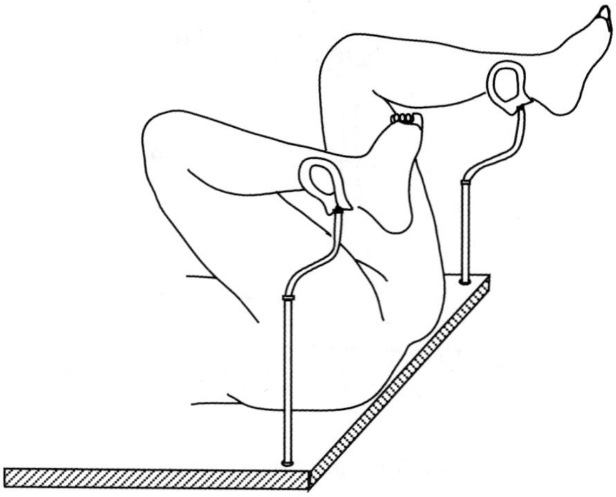

Fig. 9-3 Lithotomy position with the legs supported by stirrups.

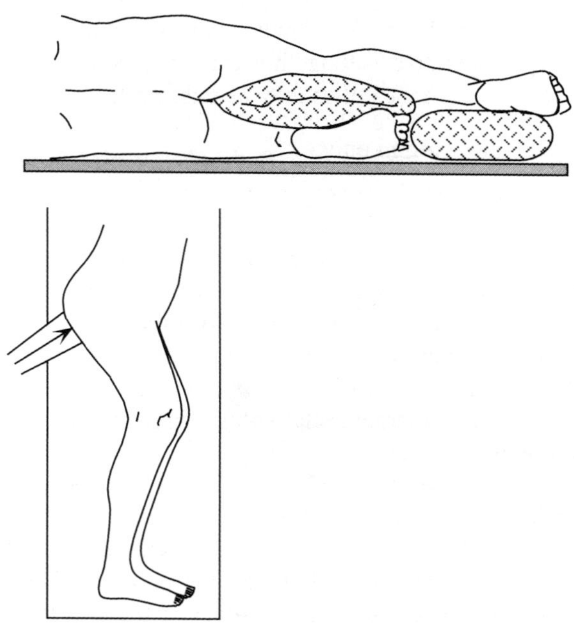

Fig. 9-4 A decubitus position with the knees bent may facilitate a perineal field.

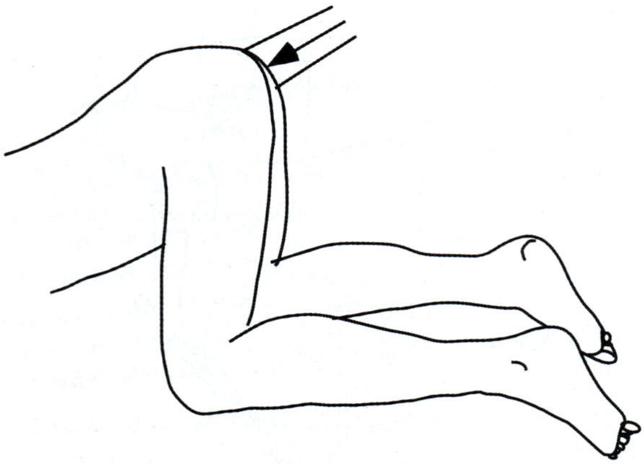

Fig. 9-5 Knee-chest position.

others the testicles are *intentionally* irradiated. Intentional irradiation of the scrotum is sometimes delivered as a boost during total-body irradiation in preparation for bone marrow transplant in patients with leukemia, since the testis appears to be a sanctuary for leukemic cells. During such intentional treatment of the scrotum, the dose to normal tissues in the vicinity can be minimized by placing the patient in the supine position with the legs separated and the knees bent (Fig. 9-6). The penis is taped superiorly, allowing an anterior/superior field to include the scrotum only.

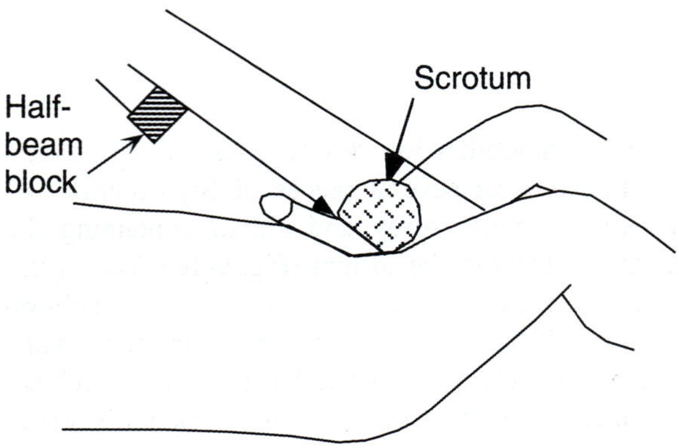

Fig. 9-6 With the legs separated, knees bent, and the penis taped superiorly, an anterior/superior half-beam blocked field can be set up to include the scrotum only.

The dose to the gonads during radiation therapy may consist of primary or scattered radiation (external or internal). In patients where preservation of fertility is desired, efforts should be made to minimize gonadal dose. Consideration of gonadal dose is discussed in Chap. 7.

IMMOBILIZATION TECHNIQUES AND DEVICES

SIMPLE AIDS

Frequently, patients undergoing radiation therapy to the pelvis and abdomen are treated in the supine or prone position without elaborate positioning or immobilization devices. A few simple aids can be used to make these patients more comfortable. For example, a support (foam rubber or regular bed pillow) under the supine patient's knees helps to relax the lower back—an important consideration when a person is lying supine on a hard surface (Fig. 6-5 in Chap. 6). For the prone patient, a pillow can be placed under the ankles to allow the knees to bend and keep the tips of the toes from resting on the tabletop (Fig. 9-7). Since treatment tables are generally narrow, leaving little or no room for the patient's arms, a Plexiglas extension, described in Chap. 6 (Fig. 6-5), can be placed on each side of the torso to support the arms. The legs of patients treated in the lithotomy position are usually supported by stirrups (Fig. 9-3).

FOOT POSITIONING AIDS

Changes in the foot position may change the position of skin and bony reference points. Skin marks

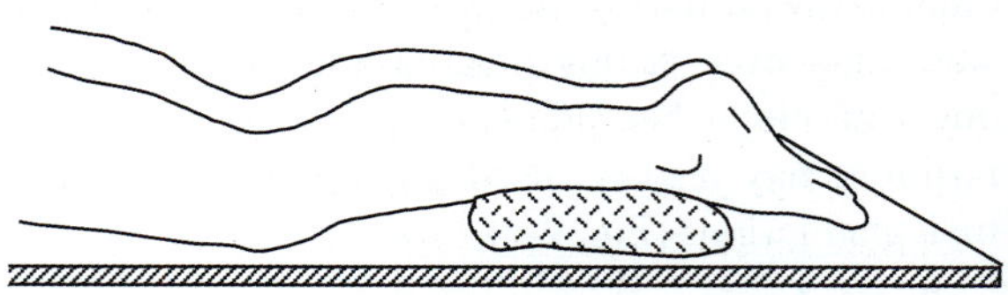

Fig. 9-7 A pillow can be placed under the ankles of a patient in the prone position to allow the knees to bend and to keep the toes from resting on the tabletop.

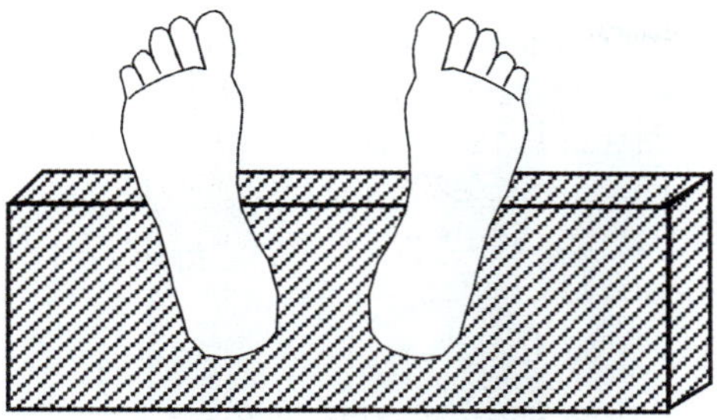

Fig. 9-8 A foot position device made from a block of Styrofoam facilitates reproducible foot separation.

are often used to set up the treatment fields and bony landmarks are typically used to assess port films. Thus, care should be taken to assure consistent foot position. To help reproduce the foot position, the feet can be held together with a rubber band or tape. Another alternative is a Styrofoam block, measuring approximately 20 × 8 × 3 in., with a groove for each foot (Fig. 9-8). A softened thermoplastic sheet can then be formed under and on the sides of the feet to prevent motion within the groove. Alternatively, a mold can be made, using a plastic bag and polyurethane foam—e.g., an Alpha Cradle™.*

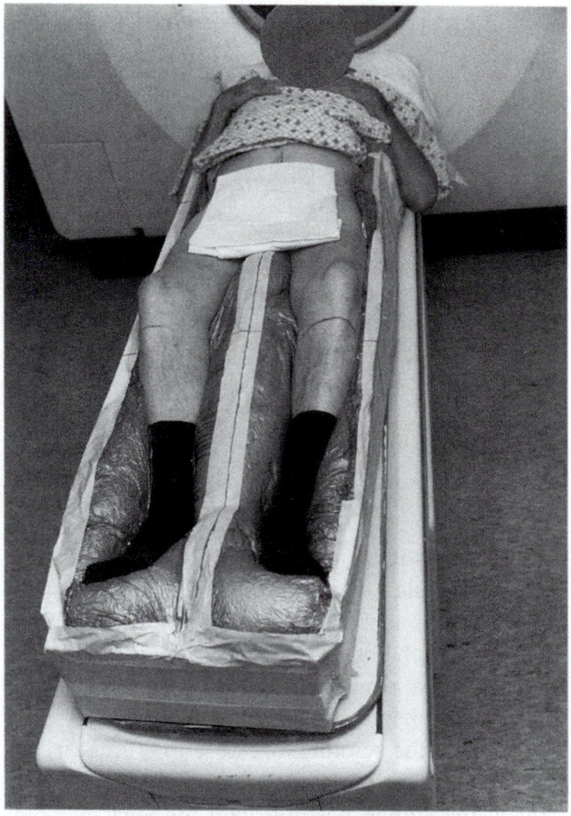

Fig. 9-9 Positioning mold for prostate treatment. The mold extends from below the feet to the lower chest area. A sagittal alignment line is marked between the patient's legs and thighs. Transverse and coronal alignment lines are made on each side of the mold. A second transverse line is marked on the mold and the patient's legs to assure that the patient is repositioned correctly in the cephalad/caudal direction.

PELVIS IMMOBILIZATION DEVICES

For patients undergoing high-dose curative radiation therapy to the pelvis, more extensive immobilization may be necessary. Two pelvic immobilization devices are described in the following section; one primarily used for the supine and one for the prone position. With minor modifications, such a device can be used for either position.

Half-Body Mold. At Duke University Medical Center, all patients undergoing 3DTP for prostate cancer are immobilized supine in an Alpha Cradle extending from the lower thoracic area to below the feet (Fig. 9-9). This mold can also be used for other pelvic or lower abdomen treatment and, with minor modifications, for prone and decubitus patients.

The immobilization device consists of foaming chemicals with several pieces of Styrofoam† that make the mold sturdy and aid in containing the foam adjacent to the patient (Fig. 9-10). The Styrofoam pieces include a base plate (approximately 60 in. long, 36 in. wide, and 1 in. thick) and three walls (approximately 6 in. high and 1 in. thick), which are fastened on each side and below the patient's feet to

*Smithers Medical Products, Inc., North Canton, Ohio.

†Dow Chemical, Midland, Michigan.

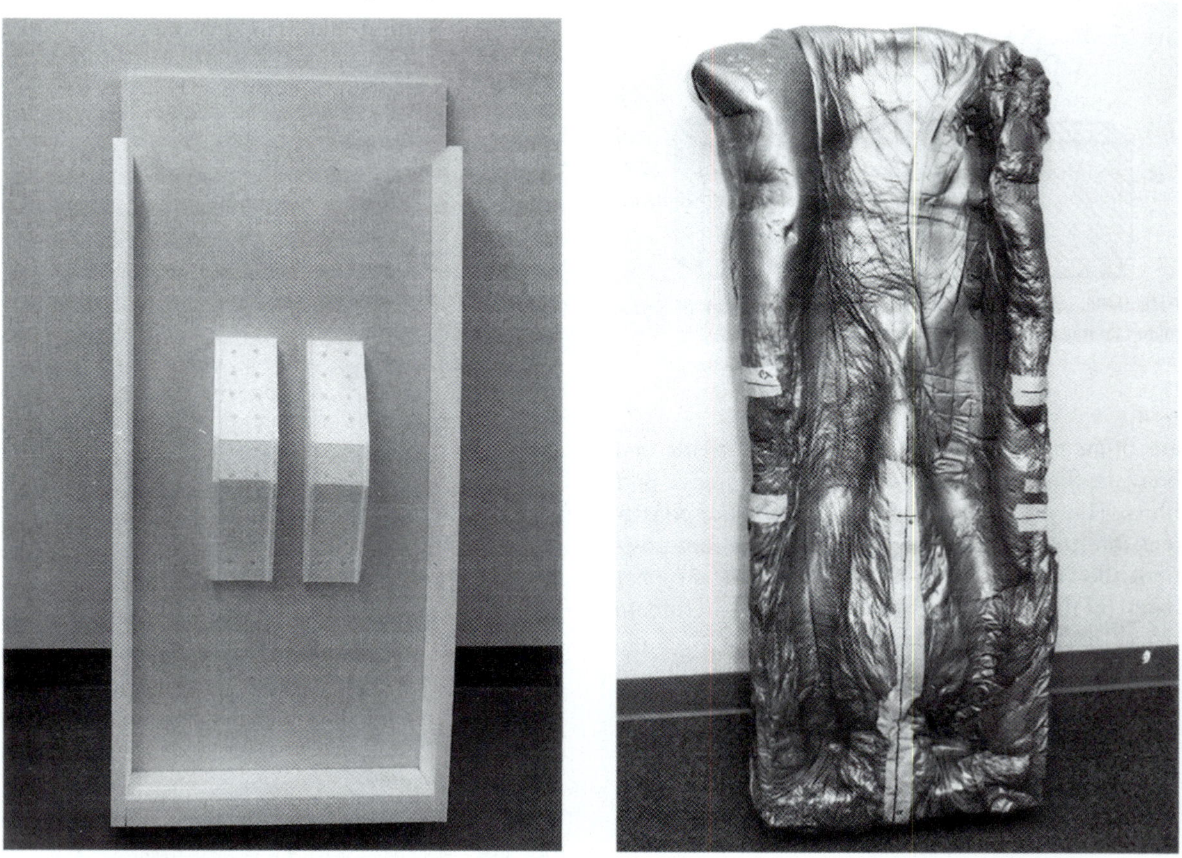

Fig. 9-10 The mold is made from a base plate, with three retaining walls and knee supports for the patient's bent knees *(left)*. This shell is placed inside a large polyvinyl bag before the foam is poured into the shell. The bag is sealed and the patient is positioned on top of the bag. The finished mold *(right)* conforms closely to the patient's skin.

form a barrier for the foam. The length of these pieces should approximate the dimensions of the base plate. Since patients appear to be more comfortable with their knees bent rather than straight on the base plate, a triangular piece of Styrofoam is fastened to the base plate under each knee.

The position of these Styrofoam pieces is determined and marked on the base plate with the patient in treatment position. The goal is to place the retaining walls as close to the patient as possible to help contain the foam close to the torso. With the patient removed, each Styrofoam piece is fastened to the base plate with adhesive tape. The excess width of the base plate is trimmed off to minimize the width of the finished mold. The trimmed-off Styrofoam pieces are broken into smaller pieces and used to fill the space between the patient's legs. This reduces the amount of foam needed to fill spaces between the patient and barriers. The entire Styrofoam shell is placed inside a polyvinyl bag, approximately 2 ft wider and 2 ft longer than the shell. Approximately 660 mL of the foaming agents is mixed, as directed by the manufacturer, and poured evenly into the prepared shell and on top of the knee supports inside the polyvinyl bag. In general, smaller amounts of foam are used for large patients, since they usually leave less space for the foam to fill.

Air is allowed to circulate inside the bag for a few seconds, following which excess air is squeezed out and the bag is securely sealed. Immediately after sealing the bag, the patient, dressed in a hospital gown only, is asked to first sit on the head end of the couch and then swing the legs up on the bag covering the shell. With the help of staff, the patient moves down into the shell until his or her feet touch the foot end. On lying down, the patient is asked to adjust his or her position until the knee supports are in the right place and he or she is straight. A visual registration of the patient's straightness should also be made by the staff. (This can also be done with fluoroscopy if available.) The hospital gown is pulled up from under the patient so that he or she lies directly on the polyvinyl bag. The polyvinyl bag is pulled up between the knees to allow the foam to expand and form an elevation for making a sagittal alignment mark. The height of this elevation is not important, since the patient enters and leaves the mold from the opposite end; thus there is no need for the patients to lift themselves over the elevation.

Since the foam is light and tends to expand in the direction of least resistance, it is often necessary to prevent foam from expanding *over* the patient's legs, preventing him or her from leaving unless portions of the finished mold are removed. Since the expanding foam tends to displace the side barriers away from the patient, adhesive tape is stretched anteriorly across the torso, pulling the two side pieces in toward the torso. This forces the foam inside the polyvinyl bag medially toward the patient as it expands and sets within approximately 7 to 10 min. An additional 10 min is needed for the foam to harden.

It is important to make the mold strong on the sides near the waist since patients will grasp onto this portion when they lift themselves into the mold. Care should be taken so that this thicker portion is not in the path of lateral treatment fields. This is most important with large separations and when relatively modest beam energies ($\leq$6 MV) are used. Skin erythema was observed in the lateral fields of one moderate-sized patient with prostate cancer when the foam was 6 to 8 cm thick and ~66 Gy were delivered via a four-field plan using 6-MV photons. During the mold-making process, the foam can be guided away from the area where lateral fields are anticipated. Removal of the sides of the mold in the region of the lateral fields is discouraged, since it is unnecessary and precludes making setup marks on the mold—the most reliable set of marks.

Small amounts of foam may leak out from the Styrofoam shell, and since the mold often is wider than the couch it is made on, the foam may form a "lip" around the couch. When the mold is later placed on a wider couch, this lip may cause an undesired tilt of the patient. To prevent this, a large sheet of hardwood, wider and longer than the mold, is placed under the base plate *prior* to making the mold to prevent any irregular surfaces from forming under the device. The hardwood sheet is removed after the foam has set and prior to obtaining a CT scan. The process of making the device requires two persons and takes approximately 30 min.

This immobilization device allows the alignment lines to be marked on the mold in addition to the patient's skin. When discrepancies arise between these marks, the staff rely on the mold marks, since the skin is mobile. The sagittal alignment line is marked on the mold between the patient's legs and thighs. The transverse and coronal alignment lines are made on each side of the mold. A second transverse line is marked on the mold and the patient's legs (just below the knees), where the skin usually is relatively immobile. The purpose of these marks is to assure that the patient is repositioned correctly in the cephalad/caudal direction in the mold.

A similar device can be made for patients in the prone or decubitus position. For the decubitus position, the anterior and posterior retaining walls need to be higher than the 6 in. suggested for the supine mold to prevent the patient from "rolling" when lying on the side (Fig. 9-11).

Thermoplastic Device. A thermoplastic pelvic immobilization device has been described for immobilization of prostate patients in prone position[41]

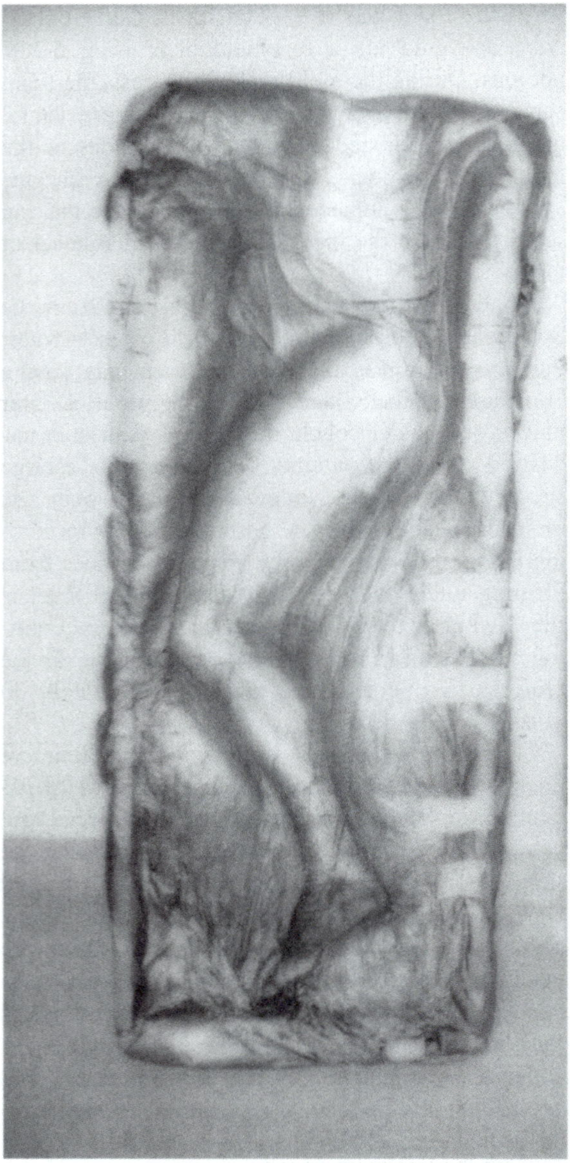

Fig. 9-11 Positioning molds for the decubitus position usually require retaining walls that are higher than the 6 in. suggested for the supine mold to prevent the patient from "rolling" when lying on the side.

but can, with minor modifications, also be used for supine patients. The patient is placed on a rigid plastic base plate and a softened thermoplastic sheet is draped over and molded to the patient from approximately midchest to midthighs (Fig. 9-12). In approximately 7 to 10 min, the thermoplastic sheet hardens and forms a rigid mold. A handle is attached to each end of the thermoplastic sheet for easier handling of the pliable material and for securing the sheet to the base plate. The sheet is fastened to the base plate on each side of the patient and between the legs with a locking-pin mechanism. The position of the side locking mechanism is adjustable to accommodate different size patients while keeping the mold in close contact with the patient's body. The base plate has a window, permitting unobstructed treatment of an anterior field of the prone patient.

WHOLE-BODY STEREOTACTIC FRAME

A whole-body stereotactic device has been developed and used for prostate irradiation at Karolinska Hospital in Stockholm (Fig. 5-16 in Chap. 5).[44] The design of this frame, described in Chap. 5, is based on a unique concept where the patient alignment is made with the patient in an upright position. The frame with the patient standing in it is placed vertically at the foot end of the treatment couch. After aligning the patient, the frame is slowly tilted backward onto the treatment couch to a recumbent patient position. Scales on each side and above the frame corresponding to CT (or MRI) indicators define the stereotactic space.

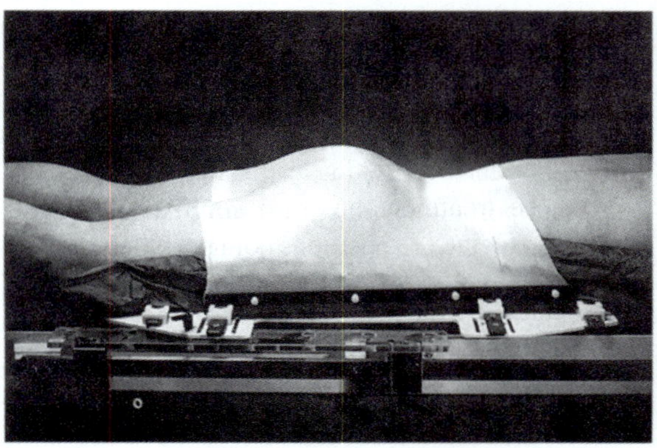

Fig. 9-12 A thermoplastic pelvic immobilization device can be used for prone or supine position. (Courtesy of MED-TEC, Inc., Orange City, Iowa.)

SMALL-BOWEL DISPLACEMENT

Radiation-induced injury to the small bowel is an important consideration during pelvic irradiation.[45-52] Letschert et al. found a 37% incidence of severe small-bowel injury following 45 to 50 Gy in 5 weeks with large opposed anterior and posterior fields versus only 6% with smaller fields and a three-field technique.[47] The authors suggest that when the small-bowel volume is increased by a factor of 2, the dose has to be reduced by 17% for the same incidence of small-bowel injury. Displacement of the small bowel out of pelvic radiation fields is thus a desirable goal and several methods to accomplish this have been described. These methods include the prone position, bladder distention, abdominal wall compression, a belly board,[22,27-34,53] and surgical displacement.[35-38]

The mobility of the small bowel varies from patient to patient. A certain displacement method effective in one patient may not be as effective in others and some patients may require a combination of methods. A prone position likely provides a benefit relative to supine in most patients since an anterior/cephalad gravitational shift may occur. The degree of benefit is likely related to the mobility of the anterior abdominal wall. Thus, one would hypothesize that small-bowel mobility (e.g., prone versus supine) would be greater in obese patients with poor abdominal muscle tone versus thin patients with good muscle tone.

Determination of the optimal displacement method(s) can be made through comparison of radiographs obtained 1 to 2 h after the patient drinks about 1 pint of barium sulfate contrast. The patients should be well hydrated and the bladder full. The films should be centered near the anticipated central axis of the treatment fields to simulate most correctly the relative positions of ports and small bowel.[22]

DEVICES AND TECHNIQUES

Belly Board. A device that eliminates the resistance of the hard tabletop on the abdomen of the prone patient is referred to as a *belly board* (Fig. 9-13).[27,31,32] Such a device offers an opportunity for unobstructed gravitational displacement of the anterior abdominal wall and small bowel. A belly board can be made from a sheet of Styrofoam approximately the size of the treatment couch and about 3 in. thick. A hole made in the Styrofoam (approximately 12 × 12 in.) facilitates a 3-in.-deep unobstructed opening for the pelvis/lower abdomen of the prone patient (Fig. 9-14*A*). To facilitate patient repositioning, an Alpha Cradle can be made with the patient in treatment position on the Styrofoam block. The mold should extend from the patient's waist to the feet. The construction of the Alpha Cradle is similar to that described above with the exception that following completion, an opening corresponding to the opening in the Styrofoam block is made in the Alpha Cradle.

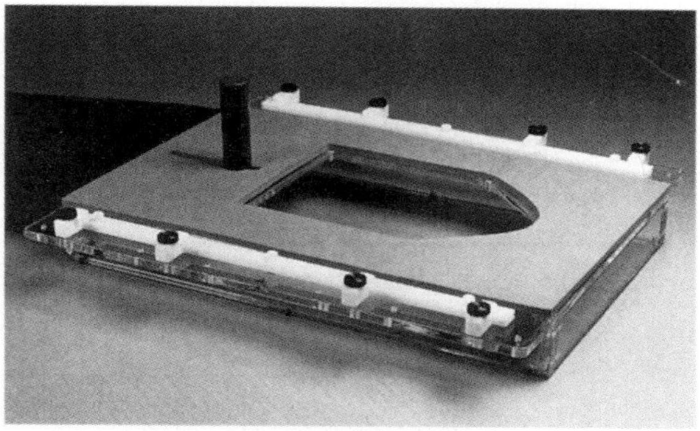

Fig. 9-13 A belly-board offers unobstructed displacement of the anterior abdominal wall and small bowel. An adjustable bar between the patient's legs facilitates repositioning on the device. (Courtesy of Bionix, Inc., Toledo, Ohio.)

As a substitute for a belly board, a simpler but perhaps less reproducible method is to place the patient's pelvis/lower abdomen over an open "window" in the treatment couch.

In obese patients, abdominal folds sometimes fall into the opening, causing an anterior treatment field to traverse an *excessive thickness* of normal tissues. The anterior contour, conformed to the opening, also becomes irregular, possibly causing an anterior field to traverse *varying thickness* of tissue (Fig. 9-15). In these patients, an anterior field should be avoided, since both the increased tissue thickness and the irregular contour can give rise to unacceptable dose heterogeneity.

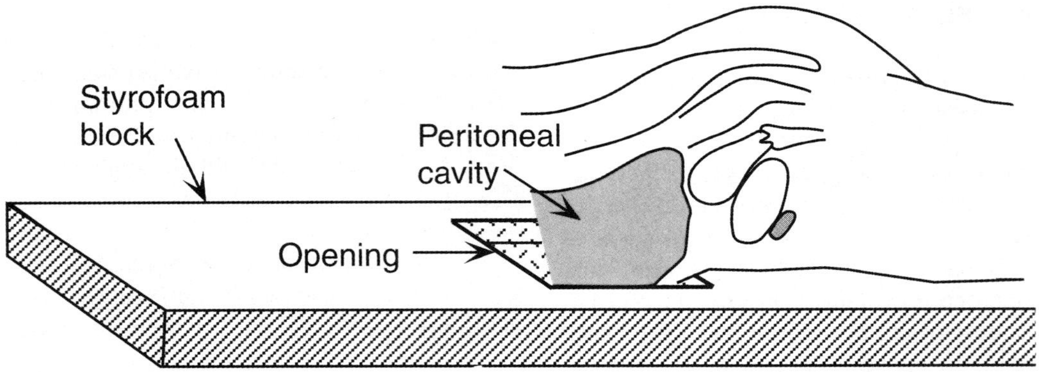

A

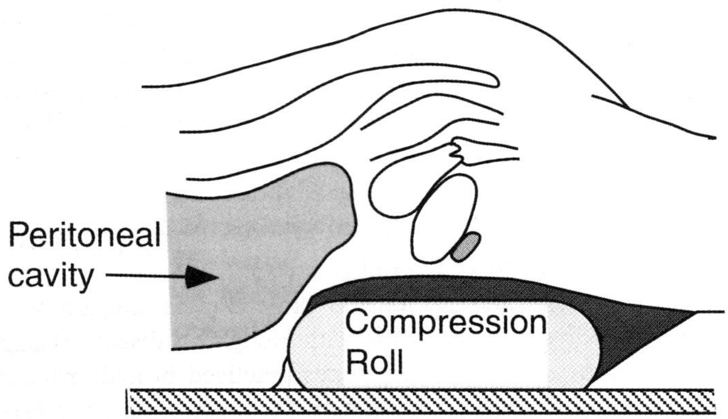

B

Fig. 9-14 *A.* A belly board can be made from a block of Styrofoam approximately 3 in. thick. An opening is made for the pelvis/lower abdomen to facilitate anterior/posterior displacement of the small bowel. *B.* A compression roll placed under the pelvis in a prone patient may cause small bowel displacement.

Abdominal Wall Compression. Small-bowel displacement may be achieved by applying pressure on the anterior pelvis in a prone patient[30,34] and by bladder distention.[33] Huh et al. have described a customized small-bowel displacement system consisting of a compression roll and foaming chemicals placed inside a plastic bag. The foam expands and forms a tight-fitting shell for positioning and immobilization. A padded Styrofoam roll (8 in. wide) placed immediately superior of the symphysis of the prone patient can also be used (Fig. 9-14*B*). If the roll is too wide, the iliac crest may rest on the roll, preventing pressure on the small bowel. The length and thickness of the roll should be approximately 3 to 4 in.; however, these dimensions may vary from patient to patient depending on specific situations and tolerance. For example, postsurgical patients or the patient with a colostomy may tolerate only a small roll or towel.

Some patients may benefit from a compression roll plus a belly board. The compression roll can then be secured to the Styrofoam block, adjacent to

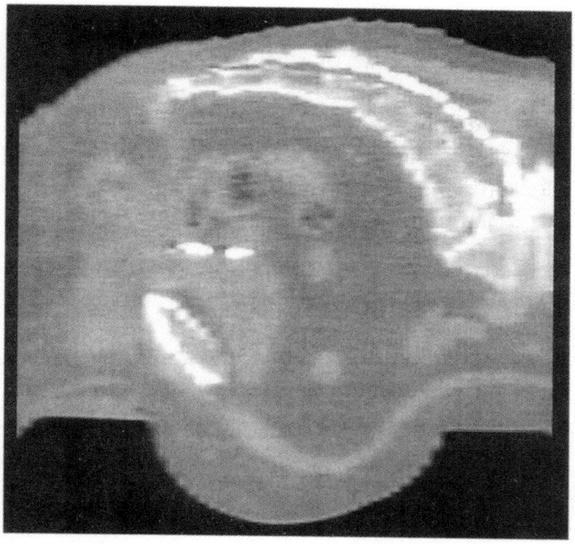

Fig. 9-15 The anterior contour may become irregular when a patient is placed on a belly board. An anterior field would traverse a large thickness of normal tissues.

the caudal side of the belly-board opening. When a customized mold is used, the compression roll can be placed inside the polyvinyl bag adjacent to the opening, thereby making a single unit that is easier to use and more reproducible.[34]

Invasive Procedures. Surgical small-bowel displacement methods include placing an absorbable mesh sling that elevates the small bowel out of the pelvis,[35,37,38,54,55] placement of a pelvic spacer,[56] use of a permanent silastic prosthesis creating a barrier for the small bowel,[57] and a temporary tissue expander that excludes the small bowel from the pelvis.[36] Devices placed surgically to displace the small bowel are usually limited to patients where a surgical procedure is necessary. It is important for the radiation oncologist to be involved in the care of multidisciplinary cases such that these interventions can be anticipated and executed during operative procedures that are already planned, thereby avoiding the possibility of a second operation.

Efficacy. In a study of 51 patients, the small-bowel volume was reduced from 50% in supine to 28% when the belly board/prone position was used. The small bowel volume was reduced from 61 in the supine position to 29% in the prone position without the belly board.[27] In another study of 30 patients using the belly board/prone position, the mean small-bowel volume within pelvic fields was reduced by 66% compared with the supine position.[32] In 13 patients without previous surgery, the small-bowel reduction was 74%. All patients were found to benefit from the prone belly-board position regardless of body habitus, weight, and age. Using the customized small-bowel displacement device described above in 55 patients, Huh et al. reported a reduction of small bowel volume of 59 and 51% within posterior and lateral whole-pelvis treatment fields, respectively.[34]

Rudat et al. reported small-bowel displacement among 22 patients using the belly-board/prone position—16 with and 6 without adhesions. Partial small bowel shifts out of the treatment field were achieved in 14 of 16 patients with adhesions and complete displacement was achieved in all patients without adhesions.[31]

TESTICULAR RETRACTOR AND SHIELDS

Gonadal protection is frequently practiced in patients with Hodgkin's disease (Chap. 7). Since it is sometimes practiced in male patients during pelvic irradiation for other diseases, a brief description is given here.

Methods to minimize scrotal dose have been described by several authors.[58–61] Most commonly, the testicles are protected by a lead cup surrounding the scrotum. Given the weight of the lead shield and the small space in which it needs to be placed, it can be difficult to position properly and may then be ineffective. The weight of the shield is supported and the position adjustable when mounted on a platform with a vertical (height adjustment) and a horizontal arm with a joint swivel (rotational adjustment) (Fig. 7-6 in Chap. 7). The shield surrounding the scrotum can also be built into an immobilization mold; thus the weight is supported by the mold and the repositioning is reliable. It is important that the internal dimensions of the lead shield be small to allow more room for thick walls. Shielding of the penis does not affect gonadal function and would increase the size of the shield. The primary purpose of this shield is to reduce the amount of internal scatter arriving at the testes during pelvic irradiation. The thickness of the lead cup is insufficient for attenuation of the primary beam.

In patients with testicular seminoma where a transscrotal resection has been performed or in patients with very extensive tumor invasion, it may be necessary to irradiate the "empty" side of the scrotum while sparing the intact testicle. In these patients, a testicular retractor may be used to retract the penis and remaining testicle to maximize the distance from the radiation field (Fig. 9-16).[60] It should be noted here that the testicular tumor bed is rarely irradiated nowadays.

Inadvertent irradiation of the testicles may occur despite heroic efforts to minimize gonadal dose. For example, the divergence of the caudal margin of a posterior pelvic field (in the opposite direction from that of an anterior) may require that a modification be made to prevent divergence into the scrotum (or the remaining testicle). Inadvertent irradiation of the testicles may occur during port filming. Routinely, port films are obtained by using a double-exposure technique where the second exposure is made with beam-shaping blocks removed and the collimator opening increased so that adjacent bony anatomy can be visualized. This may cause the primary beam

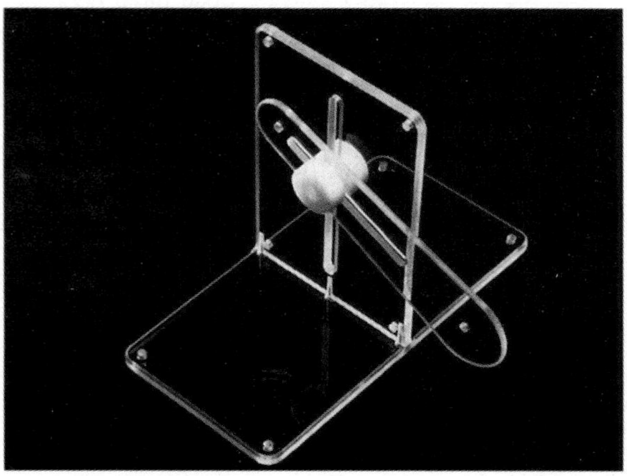

Fig. 9-16 A testicular retractor. (Courtesy of MED-TEC, Inc., Orange City, Iowa.)

to include the gonads (female and male), thus defeating the purpose of shielding. Therefore, pelvic port films in patients where gonadal shielding is practiced may need to be obtained by a single exposure of the treatment field only. Alternatively, a lead block (or independent jaw) should be placed over the gonads during the second exposure.

TREATMENT ACCURACY

It is impossible to eliminate all of the causes for field misalignments; however, it is important to intermittently assess the accuracy of treatment delivery and to develop an understanding of the source and the impact that these errors have on treatment delivery. The result of such assessment should be considered when field margins are designed, both with respect to the target and to normal tissues. Margins that are too small can result in target misses and local recurrence, while margins that are too generous may lead to higher complication rates and increased morbidity. In conformal radiation therapy of prostate cancer, where target margins generally are small, the need for accuracy and reproducibility is increased. An important potential limitation of successful conformal prostate irradiation may be related to patient repositioning and immobilization.[62,63] Thus, the frequency and magnitude of treatment field misalignments during pelvic irradiation has been extensively studied (Table 9-2).[4,12,40,42,62–77]

TRANSLATIONAL AND ROTATIONAL ERRORS

Studies Using No or Minimal Immobilization. Huddart et al. prospectively evaluated treatment accuracy in 90 patients that had CT-based treatment planning without an immobilization device.[69] The overall simulator-to-treatment differences, the number of error-free treatments, mean treatment-simulator position, and the role of systematic versus random errors was evaluated. Other variables including age, weight, and fractionation were assessed for their effect on treatment accuracy.

The mean absolute error between simulation and treatment was 0.25 and 0.32 cm in the mediolateral

Table 9-2 Mean Magnitude and Direction of Field Displacements (cm)

Author	Immobilization Device (Yes/No)	Mediolateral[a]	Anterior/ Posterior	Cephalad/ Caudad
Huddart[69]	No	0.25	0.32/0.42[b]	0.28
Bieri[42c]	No	0	0.5	0
El-Gayed[67d]				
Prostate	No	0.4 (± 2.8)	0.7 (± 2.4)	1.1 (± 1.6)
Rectum	No	1.0 (± 3.0)	1.4 (± 3.9)	0.5 (± 3.0)
Hanley[4]	Yes	0.01 (± 0.19)	0.03 (± 0.13)	0.04 (± 0.14)
Rosenthal[73d]	Yes	NA	0.3	0.2
	No	NA	0.4	0.4

[a]Standard deviations in parentheses.
[b]AP and lateral films different.
[c]Median.
[d]Average, not otherwise specified.

and cephalad/caudal directions, respectively (as seen on an anterior radiograph) and 0.42 and 0.28 cm in the anterior/posterior and cephalad/caudal directions, respectively (as seen on a lateral radiograph). On average, the field center was displaced from that intended by 0.66 cm (standard deviation, 0.34). On each treatment day, 29% of anterior and 45% of lateral port films had at least one 0.5-cm error. Overall, 59% of treatments had at least one 0.5-cm error and 9% had a 1.0-cm error. The field center was displaced more than 0.5 cm from the intended position in 66% of treatments and over 1.0 cm for 14% of treatments. Analysis of variance showed that both systematic and random errors occurred in all directions. Systematic errors were associated in the mediolateral direction with hypofractionation and in the cephalad/caudal direction with weight and age. Random errors were of similar magnitude in all directions. Conversely, systematic errors were four times greater in the anterior/posterior versus the right/left direction.

The authors conclude that a 6-mm margin is needed around the clinical target volume (CTV) to cover 95% errors in the right/left and cephalad/caudal and 9 mm in the anterior/posterior directions. The authors further suggest that each center should determine its own margin requirements based on its own practice.

Rabinowitz et al. studied field alignment errors in 71 patients undergoing radiation therapy in different sites (23 receiving pelvic irradiation) and using varying degrees of immobilization.[72] Discrepancies were slightly larger in patients irradiated to the pelvis and thorax than in other sites. The simulation-to-treatment (systematic) discrepancies were significantly greater than treatment-to-treatment (random) discrepancies.

Bieri et al. studied the reproducibility of three-dimensional conformal radiation therapy in 14 patients with prostate cancer.[42] The patients were treated in the supine position without immobilization using a six-field technique. Retrospectively, 196 anterior/posterior and lateral port films were compared by three independent observers with corresponding simulation films. No significant deviations were observed in the cephalad/caudal (0 mm median value; range, −10 to +5 mm) or lateral directions (0 mm median value; range, −4.0 to +1.0 mm). A systematic median shift of 5 mm (range, 0 to +10 mm) was observed in the anterior/posterior direction. The authors postulate that this was a consequence of the treatment couch (flexible insert) sagging under the patient's weight. Following replacement of the insert with a rigid, low-density carbon-fiber insert, no further systematic anterior/posterior shifts were observed. The authors conclude that with careful attention to details in patient positioning, excellent setup reproducibility can be achieved even without rigid immobilization. This study demonstrates that through periodic assessment of departmental procedures, deficiencies that otherwise may go undetected for a long time can be discovered and corrected.

El-Gayed et al. assessed setup deviations in 469 port films from 20 patients treated for rectal (10) and prostate carcinoma (10).[67] Translational and rotational errors were determined by superimposing the "reference" image (simulation) and the electronic portal image using a computer program. The amount and frequency of translations and rotations required to correct for displacements were recorded. Mean field placement errors up to 1.4 mm were reported, with standard deviation of 1.6 to 3.9 mm depending on the direction and treatment site. Rotational errors were negligible, 80% of the rectal patients having a rotation of <1° and 90% <2°. Random errors were smallest in the cephalad/caudal (1.7 mm) and largest in the anterior/posterior (2.8 mm) directions. Setup deviations as a function of time were also analyzed. Significant time trends were detected in 5 of 20 patients. The magnitude of displacement attributed to the time trend ranged between 4 and 11 mm. This report confirms the observation made by us[64] that displacement errors are smallest in the cephalad/caudal direction. This is logical because all of the setup marks (anterior and lateral) can be used for isocenter placement in this direction.

Dunscombe et al. analyzed 76 pairs of films from 29 prostate patients and found an average absolute error of 3.5 mm with a standard deviation of 4.5 mm.[66]

Gildersleve et al. used an electronic portal imaging system to measure setup errors in 15 nonimmobilized patients undergoing pelvic irradiation and 12 patients treated for brain tumors and immobilized with individually molded plastic shells.[68] As expected, there were more errors in the pelvic than in the brain fields. For the pelvic fields, 95% of random errors (treatment to treatment) were ≤4.5 and 87% ≤3 mm. The systematic simulation-to-treatment errors were ≤3 mm and the maximal random simulation error was ±6 mm.

Tinger et al. evaluated the relative frequency and magnitude of intra- and intertreatment field displacement in seven patients undergoing pelvic irradiation for rectal cancer in the prone position without immobilization.[76] On average, two electronic portal images were obtained of each field during each treatment (only two of four fields were treated each day), totaling 594 images. Each image was aligned with the corresponding simulation (prescription) film to determine displacements. The frequency of intertreatment displacements exceeding 10 mm was 3, 16, and 23% in the mediolateral, cephalad/caudal, and anterior/posterior directions, respectively. No intratreatment displacements greater than 10 mm were detected. The frequency of intertreatment displacements exceeding 5 mm was 40, 52, and 51% in the mediolateral, cephalad/caudal, and anterior/posterior directions, respectively. The frequency of intratreatment displacements exceeding 5 mm was 1, 5, and 7% in the same directions, respectively. In this investigation, intertreatment displacements were larger than intratreatment displacements, suggesting that patients do not move considerably during the daily treatment of pelvic fields even without immobilization devices. Thus, the authors conclude that a single electronic portal image per field may be considered representative of the treated position.

Studies Using Some Form of Pelvic Mold. The above studies demonstrate that setup deviations are generally small even when minimal or no immobilization devices are used. In four separate studies using some form of body molds, positional errors were reduced.[4,64,73,74] One additional study involving a comparison of four different devices and no immobilization reported no significant benefit of either immobilization device.

Hanley et al. retrospectively compared 300 simulation films and 1239 port films from 50 patients treated with conformal radiation therapy for prostate cancer.[4] All patients were immobilized in prone position using a thermoplastic mask (similar to that described above) extending from the midchest to the midthighs and molded to the dorsum, sides, and between the legs. Simulation and port films were digitized and imported to an image registration software program for analysis. Following alignment of the fields, skeletal reference structures were superimposed. The magnitude and direction of translations and rotations required to match the anatomy were recorded. The distribution of systematic errors (defined as the mean patient displacement for the treatment course) had a mean and standard deviation of −0.1 (±1.9) mm, 0.4 (±1.4) mm, and −0.3 (±1.3) mm in the mediolateral, cephalad/caudal, and anterior/posterior directions, respectively, and −0.1 (±0.2)° for rotational errors. The standard deviations for random errors were 2.0, 1.7, and 1.9 mm in the same directions, respectively, and for out-of-plane rotations 0.9 and 0.6° about the cephalad/caudal and anterior/posterior axes, respectively. Time-dependent displacements from 2 to 7 mm were detected in 10 of 50 patients.

Comparison with and without Immobilization. Rosenthal et al. compared setup errors among 22 patients undergoing prostate irradiation in the supine position without (12) and with (10), an immobilization device.[73] The immobilization device consisted of a mold extending from the lower thoracic area to midthigh. A total of 288 port films were retrospectively reviewed and compared with corresponding simulation films. The average simulation-to-treatment variability was 0.4 cm with and 0.6 cm without immobilization. Since a six-field technique was used, directional shifts were reported in two directions only. The immobilization device reduced the average setup deviation from 4 to 3 mm and from 4 to 2 mm in the anterior/posterior and cephalad/caudal directions, respectively. Among the immobilized patients, the treated field was within 5 mm of the simulated field in 66% (132/201 port films) compared with 43% (37/87 port films) among nonimmobilized patients. The number of setup errors >5 mm was significantly larger when no immobilization was used. The authors conclude that the use of an immobilization device significantly reduced patient positioning errors.

The two groups of patients compared in this study were treated by the same physician group but at different facilities. Some of the differences may have been due to variables such as the number of patients being treated on the machine and different technical staff.

Soffen et al., using a similar immobilization device during four-field prostate irradiation in the supine position, assessed the efficacy of the device in a prospective study.[74] They compared *daily* port films taken during 5 consecutive days of all four fields (20 films per patient) of 7 patients with *weekly* port films of 7 nonimmobilized patients (≤20 films per patient) treated in a similar fashion within the previous year. Daily variation was markedly improved when using immobilization with a median variation of 1 and 3 mm with and without immobilization, respectively. The average range of misalignments for each of the patients with and without the use of an immobilization device was 3.3 and 8 mm, respectively. The greatest benefit of the immobilization was seen in the anterior/posterior direction on lateral port films.

A noticeable difference between this and the previous study is that the immobilized patients in this report were studied *prospectively* and the port films were obtained during *consecutive* treatments. The results were then compared with data from weekly port films of retrospectively identified nonimmobilized patients treated a year earlier. One can postulate that the data may be flawed since the treating technologists, being aware that the films would be subjected to closer scrutiny, may have been more careful when setting up the treatments in the prospectively studied group. Other variables such as changes in patient weight, skin marks, and so on are more likely to occur over a 5- to 6-week period than over 5 days.

We compared setup reproducibility between using the positioning mold described above (44 patients) and without immobilization (30 patients) treated in the supine position for prostate cancer.[64] More than 1000 port films representing 540 independent isocenter placements were retrospectively reviewed. Physician-requested isocenter shifts were used as an indicator of reproducibility. The frequency of physician-requested isocenter shifts (Table 9-3) was reduced from 23.1 to 17.4% when the positioning mold was used. Most of this improvement was seen in the right/left (from 18.0 to

Table 9-3 Frequency of Requested Isocenter Shifts

	Without Mold		With Mold		
Direction	Number of Misalignments/ Number of Times Tested	%	Number of Misalignments/ Number of Times Tested	%	*p* Value
Right/left	18/100	18.0	22/180	12.2	0.30
Cephalad/caudal	6/130	4.6	12/213	5.6	0.95
Anterior/posterior	13/103	12.6	9/175	5.1	0.05
All	30/130[a]	23.1	37/213[a]	17.4	0.20

[a]Misalignments in more than one direction.

12.2%) and anterior/posterior (from 12.6 to 5.1%) directions. This improvement may in part be attributed to the ability to use alignment marks on the rigid mold rather than relying on marks on the mobile skin. The rate of setup discrepancies in the craniocaudal direction was low with and without the immobilization device, possibly due to the ability to use both anterior and lateral setup marks in this direction. The frequency of requested position adjustment in the two patient groups was compared using a two-tailed chi-square test.

Isocenter shifts <5 mm are not included in this study since isocenter shifts in our department are routinely made in 0.5-cm increments. It is assumed that smaller shifts may be difficult to detect and to make accurately, considering the thickness of setup lines and involuntary motions often encountered in the pelvis. The endpoint used in this study, the frequency of physician-requested isocenter shifts, is not ideal; however, given the large number of films reviewed it is impractical to determine precise displacement. Furthermore, it is not clear if more elaborate methods are precise, given the difficulties localizing specific bony landmarks on port films.

Song et al. performed a retrospective review of setup reproducibility without or with either of four immobilization devices in 62 supine patients receiving conformal radiation therapy for prostate cancer.[75] The five groups of patients were as follows:

(*a*) No immobilization, 20 patients
(*b*) Positioning mold extending from the waist to upper thighs, 8 patients
(*c*) Positioning mold from the hips to just below the knees, 10 patients
(*d*) Styrofoam leg immobilizer below the knees, 14 patients
(*e*) Thermoplastic cast encompassing the entire abdomen and pelvis to midthigh and a mold to the lower legs and feet, 10 patients

Only setup deviations ≥5 mm were considered misalignments in this study. Using a logistic regression model, the probability of overall and directional misalignment for each group was obtained (Table 9-4). Comparison of patient repositioning accuracy in these five groups of patients demonstrated no significant difference in the overall misalignment. However, there were significant differences when individual directions were considered. The thermoplastic immobilization device provided the best reproducibility probability among all five groups in the cephalad/caudal and anterior/posterior directions. This benefit was offset by a higher rate of displacements in the lateral direction. The authors postulate that despite their findings, other immobilization devices may still be useful.

None of the immobilization devices compared in this study extended continuously from the waist to

Table 9-4 Movement Probability

Type of Device Used	Right/ Left	Anterior/ Posterior	Cephalad/ Caudal	Overall
a. None	0.09	0.15	0.18	0.38
b. Waist-to-thigh mold	0.14	0.09	0.26	0.44
c. Hips-to-knee mold	0.17	0.13	0.19	0.41
d. Styrofoam below knees	0.11	0.10	0.16	0.30
e. Thermoplastic mold—abdomen, pelvis, thigh plus a lower leg/feet mold	0.32	0.06	0.09	0.41
Likelihood ratio test	$p < 0.001$	$p = 0.14$	$p = 0.03$	$p = 0.35$

Source: Modified from Song et al.[75]

the feet. The most extensive immobilization device (e) consisted of two separate parts—a pelvic/thigh mold and a lower leg/foot mold, leaving the knee joints free to move and possibly causing the device to be less effective than if it had been continuous. It is reasonable to apply the philosophy used by a surgeon stabilizing a fracture—use of a single rigid support that immobilizes one joint on each side of the treatment site. It has been shown in other studies that extending the immobilization device to include areas away from the treatment site improves setup reproducibility. This may in part be due to the ability to make setup marks on the device.[64,78] The issue of making setup marks on the immobilization device was not addressed in this or other studies reviewed above with the exception of our own.

Whole-Body Stereotactic Frame Positioning. Positioning accuracy in a study of 76 CT examinations in 5 patients, using the whole-body frame described above, has been reported.[44] The standard deviation of prostate motion was 1.7, 1.5, and 1.6 mm in the mediolateral, anterior/posterior, and craniocaudal directions, respectively. The results in this study are promising and this device may be a desirable immobilization option for situations where small target margins are necessary. The device is currently being developed; thus the study represent only a small number of patients.

EFFECT OF POSITIONING ERRORS ON DOSE DISTRIBUTION

Rudat et al. investigated the effect of positioning errors on three-dimensional conformal dose distributions using the mean positioning error in 194 port films from 43 nonimmobilized patients undergoing radiation therapy for tumors in the pelvis and thorax.[62] The mean two-dimensional positioning error using the data from all patients was 5.5 (±3.7) mm. Dose-volume histograms (DVH) of the CTV of each patient, with and without consideration of positioning errors, were compared using tumor control probability (TCP) estimations from DVH reduction algorithms. Inclusion of the positioning errors in the dose calculation resulted in a mean decrease in absolute TCP of 5% in prostate patients when looking at the gross target volume (GTV) and 11% when looking at the planning target volume (PTV).

Rudat et al. investigated the combined effect of position variability (nonimmobilized) and prostate motion on the dose distribution in patients undergoing conformal radiation therapy for prostate cancer.[12] Positioning errors were determined by retrospectively comparing 54 orthogonal simulation films with 125 corresponding port films from 27 patients. Prostate motion was determined retrospectively in 28 patients from weekly CT images through the treatment isocenter using a CT simulator. The standard deviation of the patient positioning error in three directions ranged from 3.1 to 5.4 mm. The prostate motion variability in the anterior/posterior and mediolateral directions was 2.8 and 1.4 mm (one standard deviation), respectively. (Their method did not facilitate determination of prostate motion in the cephalad/caudal direction.) The one standard deviation of the estimated combined error in the anterior/posterior and mediolateral direction was 6.1 and 3.6 mm, respectively. Two dose-volume histograms were calculated; one assuming no error and one modified by the combination of patient positioning error (5.4 mm) and prostate motion (3.7 mm).[12] Tumor control probabilities calculated from the DVH of the GTV were reduced by 8.3%.

Michalski et al. explored the impact of geometric treatment variations on the dose.[71] An on-line radiotherapy imaging system captured daily beam positions in 12 patients treated for head and neck, thoracic, and pelvic malignancies. Each daily portal image was aligned with the prescription image using a template of anatomic structures. The outline of each treatment field edge was superimposed on the prescription image to generate a summary "block overlap isofrequency distribution." Dose distributions were recalculated considering daily setup variations. The results were expressed in isofrequency distributions where the 100% isofrequency curve represented areas covered throughout the treatment course and the 0% curve represented the extreme limits of variation; i.e., areas outside this curve were never within the primary beam. Pelvic treatment fields had the most random variation with an average of 14 mm 0 to 100% block overlap isofrequency compared with 12 mm for thoracic and 7 mm for head and neck sites.

EFFECTS OF PATIENT PARAMETERS ON SETUP REPRODUCIBILITY

The relationship between patient parameters (e.g., age, weight, and treatment position) and the ability to reproduce the setup has been investigated.[24,40,42,69,75]

Richards and Buchler analyzed 208 port films from 28 patients treated for gynecologic malignancies using anterior and posterior fields only.[40] The patients were stratified into three groups according to body weight. They demonstrated serious errors (≥2 cm offset and/or ≥20° rotation) in 14% of port films in patients weighing <150 lb versus 37% in patients weighing >150 lb. The number of patients completing a course of radiation therapy without a documented error was 3/9, 1/8, 0/11 among patients weighing 100 to 125 lb, 126 to 150 lb, and >150 lb, respectively. Caudal and/or right shifts were most common; 28% errors were in the caudal and 31% in the right direction.

The authors made an interesting observation in trying to determine the cause of the higher error rate in the right and caudal than in the left and cephalad directions. Patients would first sit on the table from their right sides and then lie down. In patients with excess weight or flaccid skin, setup marks were pulled to the right. They also postulated that patients who were obese and lost weight during treatment may have had their marks appear to shift caudally because of sagging abdominal tissues. Thirdly, it was noted that in the treatment room, the treating staff always stood to the right and inferior to the patient. Parallax then tended to give the appearance that the light field was in the correct simulated position when in reality it was set up in a caudal/right direction from what had been simulated. This error was compounded when the patients' treatment marks were "refreshed" and parallax again caused them to be placed caudal and right. Thus, the fields may have shifted in a nonrandom direction during the treatment course.

Song et al. analyzed the effect of patient body habitus and pelvic circumference on the ability of the immobilization devices to change accuracy of patient setup. No difference was seen with obesity or in patients with pelvic circumference >105 cm.[75] In the group of patients immobilized with a thermoplastic mask extending from the abdomen to midthigh, a significantly increased amount of lateral displacement with obesity (42 versus 23%) and with pelvic girth >105 cm (33 versus 29%) was observed. Other authors report no significant effect on treatment accuracy when the patient's age and weight, site of primary tumor, and treatment position (supine or prone) are considered.[42,69]

ABDOMEN

Translational and rotational errors were assessed in 45 patients undergoing paraaortic irradiation for seminoma without an immobilization device.[79] The distribution of translational and rotational deviations ranged from 2.3 to −2.7 mm and from −0.5 to 0.3°, respectively. Deviations between the simulator and treatment were similar to those during subsequent treatment delivery, with 95% of all absolute deviations <10 mm and 4°.

DISCUSSION

The purpose of the extensive literature review presented is to give the reader a sense of the magnitude of placement errors and the vastly different methods by which the accuracy of treatment delivery is determined and presented. It is difficult to compare the studies due to methodological and reporting differences, and thus the results should be interpreted with caution. For example, some authors report translational errors only, while others include rotational errors. Some report directional changes and others report overall misalignments. Systematic and random errors are sometimes reported together while others report them separately. Differences also exist in the number of patients/treatment ports examined, the degree of patient immobilization, and patient position used (supine and prone). Most reports focus on the frequency and magnitude of field placement errors while a few focus on the effect of field placement errors on the dose.

It is interesting to note that while some studies show improvement in field placements when immobilization devices are used, others show little or no improvement. It is possible that poorly built immobilization devices can be *detrimental* to patient positioning. To achieve successful patient immobilization, several important steps need to be taken prior to building the device, including determination of the extent of the device, choosing suitable materials, and explaining the procedure to the patient. The fabrication requires cooperation of the patient and an experienced staff. In our department, patients are urged to think about how the mold feels when it is finished so that when they return they can reposition themselves correctly.

Assessment of field placement errors often relies on a visual comparison of a simulation and a port film or interpretation of electronic images. Discrepancies in detection of field placement errors using these two methods for the same treatment setup frequently occur.[77] Thus, the method used to assess field placement accuracy among the studies above should be considered when results are interpreted. In many studies, image registration methods were used to match the simulation and portal image followed by matching of anatomic landmarks. The translations and rotations required to match the anatomic landmarks were reported as displacements. Other studies, including our own, relied on a visual comparison of two films (simulation and port film). When visual comparisons are made, small inaccuracies (<5 mm) may be difficult to detect, particularly in the pelvis, where bony reference points may appear vague. The difficulties of precise matching of skeletal landmarks may also be a problem in computer-based methods since a visual interpretation may be used when images are digitized. These uncertainties should be considered when discrepancies in the pelvis are reported.

Intermittent monitoring of the ability to deliver the prescribed treatment, in terms of both dose and locale, is prudent and may lead to discovery of systematic errors that otherwise could go undetected for long periods of time. Assessing the accuracy of patient/beam alignment and the effectiveness of an immobilization device is important, and the result should be considered when field margins are designed, with respect to both the target and normal tissues.

REFERENCES

1. Chui CS, LoSasso T, Spirou S: Dose calculation for photon beams with intensity modulation generated by dynamic jaw or multileaf collimators. *Med Phys* 21:1237, 1994.
2. Ling CC, Burman C, Chui CS, et al: Conformal radiation treatment of prostate cancer using inversely planned intensity-modulated photon beams produced with dynamic multileaf collimation. *Int J Radiat Oncol Biol Phys* 35: 721–730, 1996.

3. Hunt MA, Kutcher GJ, Burman C, et al: The effect of setup uncertainties on the treatment of nasopharynx cancer. *Int J Radiat Oncol Biol Phys* 27:437–447, 1993.
4. Hanley J, Lumley MA, Mageras GS, et al: Measurement of patient positioning errors in three-dimensional conformal radiotherapy of the prostate. *Int J Radiat Oncol Biol Phys* 37:435–444, 1997.
5. Althof VG, Hoekstra CJ, Loo H: Variation in prostate position relative to adjacent bony anatomy. *Int J Radiat Oncol Biol Phys* 34:709–715, 1996.
6. Ball WS, Wicks JD, Mettler FAJ: Prone-supine change in organ position: CT demonstration. *Am J Roentgenol* 135:815–820, 1980.
7. Balter JM, Sandler HM, Lam K, et al: Measurement of prostate movement over the course of routine radiotherapy using implanted markers. *Int J Radiat Oncol Biol Phys* 31:113–118, 1995.
8. Beard CJ, Bussière MR, Plunkett ME, et al: Analysis of prostate and seminal vesicle motion. *Int J Radiat Oncol Biol Phys* 27(suppl 1):136, 1993.
9. Beard CJ, Kijewski P, Bussière M, et al: Analysis of prostate and seminal vesicle motion: Implications for treatment planning. *Int J Radiat Oncol Biol Phys* 34:451–458, 1996.
10. Hanley J, Mageras GS, Sun J, Kutcher GJ: The effects of out-of-plane rotations on two dimensional portal image registration in conformal radiotherapy of the prostate. *Int J Radiat Oncol Biol Phys* 33:1331–1343, 1995.
11. Melian E, Kutcher G, Leibel S, et al: Variation of prostate position: Quantification and implications for three-dimensional conformal radiation therapy. *Int J Radiat Oncol Biol Phys* 27(suppl 1):137, 1993.
12. Rudat V, Schraube P, Oetzel D, et al: Combined error of patient positioning variability and prostate motion uncertainty in 3D conformal radiotherapy of localized prostate cancer. *Int J Radiat Oncol Biol Phys* 35:1027–1034, 1996.
13. Schild SE, Casale HE, Bellefontaine LP: Movements of the prostate due to rectal and bladder distension: Implications for radiotherapy. *Med Dosim* 18:13–15, 1993.
14. Zelefsky MJ, Happersett L, Leibel SA, et al: The effect of treatment positioning on normal tissue dose in patients with prostate cancer treated with three-dimensional conformal radiotherapy. *Int J Radiat Oncol Biol Phys* 37:13–19, 1997.
15. van Herk M, Bruce A, Kroes AP, et al: Quantification of organ motion during conformal radiotherapy of the prostate by three dimensional image registration. *Int J Radiat Oncol Biol Phys* 33:1311–1320, 1995.
16. Roeske JC, Forman JD, Mesina CF, et al: Evaluation of changes in the size and location of the prostate, seminal vesicles, bladder, and rectum during a course of external beam radiation therapy. *Int J Radiat Oncol Biol Phys* 33:1321–1329, 1995.
17. Sandler HM, Bree RL, McLaughlin PW, et al: Localization of the prostatic apex for radiation therapy using implanted markers. *Int J Radiat Oncol Biol Phys* 27:915–919, 1993.
18. Ten Haken RK, Forman JD, Heimburger DK, et al: Treatment planning issues related to prostate movement in response to differential filling of the rectum and bladder. *Int J Radiat Oncol Biol Phys* 20:1317, 1991.
19. Ahmad NR, Huq MS, Corn BW: Respiration-induced motion of the kidneys in whole abdominal radiotherapy: Implications for treatment planning and late toxicity. *Radiother Oncol* 42:87–90, 1997.
20. Davies SC, Hill AL, Holmes RB, et al: Ultrasound quantification of respiratory organ motion in the upper abdomen. *Br J Radiol* 67:1096–1102, 1994.
21. Fontenla E, Pelizzari CA, Chen CT: Implications of 3-dimensional target shape and motion in aperture design. *Med Phys* 23:1431–1441, 1996.
22. Gunderson LL, Russell AH, Llewellyn HJ, et al: Treatment planning for colorectal cancer: Radiation and surgical techniques and value of small-bowel films. *Int J Radiat Oncol Biol Phys* 11:1379, 1985.
23. Moerland MA, van den Bergh AC, Bhagwandien R, et al: The influence of respiration induced motion of the kidneys on the accuracy of radiotherapy treatment planning, a magnetic resonance imaging study. *Radiother Oncol* 30:150–154, 1994.
24. Luchka K, Shalev S: Pelvic irradiation of the obese patient: A treatment strategy involving megavoltage simulation and intratreatment setup corrections. *Med Phys* 23:1897–1902, 1996.
25. Schwartz LH, Richaurd J, Buffat L, et al: Kidney mobility during respiration. *Radiother Oncol* 32:84–86, 1994.
26. Ten Haken RK, Balter JM, Marsh LH, et al: Potential benefits of eliminating planning target volume expansions for patient breathing in the treatment of liver tumors. *Int J Radiat Oncol Biol Phys* 38:613–617, 1997.
27. Fu YT, Lam JC, Tze JM: Measurement of irradiated small bowel volume in pelvic irradiation and the effect of a bellyboard. *Clin Oncol* 7:188–192, 1995.
28. Green N, Iba G, Smith WR: Measures to minimize small intestine injury in the irradiated pelvis. *Cancer* 35:1633, 1975.
29. Green N: The avoidance of small intestine injury in gynecologic cancer. *Int J Radiat Oncol Biol Phys* 9:1385, 1983.
30. Holst R, La Couture T, Koprowski C, Goldschmidt E: A simple manual method of repositioning small bowel during pelvic irradiation. *Med Dosim* 20:123–129, 1995.
31. Rudat V, Flentje M, Engenhart R, et al: The belly-board technique for the sparing of the small intestine: Studies on positioning accuracy taking into consideration conformational irradiation technics. *Strahlenther Onkol* 171:437–443, 1995.

32. Shanahan TG, Mehta MP, Bertelrud KL, et al: Minimization of small bowel volume within treatment fields utilizing customized "belly boards." *Int J Radiat Oncol Biol Phys* 19:469, 1990.
33. Uno T, Itami J, Shiina T, et al: Evaluation of compression radiotherapy in pelvic treatment. *Nippon Igaku Hoshasen Gakkai Zasshi* 55:501–504, 1995.
34. Huh SJ, Lim DH, Ahn YC, et al: Effect of customized small displacement system in pelvic irradiation. *Int J Radiat Oncol Biol Phys* 40:623–627, 1998.
35. Devereux DF, Chandler JJ, Eisenstat T, Zinkin L: Efficacy of an absorbable mesh in keeping the small bowel out of the human pelvis following surgery. *Dis Colon Rectum* 31:17, 1988.
36. Herbert SH, Solin LJ, Hoffman JP, et al: Volumetric analysis of small bowel displacement from radiation portals with the use of a pelvic tissue expander. *Int J Radiat Oncol Biol Phys* 25:885, 1993.
37. Kavanah MT, Feldman MI, Devereux DF, Kondi ES: New surgical approach to minimize radiation-associated small bowel injury in patients with pelvic malignancies requiring surgery and high-dose irradiation. *Cancer* 56:1300, 1985.
38. Soper JT, Clarke-Pearson DL, Creasman WT: Absorbable synthetic mesh (910-Polyglactin) intestinal sling to reduce radiation-induced small bowel injury in patients with pelvic malignancies. *Gynecol Oncol* 29:283, 1988.
39. Acker JC, Marks LB: The lack of impact of pelvic irradiation on small bowel mobility: Implications for radiotherapy treatment planning. *Int J Radiat Oncol Biol Phys* 32:1473–1475, 1995.
40. Richards MJS, Buchler DA: Errors in reproducing pelvic radiation portals. *Int J Radiat Oncol Biol Phys* 2:1017–1019, 1977.
41. Leibel SA, Heiman R, Kutcher GJ, et al: Three dimensional conformal radiation therapy in locally advanced carcinoma of the prostate: Preliminary results of a phase I dose-escalation study. *Int J Radiat Oncol Biol Phys* 28:55–65, 1993.
42. Bieri S, Miralbell R, Nouet P, et al: Reproducibility of conformal radiation therapy in localized carcinoma of the prostate without rigid immobilization. *Radiother Oncol* 38:223–230, 1996.
43. Robinson DH: Prostate immobilization survey, 1995, personal communication.
44. Näslund I, Lax I, Blomgren H, et al: New prostate repositioning paradigm—a whole body frame for conformal radiotherapy techniques, with vertical patient alignment and rotation to a horizontal position. (abstr). *Int J Radiat Oncol Biol Phys* 39(suppl 2):328, 1997.
45. Gallagher MJ, Brereton HD, Rostock RA, et al: A prospective study of treatment techniques to minimize the volume of pelvic small bowel with reduction of acute and late effects associated with pelvic irradiation. *Int J Radiat Oncol Biol Phys* 12:1565, 1986.
46. Kinsella TJ, Bloomer WD: Tolerance of the intestine to radiation therapy. *Surg Gynecol Obstet* 151:273, 1980.
47. Letschert JGJ, Lebesque JV, deBoer RW, et al: Dose-volume correlation in radiation-related late small-bowel complications: A clinical study. *Radiother Oncol* 18:307, 1990.
48. Letschert JG: The prevention of radiation-induced small bowel complications. *Eur J Cancer* 31:1361–1365, 1995.
49. Palmer JA, Bush RS: Radiation injuries to the bowel associated with the treatment of carcinoma of the cervix. *Surgery* 80:458, 1976.
50. Potish RA, Jones TK, Levitt SH: Factors predisposing to radiation-related small-bowel damage. *Radiology* 132:479, 1979.
51. van Nagell JR, Maruyama Y, Parker JC, Dalton WL: Small bowel injury following radiation therapy for cervical cancer. *Am J Obstet Gynecol* 118:163, 1974.
52. Yoonessi M, Romney S, Dayem H: Gastrointestinal tract complications following radiotherapy of uterine cervical cancer: Past and present. *J Surg Oncol* 18:135, 1981.
53. van Kampen M, Wulf J, Eble M, et al: Three-dimensional planned radiotherapy in rectal cancer: Feasibility study and preliminary clinical results. *Strahlenther Onkol* 171:87–93, 1995.
54. Feldman MI, Kavanah MT, Devereux DF, Choe S: New surgical method to prevent pelvic radiation enteropathy. *Am J Clin Oncol* 11:25, 1988.
55. Rodier JF, Janser JC, Rodier D, et al: Prevention of radiation enteritis by an absorbable polyglycolic acid mesh sling. *Cancer* 68:2545, 1991.
56. Durig M, Steenblock U, Heberer M, Harder F: Prevention of radiation injuries to the small intestine. *Surg Gynecol Obstet* 159:162, 1984.
57. Sugarbaker PH: Intrapelvic prosthesis to prevent injury of the small intestine with high dose pelvic irradiation. *Surg Gynecol Obstet* 157:269, 1983.
58. Bentel GC: *Radiation Therapy Planning,* 2d ed. New York: McGraw-Hill, 1996.
59. Fraass BA, Kinsella TJ, Harrington FS, Glatstein E: Peripheral dose to the testes: The design and clinical use of a practical and effective gonadal shield. *Int J Radiat Oncol Biol Phys* 11:609, 1985.
60. Harter DJ, Hussey DH, Delclos L, et al: Device to position and shield the testicle during irradiation. *Int J Radiat Oncol Biol Phys* 1:361, 1976.
61. Kubo HD, Shipley WU: Reduction of the scatter dose to the testicle outside the radiation treatment field. *Int J Radiat Oncol Biol Phys* 8:1741, 1982.
62. Rudat V, Flentje M, Oetzel D, et al: Influence of the positioning error on 3D conformal dose distributions during fractionated radiotherapy. *Radiother Oncol* 33:56–63, 1994.
63. Verhey LJ: Immobilization and positioning patients for radiotherapy. *Semin Radiat Oncol* 5:100–114, 1995.

64. Bentel GC, Marks LB, Sherouse GW, et al: The effectiveness of immobilization during prostate irradiation. *Int J Radiat Oncol Biol Phys* 31:143–148, 1995.
65. Bijhold J, Lebesque JV, Hart AAM, Vijbrief RE: Maximizing setup accuracy using portal images as applied to a conformal boost technique for prostatic cancer. *Radiother Oncol* 24:261, 1992.
66. Dunscombe P, Loose S, Leszczynski K: Sizes and sources of field placement error in routine irradiation for prostate cancer. *Radiother Oncol* 26:174–176 1993.
67. El-Gayed AA, Bel A, Vijlbrief R, et al: Time trend of patient setup deviations during pelvic irradiation using electronic portal imaging. *Radiother Oncol* 26:162–171, 1993.
68. Gildersleve J, Dearnaley DP, Evans PM, Swindell W: Reproducibility of patient positioning during routine radiotherapy, as assessed by an integrated megavoltage imaging system. *Radiother Oncol* 35:151–160, 1995.
69. Huddart RA, Nahum A, Neal A, et al: Accuracy of pelvic radiotherapy: Prospective analysis of 90 patients in a randomised trial of blocked versus standard radiotherapy. *Radiother Oncol* 39:19–29, 1996.
70. Hunt MA, Schultheiss TE, Desobry GE, et al: An evaluation of setup uncertainties for patients treated to pelvic sites. *Int J Radiat Oncol Biol Phys* 32:227–233, 1995.
71. Michalski JM, Wong JW, Gerber RL, et al: The use of online image verification to estimate the variation in radiation therapy dose delivery. *Int J Radiat Oncol Biol Phys* 27:707–716, 1993.
72. Rabinowitz I, Broomberg J, Goitein M, et al: Accuracy of radiation field alignment in clinical practice. *Int J Radiat Oncol Biol Phys* 11:1857, 1985.
73. Rosenthal SA, Roach M III, Goldsmith BJ, et al: Immobilization improves the reproducibility of patient positioning during six-field conformal radiation therapy for prostate carcinoma. *Int J Radiat Oncol Biol Phys* 27:921, 1993.
74. Soffen EM, Hanks GE, Hwang CC, Chu JCH: Conformal static field therapy for low volume low grade prostate cancer with rigid immobilization. *Int J Radiat Oncol Biol Phys* 20:141, 1991.
75. Song PY, Washington M, Vaida F, et al: A comparison of four patient immobilization devices in the treatment of prostate cancer patients with three-dimensional conformal radiotherapy. *Int J Radiat Oncol Biol Phys* 34:213–219, 1996.
76. Tinger A, Michalski JM, Bosch WR, et al: An analysis of intratreatment and intertreatment displacements in pelvic radiotherapy using electronic portal imaging. *Int J Radiat Oncol Biol Phys* 34:683–690, 1996.
77. Valicenti RK, Michalski JM, Bosch WR, et al: Is weekly port filming adequate for verifying patient position in modern radiation therapy? *Int J Radiat Oncol Biol Phys* 30:431–438, 1994.
78. Bentel GC, Marks LB, Krishnamurthy R, Prosnitz LR: Comparison of two repositioning devices used during radiation therapy for Hodgkin's disease. *Int J Radiat Oncol Biol Phys* 39:791–795, 1997.
79. Kortmann RD, Hess CF, Meisner C, et al: Accuracy of field alignment in abdominal radiation therapy. *Int J Radiat Oncol Biol Phys* 35:779–783, 1996.

PROBLEMS

9-1 Pelvic organ motion related to prostate irradiation is
(*a*) not of concern since the treatment fields are small
(*b*) not of concern because the patients are always treated in the prone position
(*c*) important to be aware of since the target margins frequently are small and the dose high
(*d*) important to be aware of since the complication rates in the bladder are very high

9-2 Prostate motion is generally
(*a*) in excess of 10 mm
(*b*) in excess of 5 mm
(*c*) less than 5 mm
(*d*) between 5 and 10 mm

9-3 Patients irradiated for rectal carcinoma are often treated
(*a*) in the prone position to reduce skin reaction in the gluteal fold
(*b*) in the supine position to reduce skin reaction in the gluteal fold
(*c*) in the prone position to reduce small bowel volume within the pelvis
(*d*) in the decubitus position to reduce small bowel volume within the pelvis

9-4 Small-bowel displacement can be achieved by placing the patient
(*a*) in the supine position and exerting pressure over the pelvis
(*b*) prone and giving small bowel contrast
(*c*) prone with the pelvis over an opening in a belly board
(*d*) in decubitus position and asking him or her not to breathe

9-5 Patients with abdominal skin folds and morbidly obese patients may benefit from
(*a*) a prone position with the folds pulled away from the treatment fields
(*b*) a prone position because it flattens the abdomen
(*c*) a prone position because it allows field marks to be made on the less mobile posterior skin surface
(*d*) all of the above are true
(*e*) none of the above are true

9-6 Reproducing the foot position during pelvic irradiation is
(*a*) important as the appearance of pelvic bony anatomy on port films may change
(*b*) important for patient comfort
(*c*) irrelevant because it makes no difference to the treatment
(*d*) important for realigning the patient with pelvic skin marks

9-7 When a half-body positioning mold is made
(*a*) a support is placed under the patient's bent knees
(*b*) the foam is guided up between the patient's legs
(*c*) the mold is made thick and strong on each side of the waist
(*d*) when beam energies of $\leq$6 MV photons are used for lateral fields, the mold is made thin where the lateral beams traverse
(*e*) all of the above are true
(*f*) none of the above are true

9-8 Using a half-body positioning mold during prostate irradiation
(*a*) is detrimental to the treatment because only anterior setup marks can be made on the patient's skin
(*b*) is beneficial because setup marks can be made on the mold
(*c*) is beneficial because higher beam energies can be used
(*d*) is beneficial because higher doses can be delivered

9-9 When morbidly obese patients are placed prone on a belly board
(*a*) it is easy to see how the small bowel falls into the opening in the belly board
(*b*) an anterior field may be precluded because the beam would pass through an excess volume of normal tissue
(*c*) the small bowel is always displaced away from the pelvis
(*d*) the patient's position may be more reproducible

9-10 The ability to displace the small bowel away from pelvic radiation fields
(*a*) depends on what the patient ate for breakfast
(*b*) may be reduced in patients who had previous pelvic surgery
(*c*) depends on whether the patient had previous radiation therapy
(*d*) is irrelevant of previous surgery, radiation therapy, age, weight, and body habitus

9-11 In patients where preservation of fertility is desired and gonadal shielding is used

(*a*) it may be necessary to remove the testicular shield when port films are obtained so that the anatomy in the vicinity can be visualized

(*b*) port films should never be obtained of pelvic fields

(*c*) port films may need to be omitted after the initial set of films has been approved

(*d*) it may be necessary to modify the routine port film procedure by obtaining a single exposure of the irradiated field only

9-12 In evaluating the accuracy of pelvic field setup

(*a*) small discrepancies should be ignored

(*b*) everyone in the department should be told that the accuracy will be determined and results published

(*c*) comparison of simulation films and treatment port films is the only method used

(*d*) comparing simulation films with port films or electronic portal images can be used

9-13 In evaluating the accuracy of pelvic field setup, the results may vary depending on

(*a*) whether the study is prospective or retrospective

(*b*) the number of setups rather than the number of port films evaluated

(*c*) whether systematic and random errors were considered together or separately

(*d*) whether translational and rotational errors were considered together or separately

(*e*) all of the above are true

(*f*) none of the above are true

9-14 Using an immobilization mold during prostate irradiation

(*a*) appears to be detrimental for setup reproducibility

(*b*) appears to be beneficial for setup reproducibility

(*c*) has never been proven to improve setup reproducibility

(*d*) improves survival rates

CHAPTER

10

Extremities

INTRODUCTION

The most frequently occurring malignancies in the extremities that require radiation therapy include soft tissue sarcoma, Ewing's sarcoma, osteosarcoma, and metastatic disease. Soft tissue sarcomas are locally aggressive, not encapsulated, and usually infiltrate beyond the clinically evident tumor. They usually spread locally along muscle planes and tendinous attachments within their tissue compartments. Bone, interosseous membranes, and major fascial planes may provide a barrier for spread outside the compartment. Radiation therapy fields generally extend well beyond the tumor mass in the direction of the muscle compartment.

It is usually desirable not to irradiate the full circumference of an extremity in order to reduce the risk of edema distal to the radiation fields. The design of treatment fields that encompass a long muscle compartment while sparing a strip of tissue along the entire extremity can be difficult. This is particularly true when the beam orientation is oblique with respect to the extremity. It becomes more complicated when the tumor is in the proximal thigh and the fields need to extend into the pelvis. The optimal beam orientation for the thigh portion may be inappropriate for avoiding pelvic organs. Utilization of three-dimensional treatment-planning (3DTP) tools in these situations is usually helpful.

In this chapter, emphasis is placed on positioning and immobilization of patients irradiated for soft tissue sarcomas. However, these techniques apply to the treatment of other malignancies in the extremities. The most common extremity lesions irradiated are bone metastases. In such palliative situations, the issues of position and immobilization are usually not considered, since margins are often generous, the dose moderate, the treatment duration short, and long-term morbidity is not a concern. However, suboptimal positioning may increase acute effects and make further palliative radiation therapy of an adjacent site difficult. In irradiating bone metastases, care should be taken to minimize skin folds within the field and to orient and position field borders in a way that foresees possible future radiation therapy to an adjacent site. An immobilization device may occasionally be used to achieve these goals.

POSITIONING

The desired position is driven by efforts to avoid unnecessary irradiation of normal tissue, especially joints, and the need to leave a strip of unirradiated tissue along the entire extremity. When the target lies close to a joint, attempts should be made to spare at least a portion of the joint to preserve long-term function of the extremity.[1] Delivering high doses of irradiation to the entire circumference of an extremity may cause obstruction of lymphatic return, resulting in distal swelling (edema) that can be severe. In children requiring radiation therapy, it is also extremely important to consider avoiding the epiphyseal growth plates.

In computed tomography (CT)-based treatment planning, patient position may be limited by the physical diameter of the CT aperture and by the smaller CT image reconstruction area (Fig. 10-1).

Beam orientation relative to the patient depends on the target size, location, adjacent normal tissues, ability to move the opposite extremity away from the beams, the patient's agility, and collimator/couch/patient clearance; it is thus individualized. The desired orientation can be achieved by adjusting either the patient's position, machine settings, or both. Thus, it is important that the treatment planning team be aware of the anticipated beam arrangement prior to determining a feasible patient position and fabricating an immobilization device.

The extremity should be positioned such that its long axis is perpendicular to the beam's central axis in an effort to produce a uniform dose distribution (Fig. 10-2). If this is not done, the source-surface distance (SSD) may vary considerably across the field, leading to excess dose heterogeneities. The dose uniformity is also affected by the thickness of the limb.

UPPER EXTREMITIES

When the upper extremity is irradiated, it is desirable to extend the arm away from the torso to re-

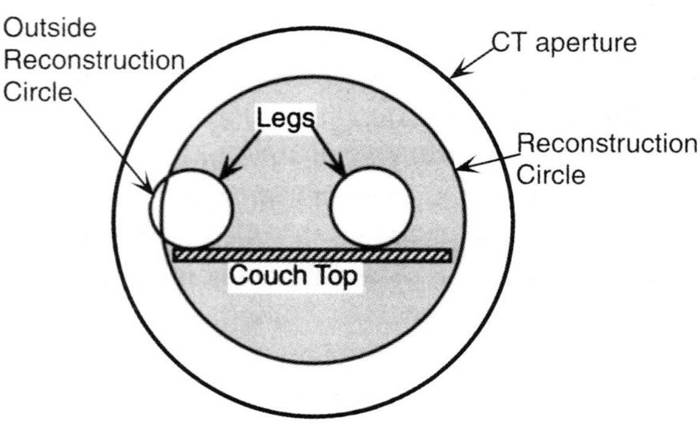

Fig. 10-1 The diameter of the image reconstruction circle on a CT unit is usually approximately 20 cm smaller than the aperture of the unit. In this illustration, part of one leg lies outside the reconstruction circle.

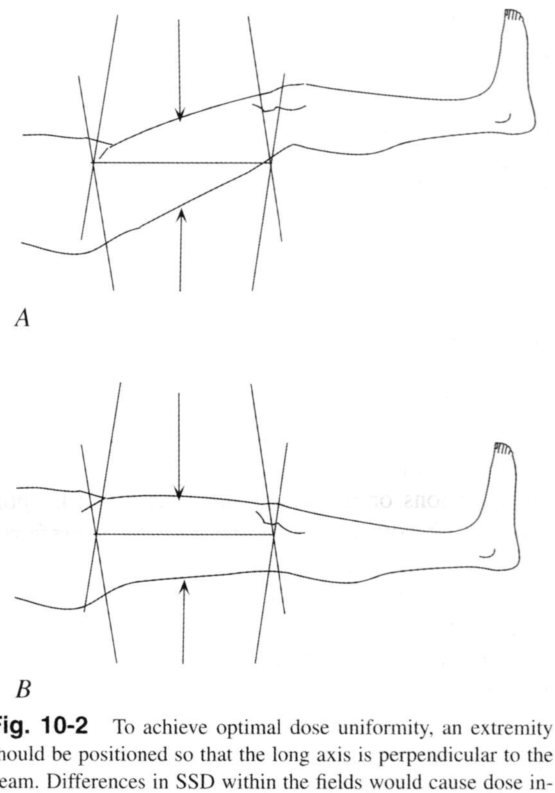

Fig. 10-2 To achieve optimal dose uniformity, an extremity should be positioned so that the long axis is perpendicular to the beam. Differences in SSD within the fields would cause dose inhomogeneties (*A*). When the long axis of the extremity is perpendicular to the beam, the dose uniformity is improved but is still affected by the variations in thickness of the limb (*B*). (From Bentel,[2] with permission. Courtesy of McGraw-Hill, New York.)

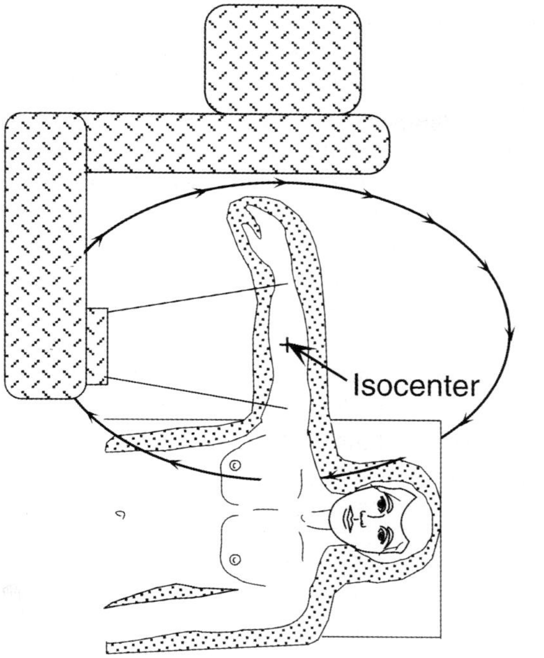

Fig. 10-3 When tumors in the lower arm or hand are treated, the arm can be abducted 90°. With the couch rotated 90°, the gantry can be rotated 360° without a collision. (From Bentel,[2] with permission. Courtesy of McGraw-Hill, New York.)

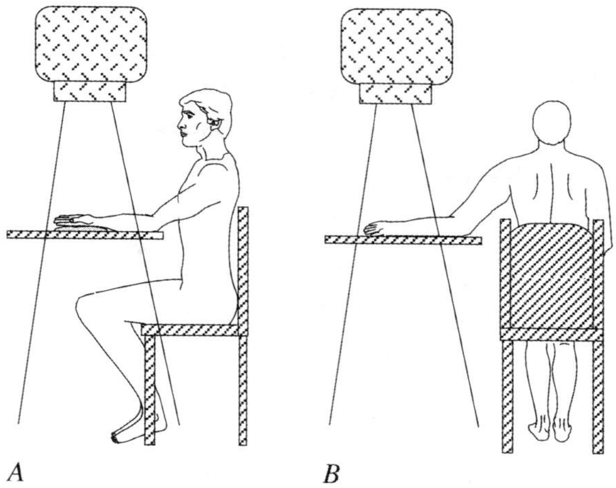

Fig. 10-4 When the patient is sitting during the treatment of the lower arm or hand, care should be taken to prevent the beam from exiting in the legs and feet (*B*).

duce axillary skin folds and reduce incidental irradiation of nontarget tissues. When tumors in the forearm or hand are treated, the arm can be abducted 90° and the couch turned 90° (Fig. 10-3).[2] With this setup, the possible beam orientations are practically unlimited, since the gantry can be turned 360° without collisions or interceptions of the beam by portions of the couch. The supine position is preferred over the prone because it usually is more comfortable and offers more freedom of arm positioning. A disadvantage of extending the arm away from the torso is the difficulty in obtaining a CT scan in the treatment position. Alternatively, when the tumor is in the forearm or hand, a scan could be obtained with the patient sitting or standing with the arm extended into the scanning aperture. This position can also be used for treatment delivery. However, care should be taken to prevent the exiting beam from diverging into the patient's legs (Fig. 10-4).

Tumors in the forearm and hand can usually be treated with opposed beams at some desirable oblique angle achieved by a combination of gantry angle and arm rotation. Selection of the precise rotation and translational position of the arm and the hand in these treatments is important due to the proximity of joints (elbow, wrist, fingers). Small arm/wrist rotations change the relative position of the ulna and radius and have a large effect on the relative position of bone/soft tissues/skin. In previous chapters, the problem of skin marks moving with respect to underlying tissues has been stressed. In this location (and the lower extremities) the situation is comparable, as the soft tissues move with respect to the skin marks.

When the medial portion of the arm is irradiated, the arm should be moved away from the torso to avoid unintentional inclusion of the chest or breast. In patients where the field includes the axilla, the arm should be moved away to reduce skin folds in the axilla and maintain skin sparing.

When the tumor is located in the upper arm and shoulder, raising the arm above the head in either the prone or supine position may facilitate desired beam orientations and a CT scan in treatment position (Fig. 10-5).

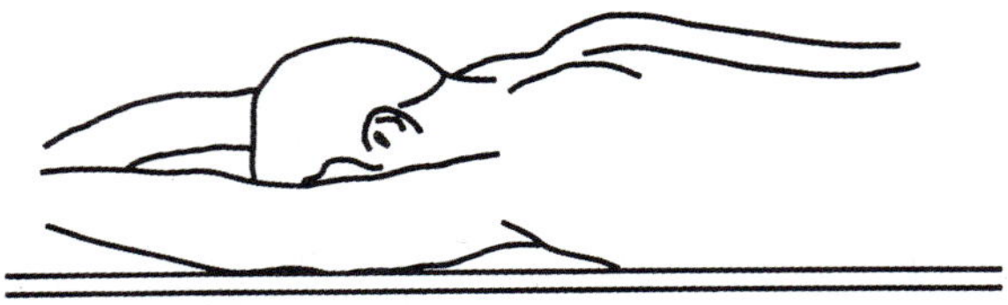

Fig. 10-5 A supine or prone position with the arms raised above the head can be used in irradiating tumors in the arm and shoulder. This position usually facilitates CT imaging.

LOWER EXTREMITIES

Radiation therapy of the lower extremities is often complicated by the need to move the unaffected leg away to facilitate a wider range of possible treatment angles. In patients where a CT scan is desired, the range of leg separation may be compromised by the limitations of the CT unit (Fig. 10-1). This can be addressed by moving the unaffected leg closer to the affected leg only for the CT scan. This move should be done carefully so that it does not change the position of the irradiated leg. Preferably, an immobilization device is made first (with the patient in desired treatment position), and then the contralateral leg is moved to facilitate movement through the CT aperture. Large leg separations may limit gantry clearance in the treatment room.

When tumors in the foot and lower leg are irradiated, the direction in which the unaffected leg is moved depends largely on the beam orientation needed to treat the affected leg. Tumors in the anterior and lateral muscle group compartments can generally be treated with the patient in supine position (Fig. 10-6). Opposed anteromedial/posterolateral fields can often be used in irradiating tumors in the anterior muscle group and opposed anterior/posterior fields for the lateral group. Tumors in the posterior muscle group compartment can usually be treated via opposed lateral fields. To avoid the unaffected leg, the patient can be placed in a decubitus position, with the legs separated in the anterior/posterior direction (Fig. 10.7*A*) and beams directed laterally, e.g., vertically. A decubitus position may be unstable for some patients and the supine position may therefore be preferred. In this case, the legs can be separated by elevating the affected leg, and the beam orientation, still lateral, would be horizontal

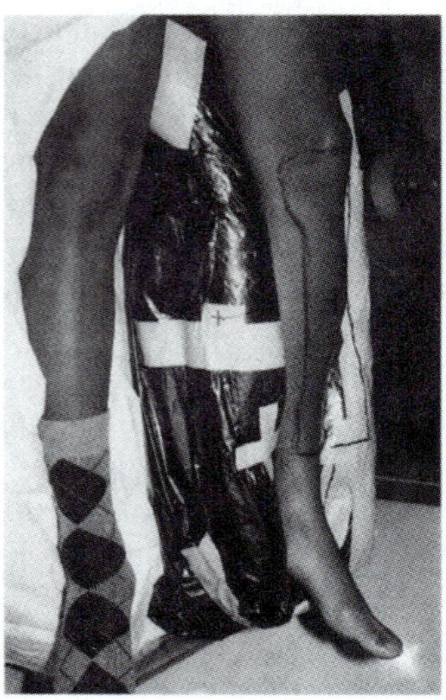

A

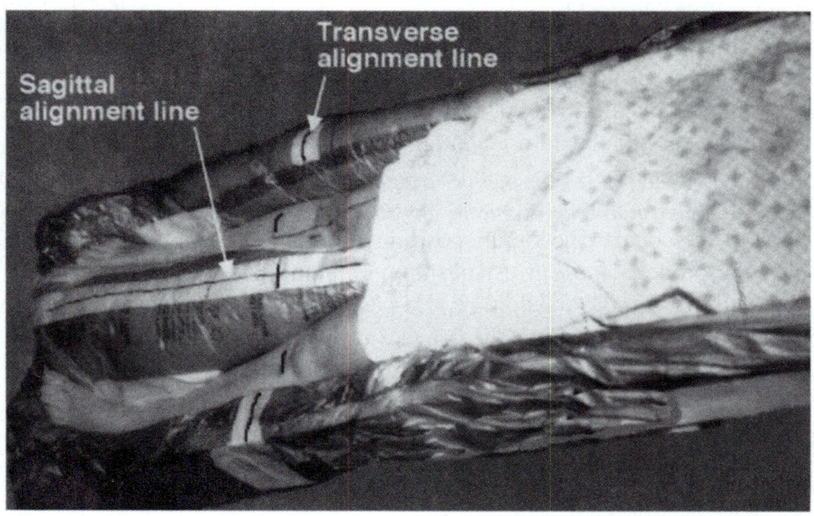

B

Fig. 10-6 *A* and *B*. Tumors in the anterior or lateral muscle groups can usually be treated with the patient in the supine position.

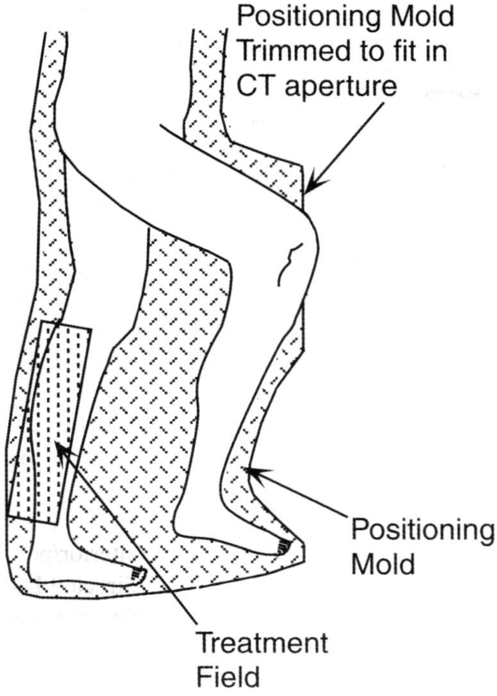

A

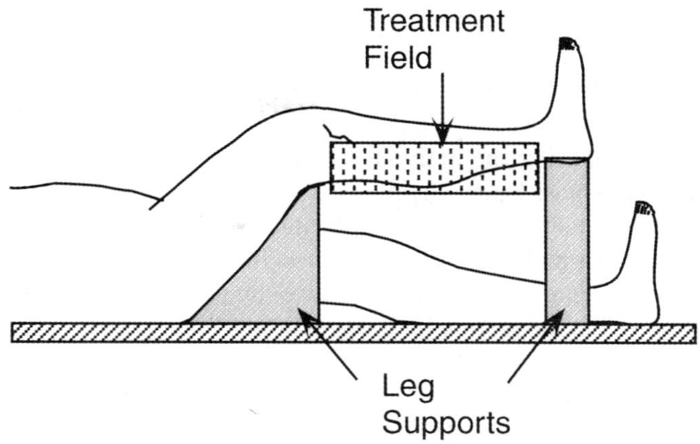

B

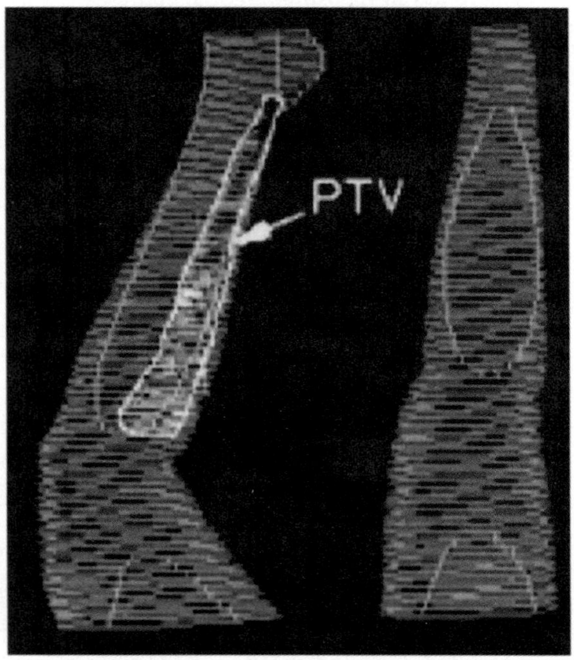

C

Fig. 10-7 For tumors in the lower leg, it is often possible to separate the legs, either by placing the patient in a decubitus position (*A*) or in the supine position with one leg elevated (*B*). Alternatively, the patient can be in the supine position with the knee of the affected leg bent and the foot rotated laterally (*C*). This patient is reversed on the treatment couch since couch motion in the in/out direction is limited. The positioning mold may need to be trimmed to facilitate CT scanning (*A*).

(Fig. 10.7*B*). Alternatively, the patient can be in the supine position with the knee of the affected leg bent and the foot rotated laterally (Fig. 10.7*C*).

Analogous to the arm/wrist rotation in the upper extremity, leg/foot rotation may cause changes in the relative positions of bone/soft tissues/skin in the lower extremity.

IMMOBILIZATION

During treatment of the extremities, where the diameter of the limb often is small relative to the target and efforts are made to spare a strip of soft tissue, the setup requires precise rotational accuracy. Utilization of effective patient immobilization devices is therefore important in the treatment of extremities.[3–5]

Prior to making an immobilization device, it is critical that the anticipated beam orientation be known and that the optimal patient position to implement those beam directions be determined. For example, there may be some beam directions that cannot be implemented due to machine limitations when the patient is supine (e.g., couch/gantry collision, beam attenuation by portions of the couch). In this situation, prone or decubitus positions should be considered.

The extremities are mobile; there are a large number of joints that can be flexed, extended, and rotated. To aid in repositioning, the entire extremity should be immobilized in such a way that flexion and rotation are prevented, thus assuring the relative position of bone/soft tissues/skin. Fixation of the extremity position relative to the torso reduces motion and aids in repositioning the extremity with respect to the radiation beam, e.g., the alignment system. Immobilization of both lower extremities should be considered, since a small change in the position of the unaffected leg may cause a small discrepancy in the position of the irradiated leg (Fig. 10-8). Immobilization of both upper extremities may not be necessary, since motion of one arm is unlikely to cause motion of the other; however, most patients probably would feel more comfortable if both arms were immobilized. When CT-based treatment planning is used, the width of an immobilization device including both upper extremities may be prohibitive.

The position of patients undergoing radiation therapy to the lower extremities usually needs to be reversed on the treatment couch due to motion limitations of the couch. Therefore, extreme care should be used when labeling documents pertaining to the treatment, since some of the setup directions are reversed from the routine. The labeling should include whether the right or left limb is treated.

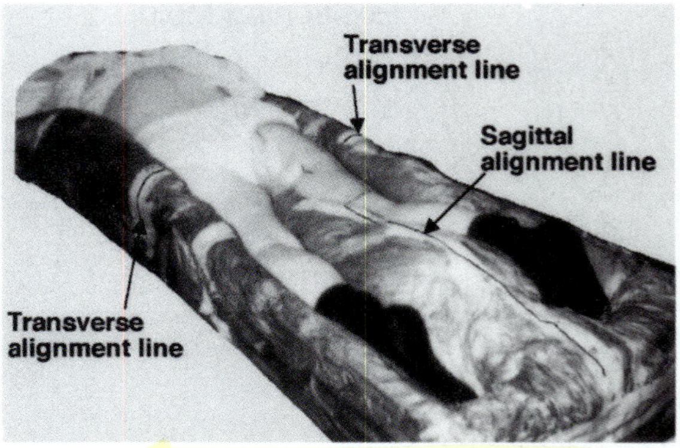

Fig. 10-8 When extremities are irradiated, it is important to immobilize the entire limb and fix the leg or arm position with respect to the torso. Setup marks are made on the immobilization device.

POSITIONING MOLDS

Patients irradiated for primary tumors of the extremities at Duke University Medical Center are usually immobilized in a customized Alpha Cradle™* including both legs and extending from below the feet to the waist for lower extremities (Fig. 10-8) or including the hand, arm, torso, and thighs for upper extremities (Fig. 10-9). The fabrication of these molds is similar; thus only the lower extremity mold is described in detail. General principles are described for the less frequently used upper extremity mold.

The positioning device consists of a Styrofoam† base, foaming agents, and a polyvinyl bag. The Styrofoam base is approximately 5 ft long, 2 ft wide, and about 1 in. thick and the polyvinyl bag is approximately 2 ft longer and 2 ft wider than the base. Before the mold is actually made, the patient, undressed below the waist and in a hospital gown, lies down on the base plate in treatment position (usually supine) for assessment of the needed leg position. Several pieces of Styrofoam are fastened to the base plate to support the patient's position and to form barriers to prevent the expanding foam from escaping. These pieces of Styrofoam become integral parts of the finished positioning device (i.e., they cannot be removed). The position of each piece of Styrofoam is determined with the patient on the base but without the foam.

*Smithers Medical Products, Inc., North Canton, Ohio.
†Dow Chemical, Midland, Michigan.

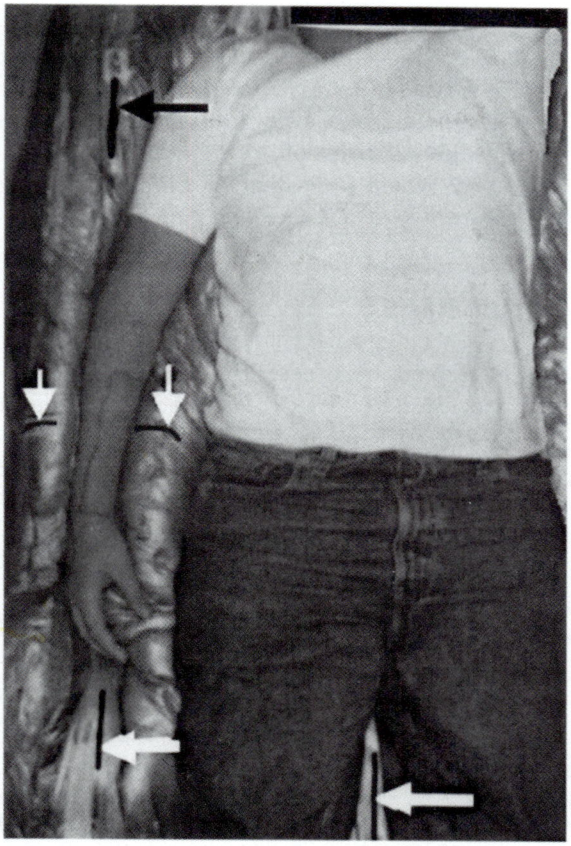

Fig. 10-9 An immobilization device used for irradiation of a tumor in the arm. The device includes both arms, the head, and the torso. It extends to the knees, thus fixing the relative position of the extremity and the torso. Setup marks are made on the mold (*arrows*).

A retaining wall of Styrofoam is added to each side and at the foot end of the base plate to contain the foam in close proximity to the patient. The legs are generally separated and the space between the legs is filled with scrap pieces of Styrofoam to reduce the amount of foam needed to make a tight-fitting mold. The affected leg is positioned such that it is approximately horizontal by placing small pieces of Styrofoam under the foot. If the separation of the legs requires that one leg be elevated rather than moved to the side, supports are added under this leg. A wedge-shaped piece of Styrofoam is placed under the thigh with the thick portion under the knee, and a large rectangular piece of Styrofoam is placed under the heel. The space under the lower leg (knee to heel) can be left unsupported in anticipation of treatment fields. The size of the foot support depends on how high the leg needs to be elevated but is often approximately 15 to 17 in. Prior to actually making the mold, this position is not very comfortable or stable; however, when the foam is added, it will aid in securing the supports to the base and form a mold under and on the sides of the foot.

With the patient removed, each piece of Styrofoam is fastened to the base plate, using masking tape. The Styrofoam shell is placed inside the large polyvinyl bag and approximately 660 mL of foaming chemicals, after being mixed and prepared as directed, is evenly distributed in the shell inside the protective bag. After the air is allowed to circulate inside the bag for a few seconds, it is squeezed out and the bag is sealed. The patient is returned to the shell by first sitting at the head end of the couch and then, with the help of staff, returns to the shell and assumes the treatment position. The foam expands inside the bag and fills the space between the barriers of the shell and the patient. The hospital gown is pulled up from under the patient such that the patient lies directly on the polyvinyl bag. The polyvinyl bag is pulled up around the legs and the foam is guided up on the sides of each foot and leg to form a tight-fitting mold preventing the foot from rotating. Similarly, in making a mold for the upper extremity, it is important to guide the foam up between the arm and chest and between the fingers. To make an effective mold, it is important that the polyvinyl bag be large to allow space for the foam to expand without being restricted by the bag. Masking tape, fastened to each side of the shell and stretched anteriorly across the patient's pelvis, forces the foam medially toward the patient, forming a tight-fitting mold. The foam stops expanding after approximately 7 to 10 min but requires an additional 10 min to become firm.

When the leg is elevated, the immobilization device is also made with a base plate and barriers placed inside a large polyvinyl bag. To contain foam near the elevated heel, the heel support can be placed inside a separate smaller bag with about 150 to 200 mL of foam. The smaller bag is placed inside the larger bag and, as the foam expands, it is guided up around the sides of the heel and foot, where it will set and form an excellent foot immobilization within a few minutes. The separate bag becomes an integral part of the device (i.e., it cannot be removed). A similar arrangement can be used when it may be desired to extend the patient's arm and raise the hand in treating an upper extremity.

A flat hardwood board, wider and longer than the mold and placed on top of the couch *before* the fabrication is initiated, is used to prevent leaking foam from forming a lip over the couch. Such a lip or other irregular surface under the mold can cause the immobilization device to tilt, potentially giving rise to field misalignments.

In patients where the legs are widely separated and the unaffected limb is temporarily displaced for a CT scan, the empty indentation should be indicated with radiopaque markers to give a better understanding of the limb's position during treatment. This aids in determining the range of acceptable beam directions that do not incidentally include the unaffected leg. For patients where the unaffected leg needs to be displaced during the CT scan, it is usually necessary to trim the width of the positioning mold such that it fits inside the CT aperture (Fig. 10-7*A*). The leg position should be selected prior to the mold fabrication such that minimal trimming is necessary.

Obtaining a CT scan may not be possible when the *affected* leg is elevated, since this leg position should not be changed. However, if the *unaffected* leg is elevated, it can temporarily be positioned straight during the CT scan. The height of the foot support should be limited such that it will clear the CT aperture while the leg is displaced.

In patients where a scrotal shield is anticipated, it should be in place during the mold making so that an indentation for its position is formed. When external male genitalia need to be displaced during treatment, a retractor (Fig. 9-16, Chap. 9) or an athletic support should be used during the mold making. In some patients it is also possible to guide the foam such that, when it hardens, it creates a displacement barrier for the external genitalia. Likewise, in making a mold for the upper extremity, it may be possible to use the foam to create a barrier to displace the breast away from the arm so as to avoid incidental radiation to the breast. Some patients may benefit from wearing a brassiere during the treatment to displace the breast medially.

SETUP MARKS

The positioning mold described above is an excellent repositioning device that allows alignment marks to be made on the mold—an important consideration in treating an extremity (Figs. 10-6 and 10-8). Small motions of the distal portion of the extremity may cause skin marks and underlying tissues to move. For successful patient/beam alignment, it is extremely important that the limb be repositioned precisely with respect to the sagittal alignment line for each treatment. The same is certainly true for the coronal line; however, this is hopefully achieved by placing the mold on the same flat tabletop each day.

When CT-based treatment planning is utilized, the sagittal alignment line is marked on the mold between the legs from the thighs to the feet (above the head and between the knees for upper extremity). The transverse alignment line is marked on each side of the mold and on the patient's legs. The skin just below the knees is usually relatively immobile and therefore is an excellent location for alignment marks. These marks help in assuring that the patient is returned to the mold correctly in the cephalad/caudal direction. These marks may not necessarily represent the isocenter but are merely to align the patient correctly on the couch. Of course, it is necessary that the couch be set at the 0° position when these lines are marked. During treatment simulation, the central axis and treatment fields are marked on the mold and on the patient's skin.

Reports pertaining to setup reproducibility during extremity irradiation are largely nonexistent; however, one might postulate that using an immobilization device provides an advantage.

REFERENCES

1. Stinson SF, DeLaney TF, Greenberg J, et al: Acute and long-term effects on limb function of combined modality limb sparing therapy for extremity soft tissue sarcoma. *Int J Radiat Oncol Biol Phys* 21:1193–1199, 1991.
2. Bentel GC: *Radiation Therapy Planning,* 2d ed. New York: McGraw-Hill, 1996.
3. Niewald M, Berberich W, Schnabel K, et al: A simple method for positioning and fixing the extremities during the radiotherapy of soft-tissue sarcomas. *Strahlenther Onkol* 166:295–296, 1990.
4. Perez CA, Brady LW: *Principles and Practice of Radiation Oncology,* 2d ed. Philadelphia: Lippincott, 1992.
5. Tepper J, Rosenberg SA, Glatstein E: Radiation therapy technique in soft tissue sarcoma of the extremity—policies of treatment at the National Cancer Institute. *Int J Radiat Oncol Biol Phys* 8:263–273, 1982.

PROBLEMS

10-1 Soft tissue sarcomas
- (*a*) usually spread through several muscle compartments
- (*b*) usually spread locally along muscle planes and the tissue compartments from which they originate
- (*c*) usually spread along muscle planes in the compartments from which they originate toward the nearest joint
- (*d*) spread, promoted by gravity, toward the distal joint

10-2 When extremities are irradiated, it is important to spare
- (*a*) a strip of soft tissue along the entire extremity to prevent obstruction of blood flow from the distal portion of the limb
- (*b*) a strip of a bone in the limb to prevent obstruction of lymphatic flow from the distal portion of the limb
- (*c*) a strip of soft tissue along the entire extremity to prevent obstruction of lymphatic flow from the distal portion of the limb
- (*d*) a muscle compartment on each side of the affected muscle to prevent obstruction of blood flow from the distal portion of the limb

10-3 When tumors in the hand and forearm are irradiated
- (*a*) the patient should be sitting with the arm on the couch and facing the treatment couch with the other arm on the knee under the couch
- (*b*) the patient should be supine on the treatment couch with the arm as close to the torso as possible
- (*c*) the patient should be standing as close to the couch as possible with the affected arm on the couch and the other arm under the couch
- (*d*) the patient should be supine on the treatment couch with the affected arm extended out 90° and the couch turned 90°

10-4 When soft tissue sarcomas in the posterior lower extremities (calf of the leg) are irradiated
- (*a*) the opposite leg can be resting comfortably close to the affected leg
- (*b*) the patient should be in decubitus position with the opposite leg elevated as high as possible
- (*c*) the patient should be in prone position with both legs together
- (*d*) the patient should be in decubitus position with the unaffected leg moved as far posterior as possible

10-5 When soft tissue sarcomas in the extremities are irradiated, immobilization devices
(*a*) are unnecessary because the target is easily identified
(*b*) are unnecessary because the patients can hold the limb very still
(*c*) should be used because patients with tumors in an extremity tend to move more
(*d*) should be used because it is important to spare normal tissues and therefore the target margins are often small

10-6 When soft tissue sarcomas in the calf of the leg are irradiated
(*a*) only the affected area below the knee needs to be immobilized
(*b*) the limb should be immobilized from the midthigh to below the foot
(*c*) booth legs need to be immobilized from the waist to below the feet
(*d*) only the foot of the affected extremity needs to be immobilized

10-7 Using a positioning mold for patients irradiated for soft tissue sarcomas in the extremities
(*a*) allows setup marks to be made on the mold
(*b*) precludes having to make setup marks on the skin
(*c*) precludes the need for a treatment-planning CT scan
(*d*) allows a treatment-planning scan to be made on every patient

CHAPTER

11

Unconventional Treatment Positions

INTRODUCTION

There are some situations in radiation therapy where the customary horizontal patient position on the treatment couch is not used. This may be because the patient's weight exceeds the tolerance of the table, the patient is unable to lie down (e.g., shortness of breath), an erect position is preferred, or large field sizes (e.g., extended treatment distances) are needed. In some patients, an unconventional treatment position may be necessary due to more than one of these reasons.

Patients whose weight exceeds the couch tolerance may be treated while lying on an alternate bed (stretcher, hospital bed) or while sitting in a chair. When the head, chest, or upper extremities need to be irradiated in patients unable to lie down or where an erect position is desirable, the treatment may be delivered with the patient seated. When the abdomen, pelvis, or lower extremities need to be irradiated, a sitting position may not be possible and the patient may be standing. Patients who do not exceed the weight restriction of the couch but require an erect position may be treated while seated on the treatment couch. This facilitates utilization of the couch motions when setting up the treatment fields, an advantage when setting up complex field arrangements (Fig. 8-11, Chap. 8). In some situations, the needed treatment distance cannot be achieved when the patient is lying on the treatment couch. In these situations, the treatment may be delivered with the beam directed horizontally across the room and the patient standing or lying on an alternate bed at an appropriate distance. Alternatively, the beam may be directed vertically with the patient lying on the floor.

SITTING POSITION

A sitting position is sometimes preferred in patients with Hodgkin's disease to reduce the width of the mediastinal mass. A sitting position may also be necessary in patients with vena cava obstruction and/or congestive heart failure. These patients frequently have shortness of breath that worsens when they are lying flat, requiring an erect or semirecumbent position. After a few treatments, the vena cava obstruction often subsides and the remaining treatments may be delivered with the patient in the conventional horizontal position. A semirecumbent position can be achieved by having the patient sit up in the hospital bed; however, this would preclude a posterior field. Alternatively, the patient can be seated in a chair with or without a removable back support for unobstructed treatment of the posterior field. Such a chair ideally should move vertically to facilitate appropriate height, since the machine's isocenter is fixed in space at a given distance above the floor. Casters under the chair would facilitate moving the patient to the desired position in the beam. This type of chair, (Fig. 7-3, Chap. 7) has been described by Marcus et al.[1] Other chairs offer support for the raised or lowered arm positions (Fig. 11-1).

If no dedicated treatment chair is available, the patient can sit on a straight chair with arm rests.[2] Alternatively, the arms can rest on the backs or sides of other chairs. For the posterior field, the patient may need to reverse the position and face the back rest to facilitate unobstructed treatment of the posterior field. Alternatively, the patient can be seated sideways on a chair, resting one arm on the same chair and the other arm on another chair placed alongside (Fig. 11-2). In this arrangement, height adjustment and movement into the radiation beam are limited and the setup is relatively difficult to reproduce.

HALF-BODY IRRADIATION

Half-body irradiation is typically used to treat diffuse bony metastases.[3–5] These treatments usually require large treatment fields and hence long treatment distances. Patients requiring large-field irradiation are therefore usually positioned on a cushion on the floor, alternating between the supine and prone position for anterior and posterior fields, respectively. Many of these patients are in pain and

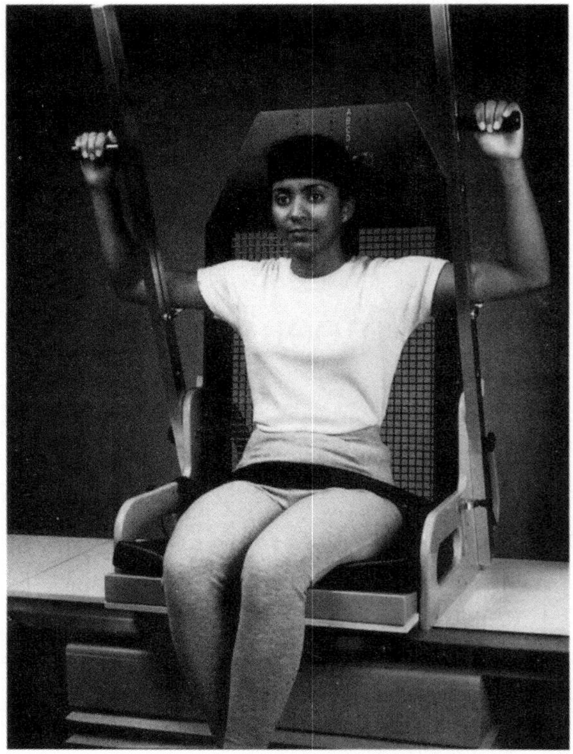

Fig. 11-1 A treatment chair offering support for the raised or lowered arm position. (Courtesy of MED-TEC, Inc., Orange City, Iowa.)

may also have fragile bones, making it difficult or impossible to lie down on or rise from the floor. Alternatively, the patient can be placed on a special platform fitted with casters that has a rigid surface and adjustable height.

Some modern treatment couches are capable of large vertical motion; thus the required field size may be obtained with the patient on the couch. The size of the treatment area can be increased by angulating the beam a few degrees cephalad or caudal for the upper or lower half-body, respectively (Fig. 11-3). When this angle is equal to the angle of the diverging field edge, the field edge will transect the patient vertically, facilitating reliable field matching with potential future fields. Another method to achieve larger coverage is to turn the collimator 45° to take advantage of the larger field dimension

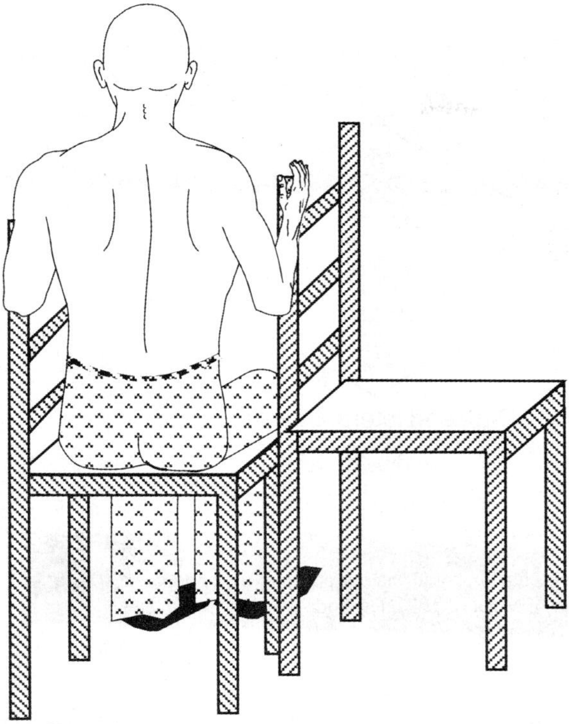

Fig. 11-2 The position of a sitting patient may be more stable when a second chair is provided for support. (From Bentel,[2] with permission. Courtesy of McGraw-Hill, New York.)

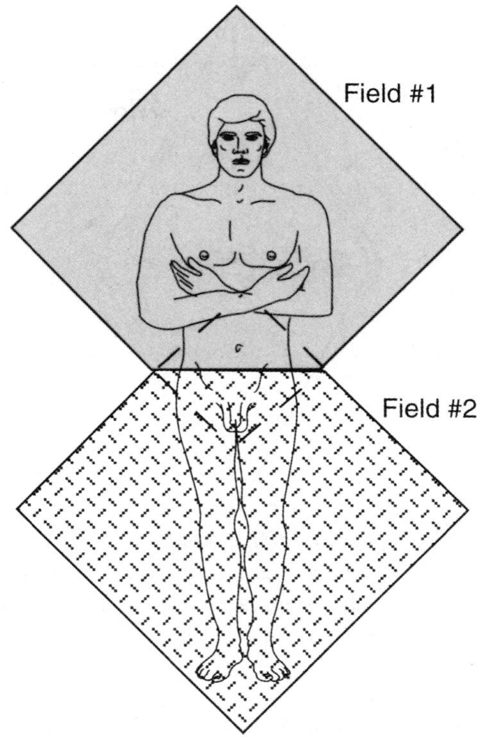

Fig. 11-4 The collimator can be turned 45° to take advantage of the larger diagonal dimensions of the field. Caution should be used, since the corners of the light field may be outside the radiation beam. (From Bentel,[2] with permission. Courtesy of McGraw-Hill, New York.)

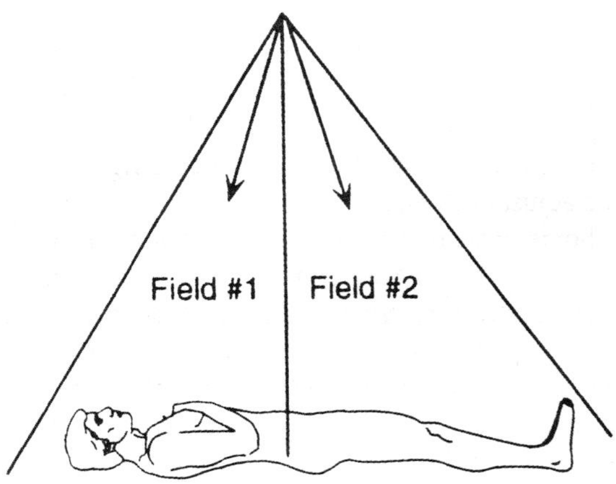

Fig. 11-3 To achieve a larger field in half-body irradiation, the gantry can be angled a few degrees. The angle should be away from the unirradiated portion of the body, facilitating potential future field matching. (From Bentel,[2] with permission. Courtesy of McGraw-Hill, New York.)

(Fig. 11-4). Caution should be used, since the corners of the light field may be outside the radiation beam.

TOTAL-BODY IRRADIATION

In total-body irradiation (TBI), very large treatment fields and long treatment distances are needed. Different treatment techniques have been described.[5–12] The choice of treatment position is largely dependent on the size of the treatment room, available equipment, whether lung shielding is required, and whether the patient is a child or an adult (Fig. 11-5). A small child may be treated on the treatment couch

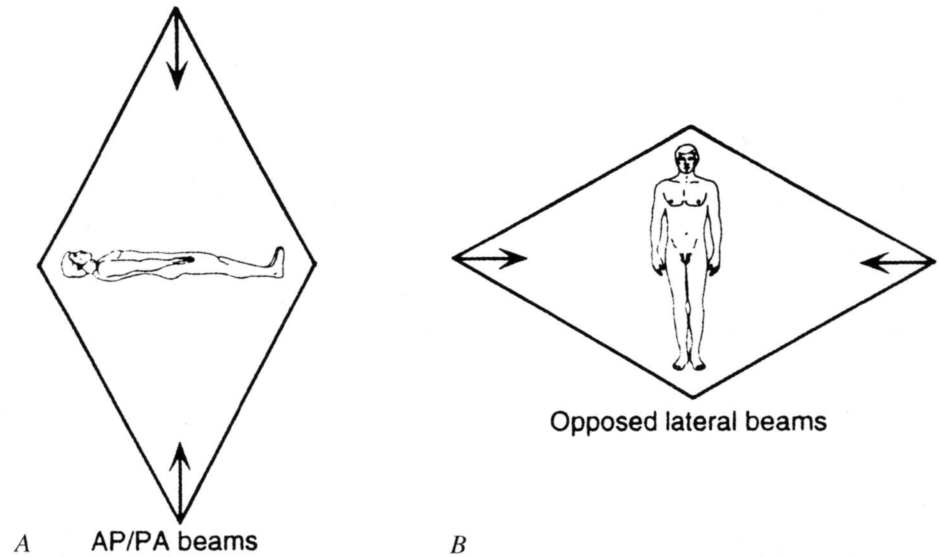

Fig. 11-5 Total-body irradiation is usually delivered via either opposed anterior/posterior (*A*) or opposed lateral fields (*B*). (From Bentel,[2] with permission. Courtesy of McGraw-Hill, New York.)

utilizing either field arrangement. The position may be supine and the gantry turned 180° for opposing fields. The ability to irradiate a child on the treatment couch is limited by the size (length) of the patient and the range of couch motion. When lateral fields are used and the patient is supine on the treatment couch, the distance, and hence the field size, can be increased by lateral motion of the couch. The anterior and posterior field sizes are increased by lowering and raising the treatment couch, respectively. However, for the posterior field, the couch often cannot be raised sufficiently to achieve the same field size. The child can be elevated (increasing the distance) on a cushion or platform placed on top of the couch (Fig. 11-6). These methods are not isocentric; however, the rotational capabilities of the machine and the laser alignment system can be used to achieve the needed treatment conditions.

Total-body irradiation of older children and adults usually requires very long treatment distances (~3 to 4 m), precluding treatment with the patient on the treatment couch. Other techniques have therefore been developed. When lateral fields are used, the patient is often placed supine in a semirecumbent position with the knees bent so that the beams can encompass the entire body (Fig. 11-7). The position of the bed and patient is reversed for the opposing lateral field. In this technique, the arms are placed over the lungs in the beam's-eye view to

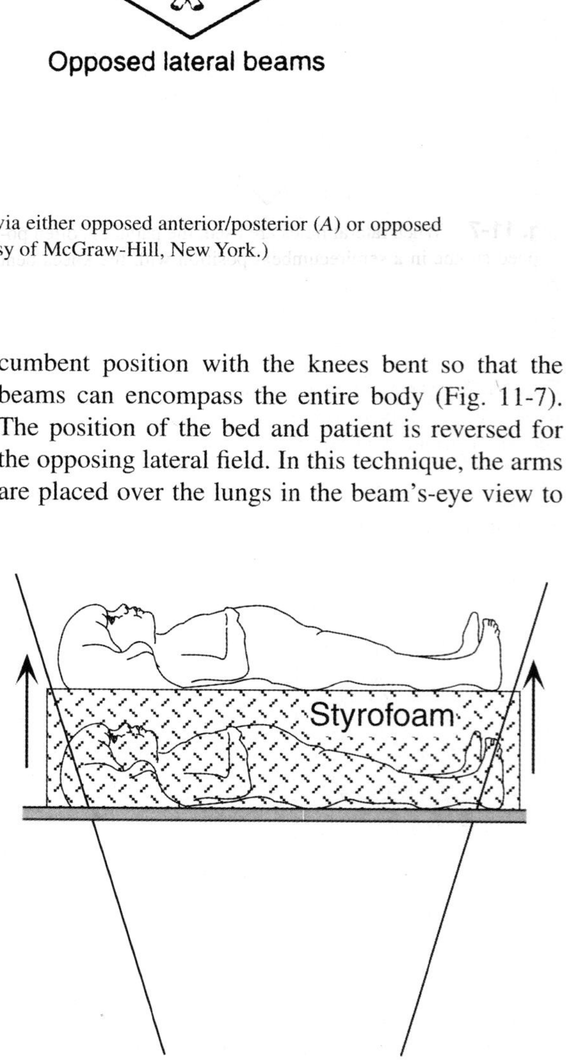

Fig. 11-6 The size of the posterior field can be increased by elevating the patient above the couch on a sheet of Styrofoam.

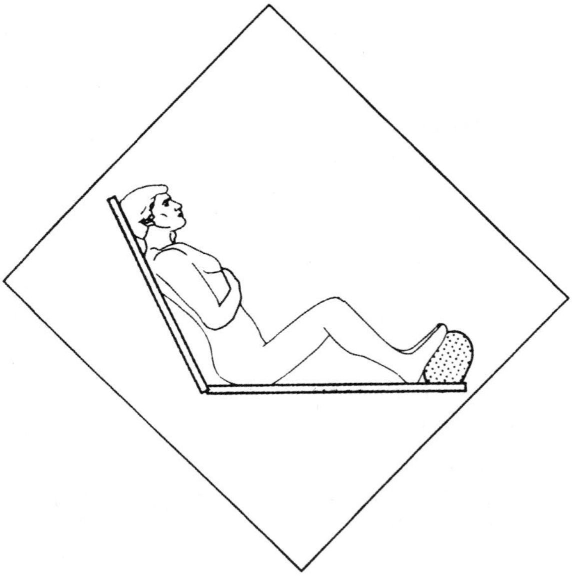

Fig. 11-7 When lateral fields are used, the patient is often positioned supine in a semirecumbent position with the knees bent in order to encompass the entire body within the beams. (From Bentel,[2] with permission. Courtesy of McGraw-Hill, New York.)

partly compensate for the lower lung density, which leads to an increased lung dose. For patients whose knees are bent, it is important to provide a brace to prevent the feet from slipping and possibly extending outside the radiation beam.

When opposed anterior and posterior fields are used, the patient may need to be treated in an erect position. Partial transmission lung-shielding blocks are sometimes used; hence the patient's position within the beams is extremely important. Concerns regarding the positional stability of the patient are therefore related to the need for the patient to remain fixed with respect to the beam-modifying devices. Every attempt should be made to immobilize the patient. One approach is to use a bicycle-type seat to rest on and adjustable handlebars to reduce risks of motion within the beams. Many patients' physical strength tends to diminish during the treatment course (only a few days) and a standing position, even with supports, may therefore not be practical.

In the treatment techniques described above, both the patient and the treatment beam are stationary. A technique where the patient moves horizontally under a stationary beam has also been described (Fig. 11-8).[13] For this approach, the patient's position is generally supine on the treatment couch.

TOTAL-SKIN ELECTRON IRRADIATION

Total-skin electron irradiation (TSEI) is sometimes used in the treatment of cutaneous diseases such as

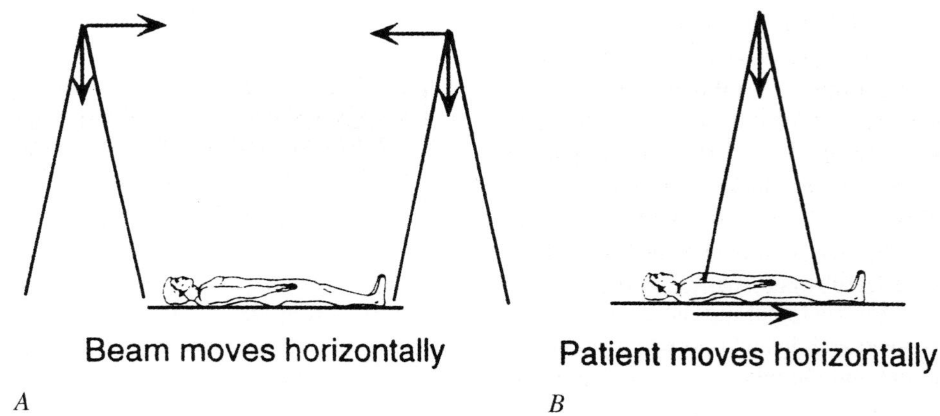

Fig. 11-8 In one technique of total-body irradiation, the beam "sweeps" over the patient (*A*) or the patient moves horizontally under a stationary beam (*B*). (From Bentel,[2] with permission. Courtesy of McGraw-Hill, New York.)

mycosis fungoides and Kaposi's sarcoma. In these diseases, a therapeutic dose is needed in approximately the first centimeter of tissue over the whole body while the underlying tissues should be spared.

Treatment techniques to achieve TSEI were developed at Stanford University during the 1950s. This technique, now used in many other centers, has undergone several modifications as new treatment equipment has been developed and more experience has been gained. Total-skin electron irradiation techniques are complex and, as in TBI, require large treatment fields and long distances. Delivering uniform doses is practically impossible due to many irregular surfaces and skin folds. For example, it is almost impossible to expose the perineum to the electron beam. Other areas where dose inhomogeneity is a problem include the hands and feet (between fingers and toes), the scalp on top of the head, ears, nose, under pendulous breasts, and the soles of the feet.

Several variations of TSEI techniques have been described.[13–22] In most techniques, the patient is standing with arms raised and legs spread to avoid self-shielding (Fig. 11-9*A*). The patient's body is turned to six different positions during each treatment; thus, the body is exposed to six fields equally spread around the circumference. Due to the higher dose in the center of the field and diminishing dose in the periphery, the treatment fields are angled up for treatment of the cephalad and down for the caudal portions of the body, respectively. Thus, the peak dose is above and below the patient—e.g., only half of the beam is irradiating the patient. Thus, 12 treatment fields are used for complete exposure: 6 for the upper and 6 for the lower half of the body. As the patient's body is turned, the arm and leg positions are also changed to expose the skin around the entire circumference of the extremities. Given the long time required to deliver the dose at such an extended treatment distance, usually only 6 fields (3 cephalad and 3 caudal) are delivered during one treatment and the other 6 on alternate treatment days (Fig. 11-9*B*).

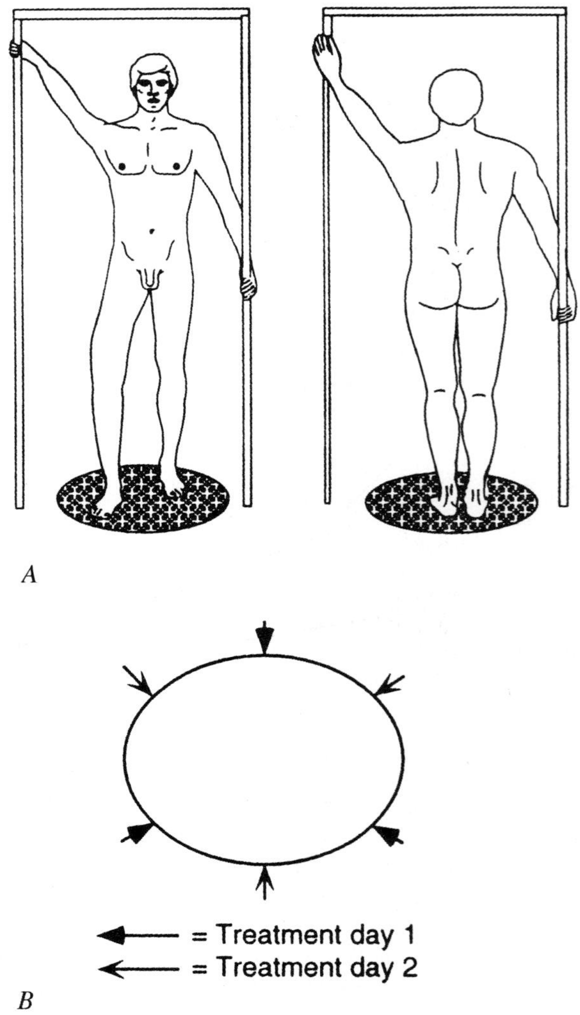

Fig. 11-9 *A*. In total-skin electron irradiation, the patient's arms are raised and legs spread to expose as much as possible of the skin surface to the beam. Six different positions are used during each treatment (*B*). (From Bentel,[2] with permission. Courtesy of McGraw-Hill, New York.)

As an alternative to the patient turning and changing position several times during the treatment, the patient may stand on a slowly rotating platform during the treatment, exposing the skin surfaces to the electron beam.[15,23] Another technique, consisting of six pendulum arcs symmetrically spread around the patient's circumference and "sweeping" in the direction of the patient's longitudinal axis, is sometimes used (Fig. 11-10).[20] In this

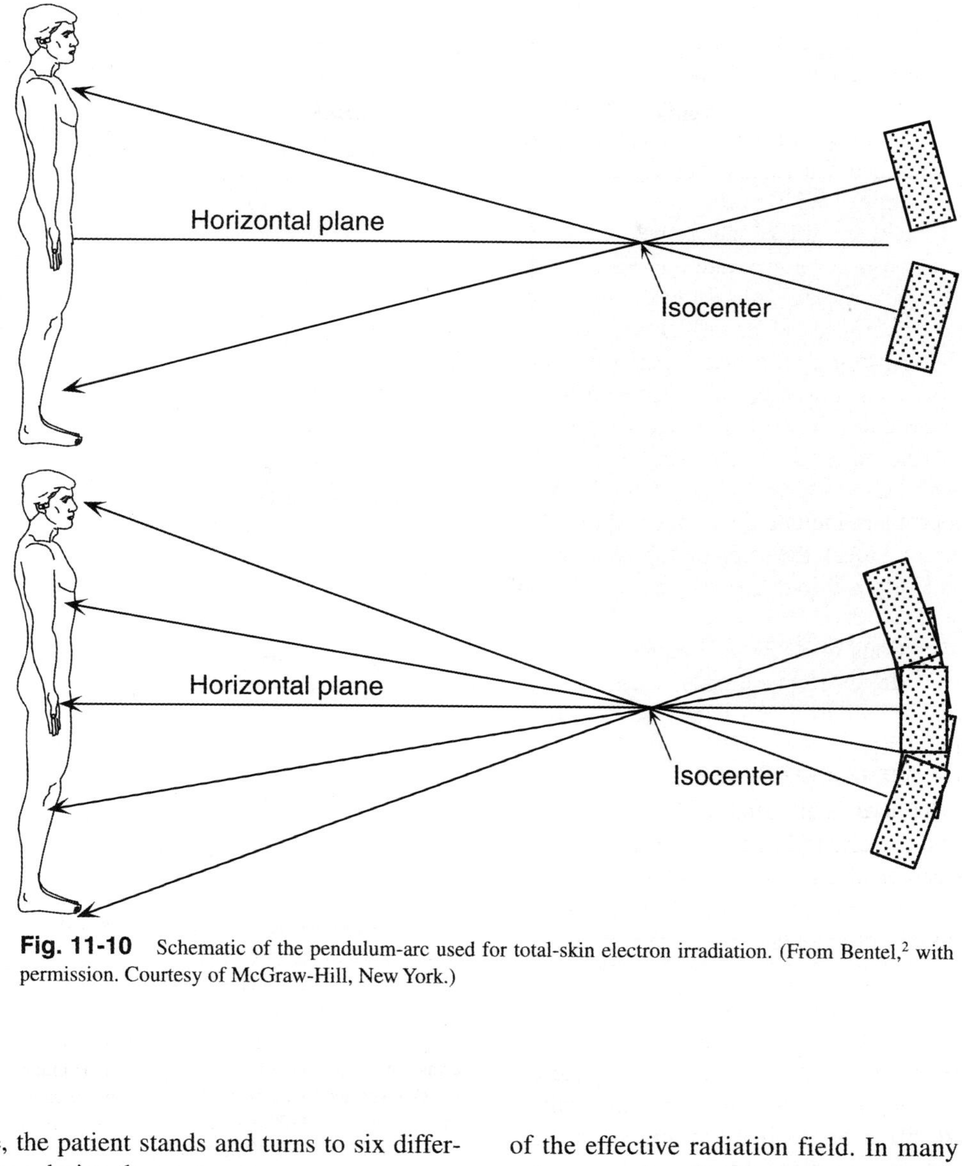

Fig. 11-10 Schematic of the pendulum-arc used for total-skin electron irradiation. (From Bentel,[2] with permission. Courtesy of McGraw-Hill, New York.)

technique, the patient stands and turns to six different positions during the treatment.

BEAM CONSIDERATIONS DURING HALF- AND TOTAL-BODY IRRADIATION

In setting up large fields (half- or total-body irradiation), consideration should be given to the penumbras of large fields and the size and shape of the effective radiation field. In many linear accelerators, the effective beam is circular when the maximum field is used, rather than square, as the field light indicates (Fig. 11-11). The circular shape originates from the fact that the primary beam collimator produces a circular field. In some linear accelerators, the secondary collimator, producing a square light field, is set to include the maximum diameter of the circle, leaving the corners unirradiated.

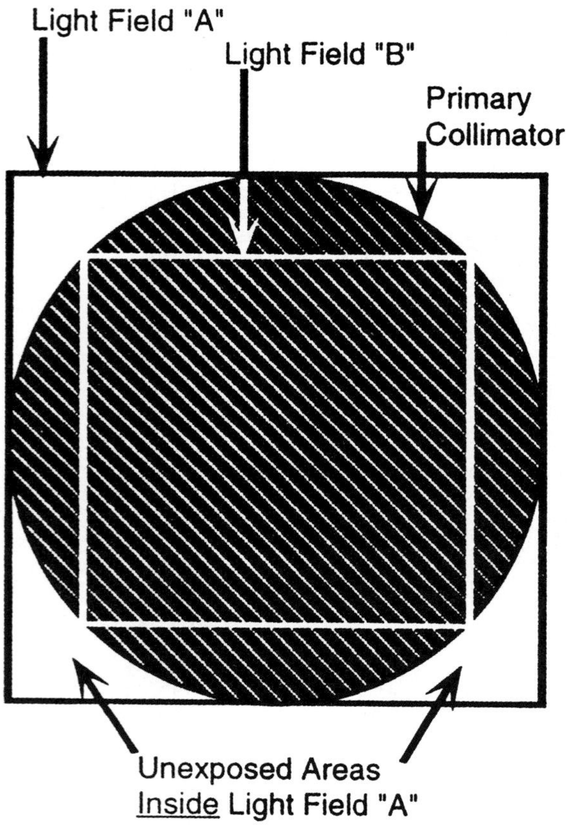

Fig. 11-11 The primary beam collimator produces a circular field. In some linear accelerators, the secondary collimator, producing a square field (light field A), is set to include the maximum diameter of the circle, leaving the corners unirradiated. In other machines, the secondary collimator is set so that the entire light field (light field B) lies within the irradiated area. In the latter scenario, the maximum field size is therefore smaller.

REFERENCES

1. Marcus KC, Svensson G, Rhodes LP, Mauch PM: Mantle irradiation in the upright position: A technique to reduce the volume of lung irradiated in patients with bulky mediastinal Hodgkin's disease. *Int J Radiat Oncol Biol Phys* 23:443, 1992.
2. Bentel GC: *Radiation Therapy Planning,* 2d ed. New York: McGraw-Hill, 1996.
3. Rider WD: Half-body radiotherapy: An update. *Int J Radiat Oncol Biol Phys* 4(suppl 2):69, 1978.
4. Salazar OM, Rubin P, Hendrickson FR, et al: Single-dose half-body irradiation for the palliation of multiple bone metastasis from solid tumors: A preliminary report. *Int J Radiat Oncol Biol Phys* 7:773, 1981.
5. Salazar OM, Rubin P, Hendrickson FR, et al: Single-dose half-body irradiation for palliation of multiple bone metastases from solid tumors: Final Radiation Therapy Oncology Group report. *Cancer* 58:29, 1986.
6. Breneman JC, Elson HR, Little R, et al: A technique for delivery of total body irradiation for bone marrow transplantation in adults and adolescents. *Int J Radiat Oncol Biol Phys* 18:1233, 1990.
7. Findley DO, Skov DD, Blume KG: Total body irradiation with a 10 MV linear accelerator in conjunction with bone marrow transplantation. *Int J Radiat Oncol Biol Phys* 6:695, 1980.
8. Galvin JM, D'Angio GJ, Walsh G: Use of tissue compensators to improve the dose uniformity for total body irradiation. *Int J Radiat Oncol Biol Phys* 6:767, 1980.
9. Khan FM, Williamson JF, Sewchand W, Kim TH: Basic data for dosage calculation and compensation. *Int J Radiat Oncol Biol Phys* 6:745, 1980.
10. Lam WC, Lindskoug BA, Order SE, Grant DG: The dosimetry of Co-60 total body irradiation. *Int J Radiat Oncol Biol Phys* 5:905, 1979.
11. Shank B: Techniques of magna-field irradiation. *Int J Radiat Oncol Biol Phys* 9:1925, 1983.
12. Van Dam J, Rijnders A, Vanuytsel L, Zhang HZ: Practical implications of backscatter from outside the patient on the dose distribution during total body irradiation. *Radiother Oncol* 13:193, 1988.
13. Umek B, Zwitter M, Habic H: Total body irradiation with translation method. *Radiother Oncol* 38:253–255, 1996.
14. Almond PR: Total skin/electron irradiation technique and dosimetry, in Kereikas JG, Elson HR, Born CG, eds: *Radiation Oncology Physics—1986.* New York: American Institute of Physics, 1987.
15. Freeman CR, Suissa S, Shenouda G, et al: Clinical experience with a single field rotational skin electron irradiation technique for cutaneous T-cell lymphoma. *Radiother Oncol* 24:155, 1992.
16. Gerbi BJ, Khan FM, Deibel C, Kim TH: Total skin electron arc irradiation using a reclined patient position. *Int J Radiat Oncol Biol Phys* 17:397, 1989.
17. Karzmark CJ, Loevinger R, Steel RE: A technique for large-field, superficial electron therapy. *Radiology* 74:633, 1960.
18. Karzmark CJ: Large-field superficial electron therapy with linear accelerators. *Am J Radiol* 37:302, 1964.
19. Karzmark CJ: Physical aspects of whole-body superficial therapy with electrons. *Frontiers Radiat Ther Oncol* 2:36, 1968.
20. Sewchand W, Khan FM, Williamson J: Total body superficial electron-beam therapy using a multiple-field pendulum-arc technique. *Radiology* 130:493, 1979.
21. Van Der Merwe DG: Total skin electron therapy: A tech-

nique which can be implemented on a conventional electron linear accelerator. *Int J Radiat Oncol Biol Phys* 27:391, 1993.
22. Williams PC, Hunter RD, Jackson SM: Whole body electron therapy in mycosis fungoides—successful translational technique achieved by modification of an established linear accelerator. *Radiology* 52:302, 1979.
23. Tetenes PJ, Goodwin PN: Comparative study of whole-body radiotherapeutic techniques using a 4-MeV nonangulated electron beam. *Radiology* 122:219, 1977.

PROBLEMS

11-1 A patient may need to be treated in a sitting position
(*a*) because of shortness of breath and inability to climb up on the treatment couch
(*b*) because his weight exceeds that of the treatment couch and he has claustrophobia
(*c*) because of shortness of breath or his weight exceeds the couch tolerance
(*d*) when the treatment couch is broken

11-2 When the patient is treated in a sitting position,
(*a*) treatment is generally limited to pelvic fields
(*b*) anterior whole abdominal fields only can be treated
(*c*) there is no limit; any field can be treated
(*d*) treatment is generally limited to the upper extremities and torso

11-3 Patients undergoing half-body irradiation
(*a*) are usually children with extensive disease
(*b*) are frequently positioned on a cushion on the floor
(*c*) are frequently treated while standing
(*d*) are usually unable to lie down due to pain

11-4 Adult patients undergoing total-body irradiation
(*a*) can be treated while lying supine on the treatment couch
(*b*) are often treated while in a semirecumbent position with the knees bent on a bed placed as far from the machine as the room allows
(*c*) are often treated while in a supine position on a rigid bed placed as far from the machine as the room allows
(*d*) can usually be treated at normal treatment distances

11-5 In delivering total-body irradiation
(*a*) the only concern is that the patients do not move
(*b*) immobilization devices are unnecessary, since the patients are allowed to move as much as they want as long as they remain inside the radiation field during the entire treatment
(*c*) concerns are generally limited to achieving uniform dose distribution and ensuring that the entire body remains within the radiation fields during the entire treatment
(*d*) the patients are asked to remain motionless and hold their breath

11-6 Large-field irradiation
(*a*) is easy because the fields are so large that one need not worry about small target margins
(*b*) is easy because there are usually no blocks, wedges, or compensators in these fields
(*c*) generally require long treatment distances
(*d*) should be used only in adult patients

11-7 Total-skin electron irradiation is usually delivered for the treatment of

(*a*) mycosis fungoides and basal cell carcinoma of the skin
(*b*) mycosis fungoides and squamous cell carcinoma of the skin
(*c*) squamous cell and basal cell carcinoma of the skin
(*d*) mycosis fungoides and Kaposi's sarcoma

11-8 Total-skin electron irradiation is usually done with the patient

(*a*) standing with the arms raised and legs spread
(*b*) sitting in a chair and resting the arms on a chair in front
(*c*) standing with the back toward the machine
(*d*) standing on a platform and turning to four different positions during each treatment

Answers to the Problems

Answers to the Problems

CHAPTER 1

1-1 (*b*)
1-2 (*d*)
1-3 (*a*)
1-4 (*a*)
1-5 (*c*)
1-6 (*d*)
1-7 (*b*)
1-8 (*d*)

CHAPTER 2

2-1 (*b*)
2-2 (*c*)
2-3 (*a*)
2-4 (*d*)
2-5 (*c*)
2-6 (*d*)
2-7 (*b*)
2-8 (*c*)
2-9 (*c*)
2-10 (*b*)

CHAPTER 3

3-1 (*b*)
3-2 (*d*)
3-3 (*a*)
3-4 (*b*)
3-5 (*b*)
3-6 (*c*)
3-7 (*c*)
3-8 (*b*)
3-9 (*d*)
3-10 (*b*)

CHAPTER 4

4-1 (*d*)
4-2 (*a*)
4-3 (*c*)
4-4 (*a*)
4-5 (*b*)
4-6 (*c*)
4-7 (*d*)
4-8 (*b*)
4-9 (*d*)
4-10 (*a*)
4-11 (*c*)
4-12 (*b*)

CHAPTER 5

5-1 (*c*)
5-2 (*a*)
5-3 (*b*)
5-4 (*b*)
5-5 (*d*)
5-6 (*d*)
5-7 (*c*)
5-8 (*d*)
5-9 (*a*)
5-10 (*d*)

CHAPTER 6

6-1 (*c*)
6-2 (*a*)
6-3 (*a*)
6-4 (*b*)
6-5 (*d*)
6-6 (*a*)
6-7 (*b*)

CHAPTER 7

7-1 (*c*)
7-2 (*c*)
7-3 (*a*)
7-4 (*d*)
7-5 (*a*)
7-6 (*c*)
7-7 (*b*)
7-8 (*a*)
7-9 (*d*)
7-10 (*c*)

CHAPTER 8

8-1 (*b*)
8-2 (*c*)
8-3 (*d*)
8-4 (*b*)
8-5 (*d*)
8-6 (*b*)
8-7 (*a*)
8-8 (*g*)
8-9 (*d*)
8-10 (*d*)
8-11 (*c*)
8-12 (*d*)
8-13 (*e*)
8-14 (*b*)

CHAPTER 9

9-1 (*c*)
9-2 (*c*)
9-3 (*a*)
9-4 (*c*)
9-5 (*d*)
9-6 (*a*)
9-7 (*e*)
9-8 (*b*)
9-9 (*b*)
9-10 (*b*)
9-11 (*d*)
9-12 (*d*)
9-13 (*e*)
9-14 (*b*)

CHAPTER 10

10-1 (*b*)
10-2 (*c*)
10-3 (*d*)
10-4 (*d*)
10-5 (*d*)
10-6 (*c*)
10-7 (*a*)

CHAPTER 11

11-1 (*c*)
11-2 (*d*)
11-3 (*b*)
11-4 (*b*)
11-5 (*c*)
11-6 (*c*)
11-7 (*d*)
11-8 (*a*)

Index

Index

Note: Page numbers followed by "f" indicate figures; page numbers followed by "t" indicate tables.

B

C

D

E

F

G

I

K

L

M

N

O

S

T

U

V

W

X

Y

Z

Notes

Notes

Notes

Notes

Notes

Notes

Notes

Notes

Notes